Social Indicators Research Series

Volume 78

This series aims to provide a public forum for single treatises and collections of papers on social indicators research that are too long to be published in our journal *Social Indicators Research*. Like the journal, the book series deals with statistical assessments of the quality of life from a broad perspective. It welcomes the research on a wide variety of substantive areas, including health, crime, housing, education, family life, leisure activities, transportation, mobility, economics, work, religion and environmental issues. These areas of research will focus on the impact of key issues such as health on the overall quality of life and vice versa. An international review board, consisting of Ruut Veenhoven, Joachim Vogel, Ed Diener, Torbjorn Moum, Mirjam A.G. Sprangers and Wolfgang Glatzer, will ensure the high quality of the series as a whole.

More information about this series at http://www.springer.com/series/6548

Richard J. Estes

The Social Progress of Nations Revisited, 1970–2020

50 Years of Development Challenges and Accomplishments

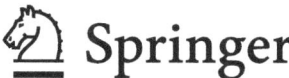 Springer

Richard J. Estes
School of Social Policy & Practice
University of Pennsylvania
Narberth, PA, USA

ISSN 1387-6570   ISSN 2215-0099   (electronic)
Social Indicators Research Series
ISBN 978-3-030-15906-1   ISBN 978-3-030-15907-8   (eBook)
https://doi.org/10.1007/978-3-030-15907-8

This Springer imprint is published by the registered company Springer Nature Switzerland AG.
The registered company address is: Gewerbestrasse 11, 6330 Cham, Switzerland

This book is dedicated to my 4 daughters, to their extraordinary husbands, and to my 12 grandchildren who already are making the world a better place to live. A special dedication goes to my grandson, Nic Payne, who helped me re-see the world through a wonder of the eyes of a child. Izzy Payne, too, has been a constant source of inspiration to me as has been Andrew Calkins, Brendan and Julia O'Connor, and Kieran Lynch.

and

To some very special caregivers who have helped me along a difficult journey:
Mellia
Stephanie
Nancy
Dawn
Paul Marcotte
Gary Walters Crooks

Preface

I began my study of comparative social development and well-being in the early 1970s as part of my doctoral studies at the University of California, Berkeley. This body of research became a central life interest and, following my graduation from Berkeley, continued to preoccupy me during my early years of employment initially as an Assistant and then Full Professor in the School of Social Work (now the School of Social Policy & Practice) of the University of Pennsylvania. My early mentors in these efforts were the late Harold L. Wilensky (1923–2011), Professor of Sociology and Organizational Intelligence in the Department of Political Science at Berkeley (Wilensky, 1975, 2002), and the late John Stewart Morgan, Professor of Comparative Social Policy at the University of Pennsylvania (Rodgers, Greve, & Morgan, 1968). Both men taught me the importance of rigor in conducting international and comparative studies and provided me with a wide range of skills for achieving that goal in my own research. They also reinforced another dimension of research for me—that of translating research findings into positive actions that would work to the benefit of others, including to the world as a whole, i.e., the foundation on which the Greek concept of *praxis* is built (Estes, 2018; Estes & Morgan, 1976).

These intellectually formative years were to shape the entirety of my professional career, even into my retirement years from Penn. In all my scholarly work, I have sought to bridge knowledge gained through research into action at all levels of social and political organization, especially as that knowledge pertains to the hundreds of millions of people living on the margins of society. I have been fortunate in the many opportunities that this area of research has opened to me including an invitation from a collaborative group of consultative nongovernmental organizations to the United Nations to develop analytical tools for measuring the underlying nature and dynamics of social development, and not just its critical economic components (United Nations Development Programme, 2018). Their goal, as was mine, was to create more valid and reliable time-series measures of development that would provide a fuller picture of the development at various units of analysis from the nation-state or country level to the planet. These organizations also were interested in the creation of new analytical tools for use in measuring the changing socioeconomic conditions of society's most vulnerable population groups—children and youth, the aged, women, persons with severe disabilities, the poor, economic and political migrants, persons with serious diseases, and the like.

I was very appreciative of the opportunity to serve these organizations while, at the same time, advancing my own research agenda as an academic and scholar. The intellectual and methodological challenges before me were many and varied; the vast array of economic tools that already were available made the task even more foreboding. The challenges, nonetheless, were met and resulted in the development of an entirely new set of analytical tools that were applied at the national, regional, and global levels (Estes & Morgan, 1976). These tools also proved to be effective in assessing the changing social status of vulnerable population groups and, over time, to be valuable for unraveling a series of conceptual issues that, at the time, had limited the area of international and comparative well-being research (Estes, 1984, 1988, 2010, 2018).

Organization

This book is divided into eight parts. *Part I* introduces the reader to some of the major challenges and accomplishments that humanity has confronted over an extended time. *Part II* lays out the methodology used to carry out the analysis summarized in this book. *Part III* begins the discussion of global social progress focusing on various units of analysis[1] starting with the world and gradually summarizing major findings for individual nations over the entire 50-year period, 1970–2020. *Part IV* uses the same approach as that adopted for Part III to perform an analysis at the regional and subregional levels, and *Part V* focuses on advances in quality of life and well-being at the country-specific level. *Part VI* focuses on the social needs and accomplishments that have occurred among the vulnerable population groups that are found in all societies, i.e., children and youth, the aged, persons with severe disabilities, the poor, disadvantaged minority groups, and others. Separate chapters focus on the changing status of women since 1970 (Chap. 8) and on poverty and its declining distribution around the world (Chap. 9). The data reported in these chapters are highly positive and provide a forward-looking analysis of the improved status of the large population groups that traditionally have functioned on the margins of male-dominated and economically advanced societies. *Part VII* comprises an overview and general discussion of some of the major findings reported in the book and puts forward a working agenda for advancing selected aspects of quality of life and well-being over the near term. *Part Backmatter* includes Appendix A, which explains the computational methods in more detail, and Appendix B, which reports country-specific scores and percent changes in the *Index of Social Progress* by major index (ISP, WISP) and for each of the ISP's 10 subindexes within the

---

[1] The **unit** of **analysis** is the major entity that is being analyzed in a study. It is the "what" or "who" that is being studied. In social science **research,** typical **units** of **analysis** include individuals (most common), groups, social organizations, and social artifacts (Wikipedia, 2018).

major sociopolitical-economic development groupings to which each country has been assigned. The data reported in Appendix B are for each 10-year period beginning 1970.

Narberth, PA, USA   Richard J. Estes

References

Council on Social Work Education (CSWE). (2010). *United States-based conceptualization of International Social Work Education*. Written by Richard J. Estes. Repository. University of Pennsylvania, PPP Papers #181. Retrieved September 15, 2018 from https://www.cswe.org/getattachment/459d3db5-d4b8-413d-9ed0-a7633e306e8c/US-Based-Conceptualization-of-International-Social.aspx

Estes, R. J. (1984). *The social progress of nations*. New York: Praeger.

Estes, R. J. (1988). *Trends in world social development: The social progress of nations, 1970–1987*. New York: Praeger.

Estes, R. J. (2018, February). The social progress of nations revisited. *Social Indicators Network News (SINET)*, #134, February, 1–7.

Estes, R. J., & Morgan, J. S. (1976). World social welfare analysis: A theoretical model. *International Social Work, 19*(2), 29–41.

Rodgers, B. N, Greve, J. & Morgan, J. S. (Eds). (1968). *Comparative social administration*. New York: Atherton Publishers.

United Nations Development Programme (UNDP). (2018). *Human development report: Statistical Annex*. New York: UNDP.

Wikipedia. (2018, March 17). Unit of analysis. In *Wikipedia, the free Encyclopedia*. Retrieved September 14, 2018, from https://en.wikipedia.org/w/index.php?title=Unit_of_analysis&oldid=830877005

Wilensky, H. L. (1975). *The welfare state and equality: Structural and ideological roots of public expenditures*. San Francisco: University of California Press.

Wilensky, H. L. (2002). *Rich democracies: Political economy, public policy, and performance*. San Francisco: University of California Press.

World Bank. (2018). *Annual report, 2018*. Washington, DC: World Bank.

Acknowledgments

A volume of the scope covered by this manuscript could not have been completed without the contributions of many people. Central among them is my friend and colleague at Virginia Tech, M. Joseph "Joe" Sirgy, with whom I have worked on many other books, seminal articles, and a full series of specialized monographs. We make a great team, and I deeply value our collegiality and friendship. In his capacity as Executive Director of the *Management Institute for Quality-of-Life Studies*, he made available to me the extraordinary research competence of David Walker, a graduate in computer science from Virginia Tech and now a specialist in data management, graphic design, and statistical analysis. David was a great help in the early stages of data collection, and I thank him for his careful attention to the many conceptual and methodological complexities involved in collecting comparable data across nations and world regions.

I would also like to acknowledge Joe's wife and the treasurer of the Management Institute for Quality-of-Life Studies, Pamela Jackson, of the Psychology Department of Radford University of Virginia, for her contributions to this volume.

I also appreciated the many and varied contributions made to this research effort by my colleagues at the United Nations, the United Nations Development Programme, the World Bank, the International Monetary Fund, and a long list of stellar colleagues employed by international governmental and nongovernmental organizations located in various regions of the world. The contributions made by these people to the current work have been substantial and reflect a richness of analysis that a single scholar could not have accomplished working alone.

Amy Hillier, Associate Professor of Social Policy and Director of the Master of Science Program in Social Policy at the University of Pennsylvania, also is acknowledged for her contribution to some of the data presentations made in this book, especially the geographic information system time-series maps that visually present the state of global development and human well-being at different time intervals.

Pamela Fried of Protext Editorial Services is acknowledged with a special thank you for her continuing efforts to help the author present his ideas more clearly and accurately. Her editorial skills have been without limits in this writing project. Thank you, Pam.

I also acknowledge the enormous contribution made by my wife and life partner, Gail Buchanan Estes, who endured long hours of my absence and distraction while I worked on this book. Gail contributed to the book in a variety of ways and, at difficult moments, provided support that sustained my continued work. Thank you, Gail.

School of Social Policy & Practice   Richard J. Estes
University of Pennsylvania
Narberth, PA, USA
October 2018

Abstract Social progress and well-being throughout the world have arrived at a critical turning point. Following decades of social losses among the world's poorest developing countries of Africa, Asia, and Latin America, the majority of these and other nations now are experiencing significant social gains. Using the author's well-established *Weighted Index of Social Progress* from 1970 to 2018 (WISP2018), the author traces the net social gains and social losses experienced by the vast majority of the world's nations over a 50-year time period, ranging from 1970 to the present. The data reported draw on the author's extensive database of historical and contemporary social indicators and link the current study to his and other reports of social progress and well-being that have been published during this time period. Data are reported at four levels of analysis, i.e., that of the world as a whole, that of the regions (continents) of the world, the world's 19 subregions using the preceding, and, finally, that of selected countries for which the changes have been most remarkable. The net social gains on the WISP18 and earlier versions of the WISP portray very positive outcomes for the 162 countries included in the study (representing 95 percent of the world's total population) for both the near and long terms.

Keywords International · Comparative · Social indicators · Quality of life · Well-being · Happiness · Development · Social development

Contents

Part VII

About the Author

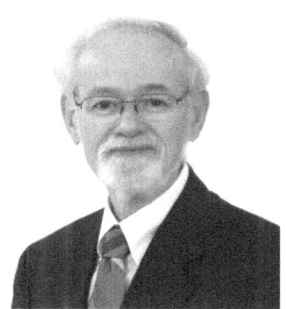

Richard J. Estes
University of Pennsylvania
School of Social Policy & Practice
3701 Locust Walk
Narberth PA 19104-6214
Cell Phone: (215) 565-5356; Skype: richard.j.estes
E-Mail: restes@upenn.edu;
Website: https://www.sp2.upenn.edu/people/view/richard-estes/

Richard J. Estes is Professor of Social Work and Social Policy at the *University of Pennsylvania* in Philadelphia. He holds an A.B. degree from *La Salle University* in Philadelphia and graduate degrees in Social Work from the University of Pennsylvania (Master of Social Work) and the *University of California* at Berkeley (Doctor of Social Welfare). He also holds a postmaster's Certificate in Psychiatric Social Work from the *Menninger Foundation* in Topeka, Kansas.

Dr. Estes' international activities have been extensive. Among other assignments, he has held visiting professorships in Iran, Norway, the People's Republic of China, Morocco, South Korea, Hawaii, Japan, Mongolia, the Russian Federation, Belgium, Sweden, Mexico, Hong Kong, and elsewhere. In the United States, he is Founding

President of the Philadelphia Area Chapter of the *Society for International Development* (SID). He is a former president of the Group for the Advancement of Doctoral Education (GADE) and is a former chair of the Council on *External Relations of the Global Commission of the Council on Social Work Education* (CSWE). In 2004, he was elected president of the *International Society for Quality-of-Life Studies* (ISQOLS).

Until 2010, Dr. Estes served as chair of the graduate concentration in *Social and Economic Development* (SED where he also directed the school's international programs until his retirement from Penn in July 2010.

Dr. Estes has been the recipient of many awards and grants for his research on international social work and comparative social development including two *Fulbright-Hays Senior Research* Awards (Iran, 1978 and Norway, 1979) and a *Fulbright Scholar Award* to Yonsei University in Seoul, Korea (1994). In 1992, he was elected Social Worker of the Year by the Pennsylvania Chapter of the National Association of Social Workers for his international activities. In 1996, he received the Alumni Recognition Award from the University of *Pennsylvania School of Social Work*. In 1997, he was awarded the *Distinguished Recent Contribution to Social Work Education Award* by the Council on Social Work Education (CSWE), the *International Rhoda G. Sarnat Award* of the National Association of Social Workers (NASW), and the Best Article in *Social Indicators Research* Award of ISQOLS. In 2002, he was appointed *Distinguished Visiting Scholar of the United College of the Chinese University of Hong Kong* where he served as an external examiner for the university's Department of Social Work until 2008. In 2005, the Global Commission of the Council on Social Work Education awarded Dr. Estes its *Partner in International Education Award*. In 2007, Dr. Estes received the *Distinguished Quality of Life Research Award* of ISQOLS and served as University Distinguished Professor at the Chinese University of Hong Kong.

In January 2014, Dr. Estes was inducted into the American Academy of Social Work and Social Welfare (AASWSW), the leading professional honorific organization for social welfare specialist in the United States. Also in 2014, the ISQOLS honored Dr. Estes in Florence, Italy, by establishing a permanently endowed lecture series in his name on international and comparative studies in quality-of-life research. In the same year, the International Consortium for Social Development honored him in Singapore for his pioneering work in international and comparative social development research.

In recent years, Prof. Estes has become interested in development patterns occurring in Islamic nations, including in factors that contribute to Islamic terrorism both internally and that directed against other nations. He has since written extensively on developing trends occurring in these nations including problems associated with Islamic militancy and terrorism.

Recent Research Publications by Richard Estes

Books

Azaola, E., & Estes, R. J. (2003). *La Infancia Como Mercancia Sexual: México, Canadá y Estados Unidos (The commercial sexual exploitation of children in Mexico, Canada and the United States)*. Mexico City, Mexico: CIEASAS & Siglo XXI Veintiuno Editores.

Cooper, S. W., Giardino, A. P., Estes, R. J., Kellogg, N. D., & Vieth, V. I. (2005). *Medical, legal & social science aspects of child sexual exploitation: A comprehensive review of child pornography, child prostitution, and internet crimes against children*. Florissant MO: STM Publishing.

Cooper, S. W., Giardino, A. P., Estes, R. J., Kellogg, N. D., & Vieth, V. I. (2007). *Child sexual exploitation: Quick reference for healthcare, social services, and law enforcement professionals*. Florissant MO: STM Publishing.

Estes, R. J. (1984). *The social progress of nations*. New York: Praeger.

Estes, R. J. (1988). *Trends in world social development: The social progress of nations, 1970–1987*. New York: Praeger.

Estes, R. J. (1992a). *Internationalizing social work education: A guide to resources for a new century*. Philadelphia: University of Pennsylvania School of Social Work.

Estes, R. J. (1992b). *Towards a social development strategy for the ESCAP region*. Bangkok, Thailand: United Nations Economic and Social Commission for Asia and the Pacific, ST/ESCAP/1170.

Estes, R. J. (2005). *Social development in Hong Kong: The unfinished agenda*. London/New York: Oxford University Press.

Estes, R. J. (2007). *Advancing quality of life in a turbulent world*. Dordrecht, The Netherlands/Berlin, Germany: Springer.

Estes, R. J. (2019). *The social progress of nations revisited: 50 Years of Development Challenges and Accomplishments*. Cham, Switzerland: Springer, in press.

Estes, R. J., & Sirgy, M. J. (2017). *The pursuit of wellbeing: The untold global history*. Dordrecht, The Netherlands/Berlin, Germany: Springer.

Estes, R. J., & Sirgy, M. J. (2018). *Advances in Well-being: Toward a better world for all*. London: Rowman and Littlefield.

Sirgy, M. J., Estes, R., Rahtz, D., & El-Aswad, E. (2019). *Combatting jihadist terrorism through nation-building*. Dordrecht, The Netherlands: Springer.

Tiliouine, H., & Estes, R. J. (2016). *Social progress in Islamic societies: Social, political, economic, and ideological challenges*. Dordrecht, The Netherlands: Springer. ISBN 978-3-319-24772-4.

Extended Book Reviews

Michalos, A. (2017). Social progress in Islamic societies: A review. *Applied Research in Quality of Life, 12*(3), 765–793.
Thin, N., Tarragona, M., Wong, P., Jarden, R. J., Bartholomeus, J., & Jarden, A. (2017). Book review: The pursuit of human well-being – The untold global history. *International Journal of Wellbeing, 7*(1), 84–92. Retrieved from https://internationaljournalofwellbeing.org/index.php/ijow/article/view/636

Selected Articles and Book Chapters

Council on Social Work Education (CSWE). (2010). *United States-based conceptualization of international social work education*. Written by Richard J. Estes. University of Pennsylvania, Repository, PPP Papers #181.
Estes, R. J. (1984). World social vulnerability: 1968–1978. *Social Development Issues, 8*(1–2), 8–28.
Estes, R. J. (1985). Toward the year 2000: The need for global action now. *Social Development Issues, 9*(1), 54–63.
Estes, R. J. (1986, November). Europe tops survey of most livable countries. *Europe*, 36–37.
Estes, R. J. (1987). Social development trends in the Pacific: Implications for the future. *Social Development Issues, 11*(2), 3–19.
Estes, R. J. (1988a). Toward a quality of life index. In J. Norwine & A. Gonzalez (Eds.), *The third world: States of mind meaning* (pp. 23–36). London: Unwin & Hyman.
Estes, R. J. (1988b). World social ranking. In G. Kurrian (Ed.), *Encyclopedia of the third world*. New York: Facts on File.
Estes, R. J. (1988c). *Trends in world social development: The social progress of nations, 1970–1987*. New York: Praeger.
Estes, R. J. (1990a). Development trends in the Asian and Pacific region: Assessing the adequacy of social provision, 1970–1987. In *Guidelines on methodological approaches to the conduct of a regional survey on the quality of life as an aspect of human resources development* (pp. 32–59). Bangkok, Thailand: United Nations ESCAP, Publication No. ST/ESCAP/886.
Estes, R. J. (1990b). Social development under different political and economic systems. *Social Development Issues, 13*(1), 5–19.
Estes, R. J. (1990c). The international index of social progress. In *Encyclopedia of social inventions* (pp. 186–188). London: The Institute for Social Inventions.
Estes, R. J. (1993a). Education for comparative social welfare research. In D. Sanders (Ed.), *Education for International Social Welfare*, a joint publication of the Council on Social Work Education and the University of Hawaii, School of Social Work (pp. 56–86). Honolulu: University of Hawaii Press.

Estes, R. J. (1993b). Toward sustainable development: From theory to praxis. *Social Development Issues, 15*(3), 1–29.

Estes, R. J. (1994). Social work in international perspective: Professional challenges for Korea at the outset of a new century. In *Proceedings of the 9th Symposium on Social Welfare* (pp. 1–36). Yonsei University.

Estes, R. J. (1995a). Social development trends in Africa: The need for a new development paradigm. *Social Development Issues, 17*(1), 18–47.

Estes, R. J. (1995b). Education for social development: Curricular issues and models. *Social Development Issues, 16*(3), 68–90.

Estes, R. J. (1996a, December). Health and development in Asia: Regional priorities for a new century. *Forum of International Development Studies, 6*, 3-31.

Estes, R. J. (1996b). Social development trends in Asia, 1970–1994: The challenges of a new century. *Social Indicators Research, 37*(2), 119–148.

Estes, R. J. (1996c). Social development trends in Latin America, 1970–1994: In the shadows of the 21st century. *Social Development Issues, 18*(1), 25–52.

Estes, R. J. (1997a). Social work, social development and community welfare centers in international perspective. *International Social Work, 40*(1), 43–55.

Estes, R. J. (1997b). The world social situation: social work's contribution to international development. In R. Edwards (Ed.), *Encyclopedia of social work* (Supplement to the 19th Edition) (pp. 343–359). Washington, DC: National Association of Social Workers.

Estes, R. J. (1997c). Trends in European social development, 1970–1994. *Social Indicators Research, 42*(1), 1–19.

Estes, R. J. (1998a). Social development trends in the successor states to the former Soviet Union: The search for a new paradigm. In K. R. Hope (Ed.), *Challenges of transformation and transition from centrally planned to market economies* (UNCRD Research Report Series No. 26) (pp. 13–30). Nagoya, Japan: United Nations Centre for Regional Development.

Estes, R. J. (1998b). Trends in world social development, 1970–1995: Development prospects for a new century. *Journal of Developing Societies, 14*(1), 11–39.

Estes, R. J. (1999). Social development trends in the Middle East, 1970–1997: The search for modernity. *Social Indicators Research, 50*(1), 51–81.

Estes, R. J. (2000). Social development trends in the Middle East, 1970–1995: Implications for social policy reform. In L. Belkacem (Ed.), *Building and sustaining the capacity for social policy reforms* (pp. 17–46). Aldershot, UK: Ashgate Publishers.

Estes, R. J. (2003a). Advancing quality of life in Hong Kong: The unfinished agenda. In P. Lee (Ed.), *Proceedings of the International Conference on quality of life in a global world*. Hong Kong, Hong Kong: Chinese University of Hong Kong.

Estes, R. J. (2003b). European social development trends: development challenges of the 'New' Europe. In J. Vogel (Ed.), *Välfärd och ofärd på 90-talet (Good times and hard times in Sweden during the 1990s)* (Report #100: Living Conditions Series) (pp. 435–468). Stockholm, Sweden: Statistics Sweden.

Estes, R. J. (2004). Development challenges of the 'New' Europe. *Social Indicators Research, 69*(2), 123–166.

Estes, R. J. (2005a). Global change and indicators of social development. In M. Weil (Ed.), *The handbook of community practice*. Thousand Oaks, CA: Sage.

Estes, R. J. (2005b). Quality of life in Hong Kong: Past accomplishments and prospects. Shek, Daniel *Quality of life in the global context: A Chinese response*, special issue of *Social Indicators Research* 71(1–3), 183-229.

Estes, R. J. (2007a). Asia and the new century: Challenges and opportunities. *Social Indicators Research, 82*(3), 375–410.

Estes, R. J. (2007b). Development challenges and opportunities confronting economies in transition. *Social Indicators Research, 83*(3), 375–411.

Estes, R. J. (2007c). *Advancing quality of life in a turbulent world*. Dordrecht, The Netherlands/Berlin, Germany: Springer.

Estes, R. J. (2008). The international dimensions of social work practice. In R. Cnaan et al. (Eds.), *A century of social work and social welfare at Penn* (pp. 333–353). Philadelphia: University of Pennsylvania Press.

Estes, R. J. (2009). *United States-based conceptualization of international social work education prepared on behalf of the Global Commission of the Council on Social Work Education (CSWE)*. Arlington, VA: CSWE.

Estes, R. J. (2010a). The world social situation: Development challenges at the outset of a new century. *Social Indicators Research, 98*, 363–402.

Estes, R. J. (2010b). Toward sustainable development: From theory to praxis. *Social Development Issues, 15*(3), 1–29.

Estes, R. J. (2012a). Economies in transition: Continuing challenges to quality of life. In K. Land, A. C. Michalos, & M. Joseph Sirgy (Eds.), *Handbook of quality of life research* (pp. 433–457). Dordrecht, The Netherlands: Springer.

Estes, R. J. (2012b). Failed and failing states: Is quality of life possible? In K. Land, A. C. Michalos, & M. Joseph Sirgy (Eds.), *Handbook of Quality of Life Research* (pp. 555–580). Dordrecht, The Netherlands: Springer.

Estes, R. J. (2012c). Global change and indicators of social development. In M. Weil (Ed.), *Handbook of community practice* (2nd ed., pp. 587–606). Thousand Oaks, CA: Sage.

Estes, R. J. (2012d). Entries in the Of Record section of the journal of Applied Research in Quality of Life Research (ARQOL).

Estes, R. J. (2014a). Disadvantaged populations. In A. C. Michalos (Ed.), *Encyclopedia of quality of life and well-being research* (pp. 1654–1658). Dordrecht, The Netherlands: Springer.

Estes, R. J. (2014b). Index of social progress. In A. C. Michalos (Ed.), *Encyclopedia of quality of life and well-being*. Dordrecht, The Netherlands: Springer.

Estes, R. J. (2014c). Social progress. In A. C. Michalos (Ed.), *Encyclopedia of quality of life and well-being research* (pp. 6146–6148). Dordrecht, The Netherlands: Springer.

Estes, R. J. (2015a). Chapter 2: Development trends among the world's socially least developed countries: reasons for cautious optimism. In B. Spooner (Ed.), *Globalization: The crucial phase globalization: The crucial phase*. Philadelphia: University of Pennsylvania Museum Press.

Estes, R. J. (2015b). Global change and quality of life indicators. In F. Maggino (Ed.), *A life devoted to quality of life festschrift in honor of Alex C. Michalos* (pp. 173–194). Dordrecht, The Netherlands: Springer.

Estes, R. J. (2015c). Trends in world social development: The search for global well-being. In G. Wolfgang (Ed.), *The global handbook of well-being: From the wealth of nations to the human well-being of nations.* Dordrecht, The Netherlands: Springer.

Estes, R. J. (2017a). The commercial sexual exploitation of children in North America. In R. Anderson (Ed.), *Alleviating world suffering: The challenge of negative quality of life* (pp. 375–394). Dordrecht, The Netherlands: Springer.

Estes, R. J. (2017b). Aurelio Pecci: Industrialist, humanist and quality of life scholar (1908–1984). *Applied Research in Quality of Life, 12*, 231–232.

Estes, R. J. (2017c). Donella H. Dana Meadows: A designer of systems for advancing quality of life (1941–2001). *Applied Research in Quality of Life, 12*, 233–235.

Estes, R. J. (2017d). Composite scores and changing rank order positions on the index of social progress (ISP/WISP), 1970–2010 (N=162). In R. J. Estes & M. J. Sirgy (Eds.), *The pursuit of well-being: The untold global history..* Appendix D and E. Dordrecht, The Netherlands: Springer.

Estes, R. J. (2017e). Pioneer in quality of life research: Daniel Bell (1919–2011). *Applied Research in Quality of Life Research., 7*(3), 331–336.

Estes, R. J. (2017f). Pioneer in quality of life research: Donald Mc Granahan (1917–2001). *Applied Research in Quality of Life Research., 7*(3), 331–336.

Estes, R. J. (2018a). Disparities and wealth. In G. Brule & C. Suter (Eds.), *Wealth and subjective well-being.* Dordrecht, The Netherlands: Springer, in press.

Estes, R. J. (2018b). Tonon, Graciela *Indicators of quality life in Latin America: A book review*, 2016. Dordrecht, The Netherlands: Springer. *Review in Applied Research in Quality of Life, 13*, 255–256.

Estes, R. J. (2018c). Views on wellbeing research, policy and practice: An interview with Dr. Richard J. Estes. *Middle East Journal of Positive Psychology, 3*(1), 12–15.

Estes, R. J. (2018d, February). The social progress of nations revisited. *Social Indicators Network News (SINET)*, #134, 1–7.

Estes, R. J. (2018e). Advances in well-being in the Middle East and Gulf States regions: Historical background and contemporary challenges. In Lambert & N. Pasha-Zaid (Eds.), *Positive psychology: A view for the Arabian Gulf* (p. xx). Dordrecht, The Netherlands: Springer, in press.

Estes, R. J. (2018f, June). Pioneer: Eduard Pestel (1914–1988): A pioneer in social indicators, world systems modeling, industrial design, politics and public policy, *Journal of Applied Research in Quality of Life, 13*(2), 525–526.

Estes, R. J. (2019a). Disparities and wealth. In G. Brule & C. Suter (Eds.), *Wealth and subjective well-being.* Dordrecht, The Netherlands: Springer, in press.

Estes, R. J. (2019b). The social progress of nations revisited, 1970–2018: A half century of promise and progress. *Social Indicators Research*, in press.

Estes, R. J., & Sirgy, M. J. (2016). Chapter 29: Is quality of life related to radical Islamic militancy and acts of terrorism? In H. Tiliouine & R. J. Estes (Eds.), *Social progress in Islamic societies: Social, political, economic, and ideological challenges*. Dordrecht, The Netherlands: Springer.

Estes, R. J., & Sirgy, M. J. (2018b). Advances in well-being in the MENA region: Accentuating the positive. In L. Lambert & N. Pasha-Zaidi (Eds.), *Advances in Well-being in the Middle East and North Africa (MENA) Region: Historical background and contemporary challenges*. Dordrecht, The Netherlands: Springer, in press.

Estes, R. J., & Tiliouine, H. (2016). Chapter 9: Social development trends in the countries of the Fertile Crescent. In *Social progress in Islamic societies: Social, political, economic, and ideological challenges*. Dordrecht, The Netherlands: Springer.

Estes, R. J., & Weiner, N. (2005). The commercial sexual exploitation of children in the United States. In S. W. Cooper, R. J. Estes, A. P. Giardino, N. D. Kellogg, & V. I. Vieth (Eds.), *Medical, legal, and social science aspects of child sexual exploitation: A comprehensive review of pornography, prostitution, and internet crimes* (pp. 95–128). Florissant, MO: STM Publishing.

Estes, R. J., & Wilensky, H. L. (1976). Life cycle squeeze and the morale curve. *Social Problems, 25*(3), 277–292.

Estes, R. J. & Zhou, H. M. (2014, December 4) A conceptual approach to the creation of public–private partnerships in social welfare. *International Journal of Social Welfare,* 348–363.

Estes, R. J., Ives, N., & Azaola, E. (2005). The commercial sexual exploitation of children in North America. In S. W. Cooper, R. J. Estes, A. P. Giardino, N. D. Kellogg, & V. I. Vieth (Eds.), *Medical, legal, and social science aspects of child sexual exploitation: A comprehensive review of pornography, prostitution, and internet crimes*. Florissant, MO: STM Publishing.

Estes, R. J., Land, K., Michalos, A., Phillips, R., & Sirgy, M. J. (2017a). Chapter 9: The history of well-being in North America. In R. J. Estes & M. J. Sirgy (Eds.), *The pursuit of well-being: The untold global history*. Dordrecht, The Netherlands: Springer.

Estes, R. J., & Morgan, J. S. (1976). World social welfare analysis: A theoretical model. *International Social Work, 19*(2), 29–41.

Estes, R. J., Sirgy, M. J., & Selian, A. (2017b). Chapter 6: How we measure well-being: The data behind the history of human well-Being. In *The pursuit of well-being: The untold global history*. Dordrecht, The Netherlands: Springer.

Estes, R. J., & Sirgy, M. J. (2014). Radical Islamic militancy and acts of terrorism: A quality-of-life analysis. *Social Indicators Research, 117*(2), 615–652.

Estes, R. J., & Sirgy, M. J. (2017a). Chapter 1: Introduction. In R. J. Estes & M. J. Sirgy (Eds.), *The pursuit of well-being: The untold global history*. Dordrecht, The Netherlands: Springer.

Estes, R. J., & Sirgy, M. J. (2017b). Chapter 20: Well-being from a global perspective. In R. J. Estes & M. J. Sirgy (Eds.), *The pursuit of well-being: The untold global history*. Dordrecht, The Netherlands: Springer.

Estes, R. J., & Sirgy, M. J. (2017c). Major empirical instruments used to measure objective and subjective well-being. In R. J. Estes & M. J. Sirgy (Eds.), *The pursuit of well-being: The untold global history*. Appendix B. Dordrecht, The Netherlands: Springer.

Estes, R. J., & Sirgy, M. J. (2017d). *The pursuit of well-being: The untold global history*. Dordrecht, The Netherlands/Berlin, Germany: Springer.

Estes, R. J., Sirgy, M. J. (2017e, December 1–5). Myths and truths of advances in well-being. *Social Indicators Network News (SINET)*.

Estes, R. J., & Sirgy, M. J. (2018c). Advances in well-being in the MENA region: Accentuating the Positive. In L. Lambert & N. Pasha-Zaidi (Eds.), *Positive psychology: A Vvew for the Arabian Gulf*. Dordrecht, The Netherlands: Springer.

Estes, R. J., & Sirgy, M. J. (2018d). Global advances in quality of life and well-being: Past present, and future. *Social Indicators Research, 141*, 1137–1164. https://doi.org/10.1007/s11205-018-1869-4, in press.

Estes, R. J., Sirgy, M. J. (2018e, November). Advances in human well-being (using the Weighted Index of Social Progress. Social Indicators Network News (SINET). Numbers 135 & 136, 1–6.

Estes, R. J., Sirgy, M. J., & Joshanloo, M. (2018). The global challenge of jihadist terrorism: A quality-of-life model (using PEW data). *Social Indicators Research, 141*, 191–215. (SOCI-D-17-00970R1), in press.

Estes, R. J., Sirgy, M. J., & Selian, A. (2017c). Major worldwide accomplishments in well-being Since 1900. In R. J. Estes & M. J. Sirgy (Eds.), *The pursuit of well-being: The untold global history.*. Appendix C. Dordrecht, The Netherlands: Springer.

Estes, R. J., Sirgy, M. J., Rahtz, D. R., & El-Aswad, E.-S. (2019). *Human well-being and policy making* (Special Monograph series). Dordrecht, The Netherlands: Springer, in preparation.

Estes, R. J., & Tiliouine, H. (2014). Islamic development trends: From collective wishes to concerted actions. *Social Indicators Research, 116*(1), 67–114.

Estes, R. J., & Tiliouine, H. (2016a). Chapter 1: Introduction. In *Social progress in Islamic Societies: Social, political, economic, and ideological challenges*. Dordrecht, The Netherlands: Springer.

Estes, R. J., & Tiliouine, H. (2016b). Chapter 6: Social progress in North Africa. In *Social progress in Islamic societies: Social, political, economic, and ideological challenges*. Dordrecht, The Netherlands: Springer.

Estes, R. J., & Tiliouine, H. (2016c). Chapter 9: Social development trends in the countries of the Fertile Crescent. In *Social progress in Islamic societies: social, political, economic, and ideological challenges*. Dordrecht, The Netherlands: Springer.

Estes, R. J., & Tiliouine, H. (2016d). Chapter 30: Reflections and conclusions. In *Social progress in Islamic societies: Social, political, economic, and ideological challenges*. Dordrecht, The Netherlands: Springer.

Estes, R. J., Wai, C. H., Fung, J., & Wong, A. (2002). Toward a social development index for Hong Kong: The process of community engagement. *Social Indicators Research, 58*(1–3), 313–347.

Gattas, G., Figaro-Garcia, C., Landini, T. S., & Estes, R. J. (2012). Commercial sexual exploitation and missing kids in the coastal region of Sao Paulo State, Brazil. *Journal of Applied Research on Children, 3*(2). Article 10.

Inoguchi, T., & Estes, R. J. (2017). The history of human well-being in East Asia. In R. J. Estes & M. J. Sirgy (Eds.), *The pursuit of well-being: The untold global history*. Dordrecht, The Netherlands: Springer.

Renima, A., Tiliouine, H., & Estes, R. J. (2016a). Chapter 3: The Islamic golden age: A story of the triumph of the Islamic civilization. In H. Tiliouine & R. J. Estes (Eds.), *Social progress in Islamic societies: social, political, economic, and ideological challenges*. Dordrecht, The Netherlands: Springer.

Renima, A., Tiliouine, H., & Estes, R. J. (2016b). Chapter 3: The changing map of the Islamic world: From the Abbasid Era to the Ottoman Empire of the 20th Century. In H. Tiliouine & R. J. Estes (Eds.), *Social progress in Islamic societies: Social, political, economic, and ideological challenges*. Dordrecht, The Netherlands: Springer.

Rhatz, D., Estes, R. J. (2019). *The universal soldier: The dynamics of gang formation among Jihadist terrorists*, in preparation.

Shaikin, D., & Estes, R. J. (2018). Advancing development in Kazakhstan: The contribution of R&D. *Social Development Issues, 40*(2), 36–55(20).

Sirgy, M. J., & Estes, R. J. (2018a). Understanding Jihadist terrorism in the MENA and Gulf States Region: Quality-of-Life implications for counterterrorism. In L. Lambert (Ed.), *Positive psychology in the middle east and north Africa: Research, policy, and practice*. Dordrecht, The Netherlands: Springer.

Sirgy, M. J. & Estes, R. J. (2018b, Fall). Advances in well-being: An essay. *Social Indicators Network News* (SINET), 1–7.

Sirgy, M. J., Estes, R. J., & Rahtz, D. R. (2018a). Combatting jihadist terrorism: A quality-of-life perspective. *Journal of Applied Research in Quality of Life., 13*, 813–837, online https://doi.org/10.1007/s11482-017-9574-z

Sirgy, M. J., Joshanloo, M., Estes, R. J., & Rahtz, D. W. (2018b). The global challenge of Jihadist terrorism: A quality-of-life model. *Social Indicators Research, 141*, 191–215. (SOCI-D-17-00970R1), in press.

YouTube and Related Live Interviews with Professor Estes

2014. Live interview with Michael Frisch relating to professional career in all aspects of my research. YouTube: https://www.youtube.com/watch?v=ZLi9xESMWgY. Posted January 2012, San Diego, CA.

2015. Live interview with Michael Frisch in Philadelphia focusing on career in quality of life and social development research: https://www.youtube.com/watch?v=4qQOMokxG70. Posted July 9, 2015, Philadelphia.

List of Acronyms and Abbreviations

CIS	Commonwealth of Independent States
DC	Developing Country
DME	Developed Market Economies
FDI	Foreign Direct Investment
IMF	International Monetary Fund
ISP	Index of Social Progress
LDC	Least Developed Countries
MENA	Middle East and North African region
MDC	Millennium Development Campaign (Goals)
OECD	Organization for Economic Cooperation and Development
SIPRI	Stockholm International Peace Research Institute
SDG	Sustainable Development Goals
UNDESA	United Nations Department of Economic and Social Affairs
UNDP	United Nations Development Programme
WHO	World Health Organization
WISP	Weighted Index of Social Progress

List of Artwork

All of the artwork included in this book was painted by **Lylia Forero Carr** of Fresno, California. She was born in Bogotá, Colombia, traveled to the United States in 1966, and moved to Fresno, California, in 1982. She holds a Master of Arts degree in art from California State University at Fresno. She also has studied with Millard Sheets, Mario Cooper, Charles Reid, Gerald Brommer, Jane Burnham, Joseph Zirker, Glen Brill, Sandro Martini, Keiji Shinohara, and C. Dillbohner.

She has worked in painting, drawing, sculpting, and printmaking. Her recent works have been in mixed media. She starts either with monotypes, collages, or *collographs* (a printmaking process in which materials are applied to a rigid substrate such as paperboard or wood) and finishes by painting or drawing. She first researches and gathers the information necessary to develop her theme. These initial ideas or images are then combined with an intuitive sense of placement, color, texture, and line, allowing the work to develop freely. She works in series, developing a theme but also giving her attention to each piece individually. She enjoys experimenting with and exploring new visual avenues in order to grow and change. All of the artwork in the volume is original. Lylia describes the eight-part series as follows:

> These are images of eight small (8 × 8) encaustic[1] works on individual wood panels, from the series titled "The Muysca Numbers." The Muysca civilization lived in the area of the Colombian Andes where the cities of Bogotá and Tunja are located today. They are not numbers as such but representations of constellations in the sky that they followed for their rituals and the planting of their crops.

---

[1] Encaustic painting, also known as hot wax painting, involves using heated beeswax to which colored pigments are added. The liquid or paste is then applied to a surface—usually prepared wood—though canvas and other materials are often used.

Each of the eight pieces of artwork included in the volume is discretely numbered and titled.

Image 1: Muysca, *Ata*
Image 2: Muysca, *Bosa*
Image 3: Muysca, *Miqa*
Image 4: Muysca, *Muyhica*
Image 5: Muysca, *Hisqa*
Image 6: Muysca, *Ta*
Image 7: Muysca, *Cuhupcua*
Image 8: Muysca, *Suhuza*

List of Figures

List of Tables

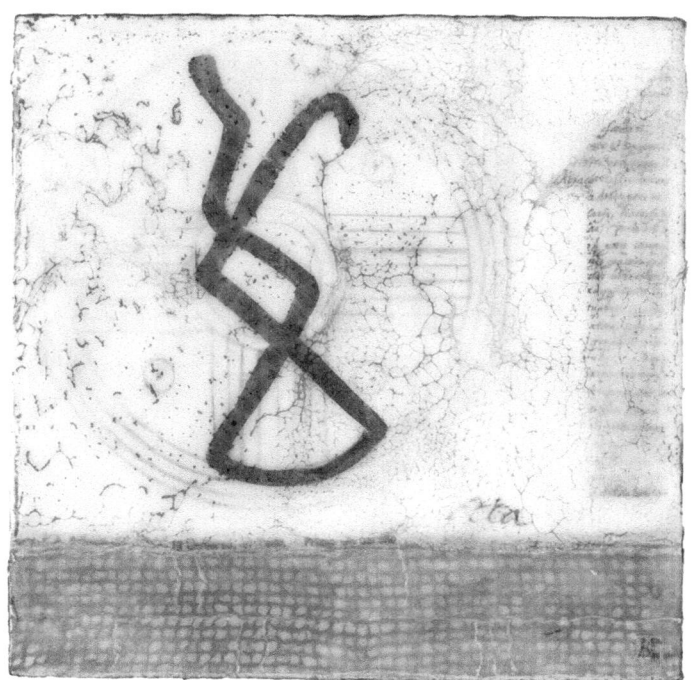

Part I

Image 1: © Lylia Ferero Carr: Muysca, Ata

Chapter 1
A Half Century of Promise and Progress

Nations are dynamic entities that are constantly changing in response to the needs of often expanding populations (Ghose, 2013; United Nations Population Division, 2018). They also change or realign existing systems in response to the complex social, economic, political, technological, and environmental needs that emerge with increased frequency and seriousness (Central Intelligence Agency, 2018; World Bank, 2018). Issues of emigration, immigration, and diversity-related social conflict also impact the capacity of nations to perform their varied functions. Though quite diverse with respect to geographic size, population characteristics, type of polity, and economic system, nations share a variety of features and functions.[1] Ranked in order by their relative importance, the most unifying characteristics of state functions are (1) recognition of their political sovereignty by other nations; (2) a coherent set of principles that guides their interactions with other sovereign states; (3) a defensible set of secure geopolitical borders; (4) the administration of justice within a system of laws to which, optimally, the governed have assented (e.g., via a written constitution and an independent judiciary); (5) the provision of a range of "public goods" designed to meet the collective needs of their populations (e.g., the creation of monetary and banking systems, road-building and other transportation networks, the development of communications infrastructure, and the provision of at least

---

[1] The concept of the "nation-state(s)" embraces two distinct components: the "state" or "states" refer to discrete political and geopolitical territories over which the state, acting as a "government," claims sovereignty; "nation" or "nations" refer to the cultural or ethnic characteristics of the people who reside in the state. The term "nation-state" implies that the two concepts coincide with one another (i.e., that the people of a given geographic territory share the same cultural, religious, and ethnic characteristics), although many modern nation-states are characterized by substantial cultural diversity even though their geopolitical borders are fully recognized and accepted by the international community (Central Intelligence Agency, 2018). Since the European Treaty of Westphalia in 1648, sovereign nation-states defer to one another as *co-equal and autonomous powers with full authority over the territories and people they govern*. The concept of sovereign nation-states constitutes the basis for membership and voting privileges in the United Nations as well as in most major nongovernmental and nonstate actor organizations, i.e., one nation, one vote.

© Springer Nature Switzerland AG 2019
R. J. Estes, *The Social Progress of Nations Revisited, 1970–2020*, Social Indicators Research Series 78, https://doi.org/10.1007/978-3-030-15907-8_1

limited health, education, and related human services); (6) special public and private initiatives designed to meet the income security and related needs of their most vulnerable inhabitants, e.g., children, the elderly, persons with chronic illnesses or disabilities, unemployed persons, families with large numbers of children (Estes & Zhou, 2014); and (7) a commitment to promoting the general well-being of the society as a whole (Estes & Sirgy, 2017a; Helliwell, Layard, & Sachs, 2017).

Within democratic societies, countries also are responsible for the conduct of fair and open elections and for the promotion of a broad range of civil liberties and political freedoms—all of which are considered necessary elements in the functioning of pluralistic, participatory societies (Freedom House, 2018; Transparency International, 2018). Further, from ancient to modern times, politically unified societies also have sought to advance the collective well-being of their citizens through the removal of, or at least reductions in, the obstacles that interfere with the pursuit of progressively higher levels of collective development. So successful has been the concept of the nation-state in the modern era that their numbers increased from 55 just prior to the collapse of the Austro-Hungarian (1867–October 31, 1918), Ottoman (July 27, 1299–October 29, 1923), and Russian (1682–1917; 1917–1991) empires to 193 politically autonomous member-states of the United Nations in 2018.

The expectation is that more territories likely will gain political sovereignty in the near term, e.g., the Palestinian territories (from Israel), the Western Sahara (from Spain and Morocco), and, very likely, the Falkland Islands (from the United Kingdom). South Sudan, which voted for independence from the Republic of the Sudan in January 2011, is now a sovereign member of the United Nations.

Additional Challenges Confronting Nations

But not all nations are created equal, and many experience severe stresses related to the national organizing principles identified above. Some nations, such as Israel, for example, experience a chronic both actual and existential threat to their right to exist whereas other nations confront especially severe challenges associated with diversity-related social conflict (the contemporary situation in Iraq and Syria). Still others are confronted with a host of serious environmental stresses that threaten their geographic integrity, e.g., recurrent flooding in Bangladesh, which plunges half of the country under sea water annually, or complete submersion of either their land or outer islands as a result of global warming—particularly those of the South Pacific's Solomon Island chain. For still others, the pace of national technological innovation compromises their capacity to resolve the fundamental challenges. Still other nations, comprising hundreds of millions of people, are further characterized by low levels of human capital and natural resource development, which slow both their development and that of associated nations—including most of the poorest nations of developing Africa, Asia, and Latin America (International Monetary Fund, 2018a, 2018b; United Nations Development Programme, 2018; World Bank, 2018).

Weak social, political, and social welfare infrastructures also challenge the internal and external capacity of many of the world's nations (Freedom House, 2018; Fund for Peace, 2017a, 2017b, 2017c; International Social Security Association, 2018). Net social gains or losses in the health, education, and income security sectors have proven to be especially predictive of the capacity of nations to satisfy both the basic and enhanced needs of their residents while also promoting development in the nation's social, political, economic, technological, environmental, and related sectors (United Nations Development Programme, 2018; World Bank, 2018). The significance of these patterns is reflected in the recently concluded United Nations' *Millennium Development Campaign* (MDC) 2000–2010 and its ambitious successor initiative of 17 *Sustainable Development Goals* (SDGs) launched in 2015 (Estes, 2000, 2005a, 2005b; Hanson, Puplampu, & Shaw, 2017).

Social Progress 1970–2018

The two figures that follow summarize major trends in world social development as the primary unit of measurement for the 50-year period that began in 1970. The figures report the highly positive improvements that have taken place during this period of worldwide social and political upheaval, including the collapse of the former Soviet Union and, with it, the emergence of more than 20 fully independent nations (Fig. 1.1). The improvements that took place occurred among the most impoverished nations of developing Africa, Asia, and Latin America. The

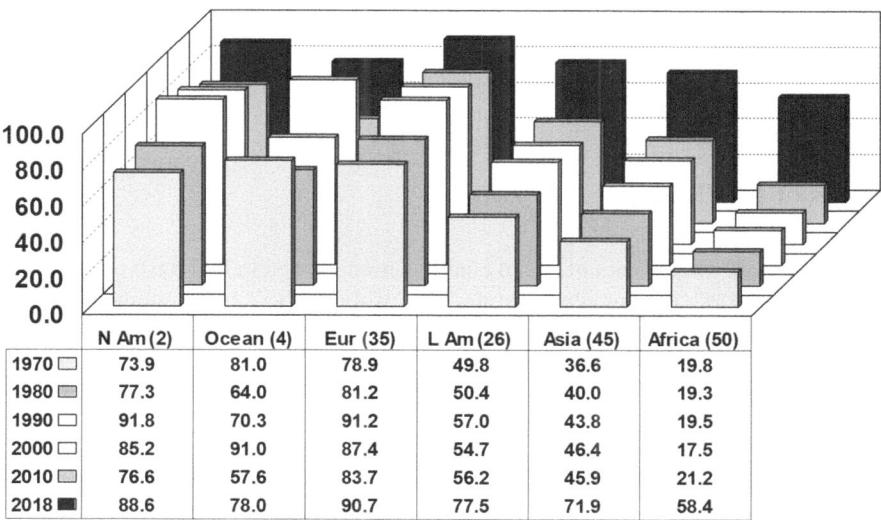

	N Am (2)	Ocean (4)	Eur (35)	L Am (26)	Asia (45)	Africa (50)
1970 ☐	73.9	81.0	78.9	49.8	36.6	19.8
1980 ▦	77.3	64.0	81.2	50.4	40.0	19.3
1990 ☐	91.8	70.3	91.2	57.0	43.8	19.5
2000 ☐	85.2	91.0	87.4	54.7	46.4	17.5
2010 ▦	76.6	57.6	83.7	56.2	45.9	21.2
2018 ■	88.6	78.0	90.7	77.5	71.9	58.4

Fig. 1.1 Average Weighted Index of Social Progress scores by continent and development decade, 1970–2018 (N = 162)

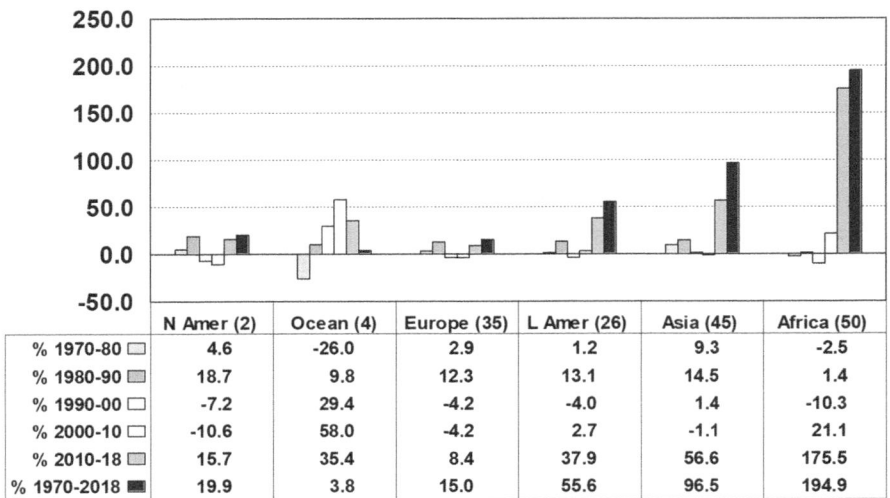

	N Amer (2)	Ocean (4)	Europe (35)	L Amer (26)	Asia (45)	Africa (50)
% 1970-80 ☐	4.6	-26.0	2.9	1.2	9.3	-2.5
% 1980-90 ▨	18.7	9.8	12.3	13.1	14.5	1.4
% 1990-00 ☐	-7.2	29.4	-4.2	-4.0	1.4	-10.3
% 2000-10 ☐	-10.6	58.0	-4.2	2.7	-1.1	21.1
% 2010-18 ▨	15.7	35.4	8.4	37.9	56.6	175.5
% 1970-2018 ■	19.9	3.8	15.0	55.6	96.5	194.9

Fig. 1.2 Percent change in average Weighted Index of Social Progress scores by continent and development decade, 1970–2018 (N = 162)

percentage of social gains reported for the nations of sub-Saharan Africa have been especially impressive since the year 2000 given their generally stagnant, even downward, trends in development during the earlier development decades (Fig. 1.2).

Many of the world's developing nations seek to emulate the social improvements of the already economically developed nations of Europe, North America, Oceania and selected countries in East Asia, which are predictably much slower and lower given their already advanced levels of development. A detailed discussion of this topic and its implications is found in Chapter 4, which focuses on an analysis of global development patterns between 1970 and 2020 (projected).

Focus of the Book

This book reviews 50 years of social challenges and progress that have occurred in 162 of the world's nations representing 95% of the world's population. The book builds on an extensive body of empirical literature previously reported by the author using five levels of analysis: (a) *the world as a whole* (Estes, 1984, 1988, 2010a, 2010b, 2015b; Estes & Morgan, 1976); (b) *major world regions and continents* (Estes, 1987, 1992a, 1992b, 1995, 1996a, 1996b, 1996c, 1997a, 1997b, 1997c, 1999, 2004, 2007a, 2007b, 2007c, 2012a; Inoguchi & Estes, 2017); (c) *major subregions of these continents* (Estes, 2012b, 2015a; Estes, Land, Michalos, Phillips, & Sirgy, 2017); (d) *selected countries* (Estes, 2002, 2005b, 2005c); and, (e) *socially vulnerable population groups* with a special focus on income disparities and poverty (Estes, 2014, 2018). Other reports of net national and global social progress have been presented in extensive analyses of the history of social progress, quality of life, and human well-being (Estes & Sirgy, 2017b, 2019; Fukuyama, 1989). A related body of empirical research using this study's methods has focused on the social, political, economic, and ideological challenges confronting the 54 predominately Islamic societies including the emergence within a subset of these countries of jihadist-inspired terrorism (Estes & Sirgy, 2014; Estes & Tiliouine, 2014; Tiliouine & Estes, 2016a, 2016b).

Organization of the Book

The content of this book is organized around five interrelated objectives:

- To briefly review the extensive history of international and comparative research on changing patterns worldwide of social development, quality of life, and well-being;
- To use primarily objective data in undertaking this review, although some attention also is given to changing patterns of subjective well-being in response to the removal of, or at least reductions in, the objective conditions of life that inhibit the pace of changes in personal and collective well-being;
- To summarize the major changes that have occurred in the objective conditions leading to subjective well-being over the 50-year period since 1970 to the present;
- To make a limited set of recommendations that consolidate and, where possible, further strengthen the drivers of well-being policies in all regions of the world, giving special attention to the widening gap in wealth disparities so that the increasingly large numbers of the absolute poor can move from poverty to at least working-class status; and, finally,
- To formulate a set of recommendations concerning the additional contributions that well-being researchers and scholars can make in accelerating the pace of social development, quality of life, and well-being at all levels of sociopolitical organization.

In response to these goals and objectives, the book is organized into seven parts. **Part I** consists of a brief introductory chapter (Chap. 1) and a chapter that discusses significant advances during the past 50 years that have influenced the drivers of social progress, technological innovation, and well-being (Chap. 2); **Part II** consists of a single chapter that summarizes the major analytic methods used throughout the book (Chap. 3); **Parts III, IV, and V** report the study's major social development patterns and trends in three chapters for countries organized by different levels of political organization for the period 1970 and 2018 and, where possible, includes projections to the year 2020—at the global (Chap. 4), regional and subregional (Chap. 5), and national (Chap. 6) levels of advances in quality of life and well-being.

Part VI directs the reader's attention to the special development needs and challenges confronting population groups that have functioned on the economic and political peripheries of many nations—both in the past and in the present. Chapter 7 identifies the major population groups at risk of social disadvantage (in education, health, access to paid jobs and to critical communications media). Chapter 8 focuses specifically on the centuries-long needs of women as well as on the enormous progress they have made toward attaining increased social parity with men during both the twentieth and opening decades of the current century. Chapter 9 focuses on the problems associated with income poverty that characterizes all nations of the world, even those that are classified in this and other studies as being the most economically advanced nations. Long after the unique needs of other vulnerable population groups are met more fully, it is likely that the problem of income poverty and the "culture" in which many of the poor live will still be with us. But substantial progress in reducing both the numbers and recurrence of poverty for many groups of people is expected to be fully resolved.

Part VII contains the book's concluding chapter (Chapter 10) and focuses on the past, the present, and the future with respect to global, regional, and national social development, quality of life and well-being. The chapter also identifies a working agenda that supplements the major international development initiatives contained in both the MDC, 2002–2015 and the recently launched SDGs, 2015–2030 with their 17 major sectors of worldwide social, political, and economic development activity that will be of central concern between 2015 and 2030. The preliminary *Agenda for Action* outlined in Chap. 10 should be read in the context of both the MDC and SDGs to arrive at a fuller understanding of the broad-based actions that are needed to fully attain our global development goals that range from improvements in health and education to protection of flora, fauna and, yes, the oceans and seas.

The last section of the book, **Part Backmatter**, contains two appendixes (**A & B**) that provide data in greater detail relating to the book's methodology (**Appendix A**) and specific data from the study's two major indexes (*Index of Social Progress* [ISP], *Weighted Index of Social Progress* ([WISP]) and for each of the study's composite 10 subindexes (**Appendix B**), e.g., *Health, Education, Demography, Social Welfare, Women, Defense Spending, Environmental Protection, the drivers of diversity-related social conflict, economics, and the changing status of women*. **Appendixes A** and **B** cover the entire 50 years of research that comprise the core content of this book.

The rich interrelationships that exist between the various sectors that contribute to advances in human quality of life and well-being are illustrated in Fig. 1.3, which identifies the major sectors and the interactions between them that result in well-being viewed more broadly. This basic framework is discussed throughout the book with an emphasis assigned to each of the component sectors of well-being, but especially to the social, political, economic, technological, environmental, and other aspects of well-being advancement in response to a broad range of drivers that inform and shape policy development in both the public and private sectors of collective and communal life.

The chapters are data rich in their philosophical and empirical presentations and confirm the validity of the major findings reported throughout the book. The volume's images, illustrations, tables, and figures have been designed to present com-

Fig. 1.3 Selected overlapping dimensions of well-being. (Illustration by David Walker, based on the writings of Hardy Stevenson and Associates Ltd)

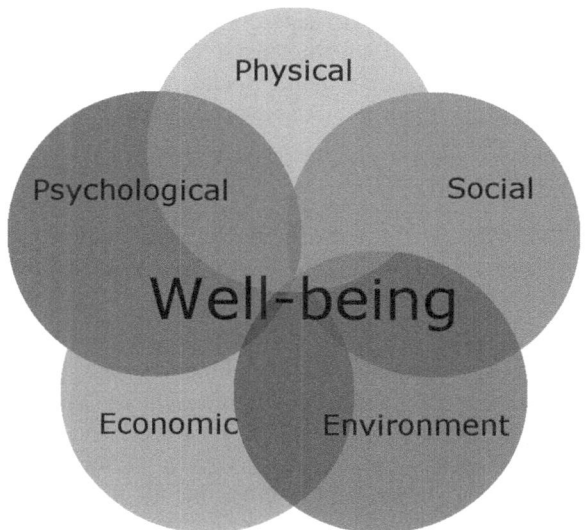

plex numbers more simply. Every effort has been made to present the volume's complex concepts, methodology and data as simply as possible so that the book would be accessible to members of the general education public and not just to scholars of social development, quality of life, and well-being. I believe that this goal has been achieved or is at least achievable with some effort on the part of persons who are not specialists in these areas that are at the center of our collective life.

One final note in this introductory chapter is that the reader should recognize that the findings reported throughout the book fluctuate considerably from one region of the world to another, among different populations, and between men and women but that the overall theme and findings are fundamentally positive as they relate to the present and future progress of the world in finally solving long-standing challenges that have prevented women and socially disadvantaged populations from participating as full and equal members of society.

The positive tone of the volume reflects the substantial progress that people and nations have achieved in advancing their development. The progress achieved has been historically unparalleled. These substantial gains in human well-being are the result of mutually supportive efforts on the part of the public and private sectors as well as people themselves working with others through their own advocacy groups. The social gains since 1970 are impressive and will provide a working roadmap for others to follow in the decades ahead. The *United Nations, the World Bank, the Organization for Economic Cooperation and Development,* and the *European Union* are providing the much-needed intergovernmental cooperation. American high-impact private philanthropists such as Warren Buffet, Bill and Melinda Gates, Michael Bloomberg, the Walton Family, George Soros, Mark Zuckerberg, Ted Turner, and many others (Wang, 2018) are contributing substantially to global social progress as are the hundreds, likely thousands today, of individuals and international development assistance organizations that are contributing generously in working with local governments to attain a broad range of goals that have proven elusive when working alone. Social progress as noted by late American Robert F. Kennedy,

> Freedom possesses many meanings. It speaks not merely in terms of political and religious liberty but also in terms of economic and social progress.

But Kennedy also warned us,

> Progress is a nice word, but change is its motivator and change has enemies. Robert F. Kennedy. *American Politician* (1968)

This book takes full cognizance of the interrelatedness of the social, political, economic, technological, and communications dynamics that shape societies. The volume also considers the contributions of history, traditions, values, and norms that form the context within which the former set of social drivers function. Taken together, each of these multiple drivers of social progress is important and each contributes to the social outcomes that all of us are seeking to improve the overall status and capacity of people worldwide. We shall explore the contribution of each of them during the 75 years that have passed since the end of the Second World War.

References

Central Intelligence Agency. (2018). *World factbook*. [Public domain]. Retrieved August 20, 2018, from https://www.cia.gov/library/publications/the-world-factbook/geos/mx.html

Estes, R. J. (1984). World social vulnerability: 1968–1978. *Social Development Issues, 8*(1–2), 8–28.

Estes, R. J. (1987). Social development trends in the Pacific: Implications for the future. *Social Development Issues, 11*(2), 3–19.

Estes, R. J. (1988). World social ranking. In G. Kurrian (Ed.), *Encyclopedia of the third world*. New York: Facts on File.

Estes, R. J. (1992a). *Internationalizing social work education: A guide to resources for a new century*. Philadelphia: University of Pennsylvania School of Social Work.

Estes, R. J. (1992b). *Towards a social development strategy for the ESCAP Region*. Bangkok, Thailand: United Nations Economic and Social Commission for Asia and the Pacific, ST/ESCAP/1170.

Estes, R. J. (1995). Social development trends in Africa: The need for a new development paradigm. *Social Development Issues, 17*(1), 18–47.

Estes, R. J. (1996a). Health and development in Asia: Regional priorities for a new century. *Forum of International Development Studies, 6*(December), 3–31.

Estes, R. J. (1996b). Social development trends in Asia, 1970–1994: The challenges of a new century. *Social Indicators Research, 37*(2), 119–148.

Estes, R. J. (1996c). Social development trends in Latin America, 1970–1994: In the shadows of the 21st century. *Social Development Issues, 18*(1), 25–52.

Estes, R. J. (1997a). Trends in European social development, 1970–1994. *Social Indicators Research, 42*(1), 1–19.

Estes, R. J. (1997b). Social work, social development and community welfare centers in international perspective. *International Social Work, 40*(1), 43–55.

Estes, R. J. (1997c). The world social situation: social work's contribution to international development. In R. Edwards (Ed.), *Encyclopedia of Social Work* (Supplement to the 19th ed., pp. 343–359). Washington: National Association of Social Workers.

Estes, R. J. (1999). Social development trends in the Middle East, 1970–1997: The search for modernity. *Social Indicators Research, 50*(1), 51–81.

Estes, R. J. (2000). Social development trends in the Middle East, 1970–1995: Implications for social policy reform. In L. Belkacem (Ed.), *Building and sustaining the capacity for social policy reforms* (pp. 17–46). Aldershot, UK: Ashgate Publishers.

Estes, R. J. (2002). Toward a social development index for Hong Kong: The process of community engagement. *Social Indicators Research, 58*(1–3), 313–347.

Estes, R. J. (2004). Development challenges of the 'New' Europe. *Social Indicators Research, 69*(2), 123–166.

Estes, R. J. (2005a). Global change and indicators of social development. In M. Weil (Ed.), *The handbook of community practice*. Thousand Oaks CA: Sage Publications.

Estes, R. J. (2005b). Quality of life in Hong Kong: Past accomplishments and prospects. In D. Shek (Ed.), *Quality of life in the global context: A Chinese response* [special issue] *Social Indicators Research, 71*(1–3), 183–229.

Estes, R. J. (2005c). *Social development in Hong Kong: The unfinished agenda*. London/New York: Oxford University Press.

Estes, R. J. (2007a). *Advancing quality of life in a turbulent world*. Dordrecht, The Netherlands/Berlin, Germany: Springer International Publishers.

Estes, R. J. (2007b). Asia and the new century: Challenges and opportunities. *Social Indicators Research, 82*(3), 375–410.

Estes, R. J. (2007c). Development challenges and opportunities confronting economies in transition. *Social Indicators Research, 83*(3), 375–411.

Estes, R. J. (2010a). The world social situation: Development challenges at the outset of a new century. *Social Indicators Research, 98*, 363–402.

Estes, R. J. (2010b). Toward sustainable development: From theory to praxis. *Social Development Issues, 15*(3), 1–29.

Estes, R. J. (2012a). Economies in transition: Continuing challenges to quality of life. In K. Land, A. C. Michalos, & M. J. Sirgy (Eds.), *Handbook of quality of life research* (pp. 433–457). Dordrecht, The Netherlands: Springer International Publishers.

Estes, R. J. (2012b, July 15). Entries in the of record. *Journal of Applied Research in Quality of Life Research, 7*(3), 331–336.

Estes, R. J. (2014). Disadvantaged populations. In A. C. Michalos (Ed.), *Encyclopedia of quality of life and well-being research* (pp. 1654–1658). Dordrecht, The Netherlands: Springer International Publishers.

Estes, R. J. (2015a). Chapter 2: Development trends among the world's socially least developed countries: Reasons for cautious optimism. In B. Spooner (Ed.), *Globalization: The crucial phase*. Philadelphia: University of Pennsylvania Museum Press.

Estes, R. J. (2015b). Trends in world social development: The search for global well-being. In W. Glatzer, L. Camfield, V. Møller, & M. Rojas (Eds.), *Global handbook of quality of life: Exploration of well-being of nations and continents*. Dordrecht, The Netherlands: Springer International Publishers.

Estes, R. J. (2018). Advances in well-being in the Middle East and Gulf States regions: Historical background and contemporary challenges. In L. Lambert & N. Pasha-Zaid (Eds.), *Positive psychology: A view for the Arabian Gulf* (pp. 285–312). Dordrecht, The Netherlands: Springer International Publishers. (in press).

Estes, R. J., Land, K., Michalos, A., Phillips, R., Sirgy, M. J (2017). The history of well-being in North America. In R. J. Estes M. J. Sirgy (Eds.), The pursuit of well-being: The untold global history (pp. 257–300). Cham, Switzerland: Springer International Publishers.

Estes, R. J., & Morgan, J. S. (1976). World social welfare analysis: A theoretical model. *International Social Work, 19*(2), 29–41.

Estes, R. J., & Sirgy, M. J. (2014). Radical Islamic militancy and acts of terrorism: A quality-of-life analysis. *Social Indicators Research, 117*(2), 615–652.

Estes, R. J., & Sirgy, M. J. (2017a). *The pursuit of human Well-being: The untold global history.* Dordrecht, The Netherlands: Springer.

Estes, R. J., & Sirgy, M. J. (2017b). *Advancing quality of life in a turbulent world.* Dordrecht, The Netherlands/Berlin, Germany: Springer International Publishers.

Estes, R. J., & Sirgy, M. J. (2019). Advances in wellbeing in the MENA region: Accentuating the positive. In L. Lambert & N. Pasha-Zaidi (Eds.), *Positive psychology in the Middle East/North Africa: Research, policy, and practise.* Dordrecht, The Netherlands: Springer International Publishers.

Estes, R. J., & Tiliouine, H. (2014). Islamic development trends: From collective wishes to concerted actions. *Social Indicators Research, 116*(1), 67–114.

Estes, R. J., & Zhou, H. M. (2014). A conceptual approach to the creation of public–private partnerships in social welfare. *International Journal of Social Welfare, 24*(4), 348–363.

Freedom House. (2018). *Freedom in the world 2018.* New York: Freedom House. Retrieved September 4, 2018 from https://freedomhouse.org/report/freedom-world/freedom-world-2018.

Fukuyama, F. (1989). The end of history? *The National Interest* No. 16 (Summer 1989), pp. 3–18.

Fund for Peace. (2017a). *Fragile states index.* Washington, DC: Fund for Peace. Retrieved September 4, 2018 from http://fundforpeace.org/fsi/data/

Fund for Peace. (2017b). *Why foreign aid and development spending is good for America.* Washington, DC: Fund for Peace. Retrieved September 4, 2018 from http://library.fundfor-peace.org/blog-20170322-usaid.

Fund for Peace. (2017c). *Human rights and business roundtable.* Washington, DC: Fund for Peace.

Ghose, T. (2013, April 29). The secret to curbing population growth. *Live Science.* Retrieved June 11, 2017, from https://www.livescience.com/29131-economics-drives-birth-rate-declines.html.

Hanson, K. T., Puplampu, K. P., & Shaw, T. M. (Eds.). (2017). *From millennium development goals to sustainable development goals.* London/New York: Routledge.

Helliwell, J., Layard, R., & Sachs, J. (2017). *World happiness report, 2017.* New York: Sustainable Development Solutions Network.

Inoguchi, T., & Estes, R. J. (2017). The history of Well-being in East Asia: From global conflict to global leadership. In R. Estes & M. J. Sirgy (Eds.), *The pursuit of human Well-being: The untold global history* (pp. 301–348). Cham, Switzerland: Springer International Publishers.

International Monetary Fund. (2018a). *IMF Data.* Retrieved July 8, 2018 from http://www.imf.org/en/Data

International Monetary Fund. (2018b). *World economic outlook, 2018.* April. Retrieved July 8, 2018 from https://www.imf.org/en/Publications/WEO/Issues/2018/03/20/world-economic-outlook-april-2018

International Social Security Association. (2018). *Social security programs throughout the world.* Geneva: ISSA. Retrieved August 24, 2018 from https://www.ssa.gov/policy/docs/progdesc/ssptw/.

Kennedy, R. J. (1968). *Social progress quote American Politician.* Cited from Brainy quotes. Retrieved December 8, 2018 from https://www.brainyquote.com/quotes/robert_kennedy_745956?src=t_social_progress

Tiliouine, H., & Estes, R. J. (2016a). Epilogue. In H. Tiliouine & R. J. Estes (Eds.), *The state of social progress of Islamic societies: Social, political, economic, and ideological challenges* (pp. 645–652). Dordrecht, The Netherlands: Springer International Publishers.

Tiliouine, H., & Estes, R. J. (2016b). Social development in north African countries: Achievements and current challenges. In H. Tiliouine & R. J. Estes (Eds.), *The state of social progress of Islamic societies: Social, political, economic, and ideological challenges* (pp. 109–136). Dordrecht, The Netherlands: Springer International Publishers.

Transparency International. (2018). *Corruptions perception index.* [Organization Web site.] Berlin: Transparency International. Retrieved August 24, 2018 from https://www.transparency. org/research/cpi/overview

United Nations Development Programme. (2018). *Human development report, 2018: Human development for everyone.* New York: United Nations Development Programme.

United Nations Population Division. (2018). *2015–17. Revision of world population prospects* (vol. 1). New York: United Nations Department of Economic and Social Affairs. [Data files]. Retrieved June 13, 2018 from https://esa.un.org/unpd/wpp/publications/files/key_findings_ wpp_2015.pdf/

Wang, J. (2018). *The greatest gives: Meet America's top philanthropists.* Forbes, October 15. Retrieved December 8, 2018 from https://www.forbes.com/top-givers/#73f5740d66ff

World Bank. (2018). *World development report, 2018: Learning to realize education's promise.* Washington, DC: World Bank. Retrieved August 19, 2018 from http://www.worldbank.org/en/ publication/wdr2018.

Chapter 2
The Past, The Present

Humanity has arrived at a dramatically different level of well-being in 2019 than that which existed 50 years ago or that which characterized people worldwide at the outset of the twentieth century. And the current century is still young and continues to reveal itself daily. The advances we have the privilege to witness reflect changes in the quality of life of people everywhere, and the forward momentum we would like to focus on continues the promise of even more significant advances in the sciences, medicine, and technology in the decades just ahead. Although distinct drivers for both contemporary and future progress in well-being are not easy to discern with clarity, the rich tapestry of the multiple stakeholders and multisector collaborations needed to bring about these changes is not. We already know the mix of public–private partnerships that are needed to bring about dramatic changes in all areas of collective life (Estes & Zhou, 2014).

With respect to additional advances in the health, education, and even economic sectors, near-term progress is apparent. One example is the dramatic nature of the changes in the average years of life expectancy: people in North America and Europe are currently living 31 years longer on average (as of 2015) than in 1900, a net increase in the average number of years of life expectancy from 47 to somewhat more than 78 years in the span of a single century. Many people live well into their 80s and 90s and increasing numbers of people enjoy healthy years of life well in excess of 100 years (World Health Organization, 2018). An increase of this magnitude is extraordinary and is the result of gains that have been achieved across a broad range of social, political, and economic sectors.

Most importantly, our children are surviving in much greater numbers the often harsh and precarious experiences of birth and early childhood encountered by earlier generations of children. Worldwide rates of infant and child mortality are now at historically low levels—down from an average of 60 deaths per 1000 live births in economically advanced societies in 1990 to an average of well below 5 or 6 infant deaths per 1000 live births in these same societies by 2015. Figure 2.1, which covers the 100-year period from 1950 to 2050, confirms that the same pattern of child

© Springer Nature Switzerland AG 2019

R. J. Estes, *The Social Progress of Nations Revisited, 1970–2020*, Social Indicators Research Series 78, https://doi.org/10.1007/978-3-030-15907-8_2

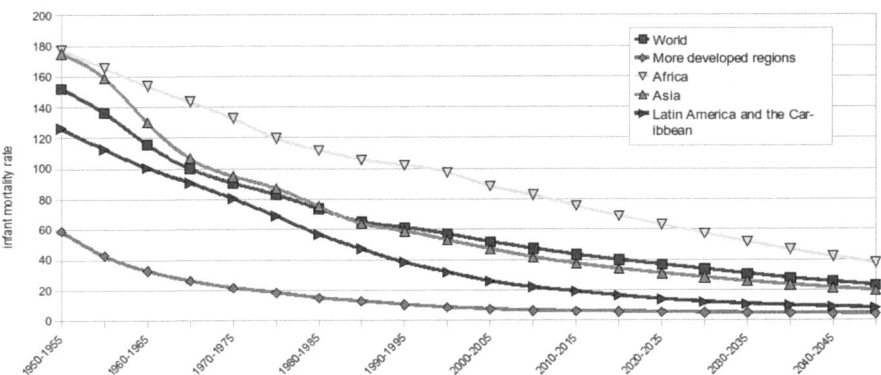

Fig. 2.1 Infant mortality rate by region, 1950–2050. (Graph by UN World Population Prospects, 2008; https://commons.wikimedia.org/wiki/File:Infant_Mortality_Rate_by_Region_1950-2050.png; Creative Commons Attribution 3.0 Unported license)

survival is occurring in all regions of the world including those that comprise the non-industrialized nations of Africa, Asia, the Caribbean, and Latin America. As with the dramatic increases in average years of life expectancy characteristic of today's adults, the contemporary high level of child survival is unparalleled in human history and will continue to increase (United Nations Children's Fund, 2018).

These gains in child and adult health have had the secondary effect of allowing families to voluntarily reduce the number of children in keeping with their financial capacity especially in situations where they have enough male children who, over the long term, are expected to support their parents in old age (van Soest & Saha, 2012). Fertility rates also are expected to drop to even lower levels because income security for the aged and other vulnerable populations is available through a combination of public and private resources. In either case, parents need no longer "expect" that some of their offspring will die before reaching the first year of life or during the years that follow.

Similarly, and increasingly, mothers are more likely to survive childbirth, a situation that at the turn of the last century took a large share of world's pregnant women who gave birth. Rates of maternal mortality have declined dramatically almost everywhere in the world as increasing numbers of pregnant women have gained access to quality pre- and postnatal care and have more secure and improved diets. Increasing numbers of pregnant women have their babies delivered under safe conditions that include access to sterile conditions and potable water supplies. The safe disposal of solid and liquid wastes is commonly available and continues to be made available to larger numbers of people living in remote rural communities, thanks to the aggressive outreach efforts of national and international nongovernmental organizations.

Similarly, better trained and more qualified midwives and other pre- and neonatal skilled health care personnel are available to pregnant women and their newborn children. In economically advanced societies, specially trained nurses, nurse practitioners, and obstetricians carefully monitor and safely deliver the babies of mothers with compromised health profiles or prior histories of miscarriages or still-born babies. Improved prenatal care in combination with the widespread availability of diagnostic and other equipment also is saving the lives of tens of thousands of children and their mothers each year. As a result, the number of maternal deaths associated with hemorrhage, infection, sepsis, genital trauma, and unsafe abortions has declined dramatically everywhere in the world by an average of at least 13% (World Health Organization, 2018). Enabling safe pregnancies and deliveries for women living in remote rural communities remains one of the greatest challenges facing humanity, but the knowledge and the resources needed to solve this challenge are gradually becoming available.

The Demographic Challenge

In the early part of the twenty-first century, more people are being born and are living longer than ever before in human history. This simple demographic reality has changed the face of our communities and will continue to do so for many decades and, in doing so, has reshaped the set of responsibilities for promoting the well-being of their growing number of citizens by both state and nonstate actors, including major national and international nongovernmental organizations. Indeed, two remarkably similar trends across societies dominated; namely, a continuing high rate of fertility in combination with high rates of aging citizens. At some point in the near term, child fertility patterns in developing countries are expected to decline as the percentages of their populations 60 years of age and older increase (Roser & Ortiz-Ospina, 2018). This trend means that today and, in the years ahead, fewer babies will be born and people will continue to live longer. Most developing countries must thus inevitably struggle with a wide range of policy issues related to rapidly increasing numbers of age-dependent persons relative to the numbers of working-age individuals (persons aged 15–64 years) who generate most of the wealth needed to build the society and support the new systems of income security available to individuals, families, and extended kinship systems (International Social Security Association, 2018).

However, the chronic joblessness of young people, often including university graduates, and uncertain income streams for the elderly are among the most frequent demographic challenges that developing countries face as they seek to increase their competitiveness in global markets while maintaining social stability at home (Tiliouine & Estes, 2016). The solutions needed to solve this challenge are not simple and require active participation by all segments of society, including the larger community of nations.

Figure 2.2 identifies two interrelated factors: (a) the population size of each of the world's 10 most populous countries and (b) the years of average life expectancy for men and women for each of these countries. The data are for midyear 2016.

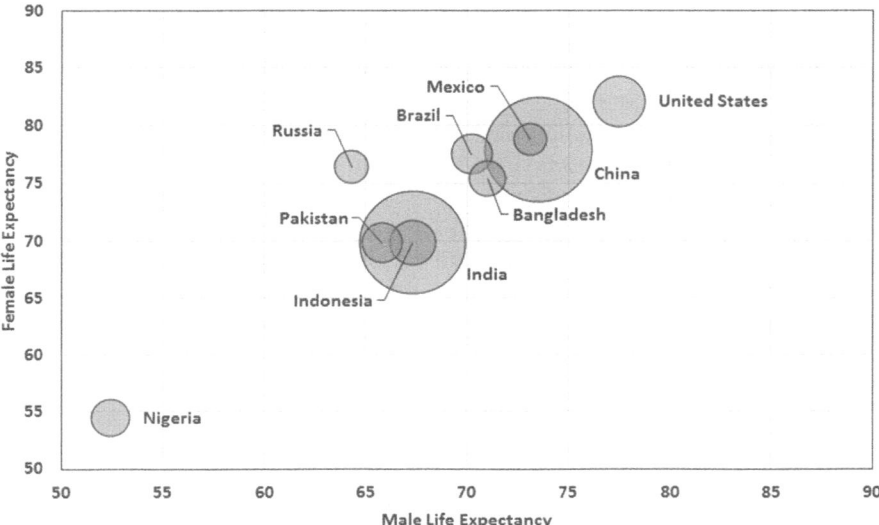

Fig. 2.2 The world's 10 most populous countries in 2016 by population size and years of average life expectancy for men and women. (Data from United Nations Population Division, 2018 illustration by David Walker)

Added together, the combined populations of these countries comprise 58% of the world's total population. Of interest is that only one of these countries, the United States, is classified as an economically advanced society; the remaining nine are classified by the World Bank as either "low-income" or "developing" countries (World Bank, 2018). All ten of these countries, though, engage in robust trade with one another, and this trade has added new resources to the economies that all the nations use in supporting a wide spectrum of advances in well-being.

Using bubbles to represent the comparative size of the population of each country, Fig. 2.2 also shows the years of average life expectancy for the men and women residing in each of the countries. The bubbles in the figure graphically summarize three variables: (1) the different population sizes of each country; (2) the average years of life expectancy by gender; and (3) gender-based disparities in average years of life expectancy. This type of data visualization makes it easier for the reader to readily discern complex patterns that are not so clearly visible when examining columns of numbers. (The authors are indebted to the late Swedish medical statistician Hans Rosling for promoting the use of such approaches for presenting complex data patterns more simply.)

The population and gender data reported in Fig. 2.2 are for mid 2016. The data confirm the relationships that exist in population size when they are disaggregated using gender as a control factor. The figure also confirms that highly populated countries, though advancing at different rates, are moving in the same direction in extending the lives of their residents and are doing so quickly. This finding is especially important because these large nations must work not only toward advancing the longevity of hundreds of millions of people but also toward establishing the means required to provide for at least their basic needs and wants. The demands placed on the governments of these nations are especially intense for improved health care, better education, and more secure employment. These are not easy well-being outcomes for even affluent nations to accomplish. At the same time, the challenge for the highly populated developing countries is to achieve the same outcomes as the more economically advanced countries but to do so with fewer material resources. Yet, the majority of the world's most populous nations have achieved this outcome, including all four of the population "super giants" shown in the figure, i.e., China, India, the United States, and Indonesia.

The data reported in Fig. 2.2 also confirm the existence of increased parity in average years of life expectancy among the 10 most populous countries. Women in each of the 10 countries, as is the case worldwide, live longer than men by an average of 4 to 5 years, but both men and women are living substantially longer on average than they did in earlier generations. This pattern is expected to continue over the near term as rich and poor countries achieve average years of life expectancy that are increasingly comparable to one another. These changes will occur most dramatically in countries with accelerated rates of economic growth, improved health conditions, and greater availability of at least a basic education. The steady introduction of reasonably secure "social safety" nets will also add to the advance in well-being among developing countries as will declines in average family size and, viewed globally, the size of the total world population (International Social Security Association, 2018).

The significant positive gains just reported are confirmed by the strikingly upward direction in which population longevity is increasing in 9 of the 10 countries. This is the case even for Nigeria, the major outlier shown in the figure, which continues to struggle with a legacy of poverty, high levels of diversity-related social conflict, classism, and political instability—all despite the great oil wealth of the country. Even so, men and women in Nigeria are living longer than they did during earlier decades despite their lagging economic and political positions.

Today, people living everywhere in the world are enjoying longer, healthier, and better educated lives than at any time in human history. In combination with emerging and already secure social safety nets that exist in most economically advanced countries, the quality of life of hundreds of millions of people has improved. In the decades just ahead, even more gains in population longevity and fertility control are expected. When that threshold is reached, the world is expected to experience a stabilization of population growth rates and, over time, an overall reduction in the total population (United Nations Population Division, 2018).

Looking ahead, Fig. 2.3 shows the expected rate of population increase for the world by developmental stage. Included with each stage are the expected patterns associated with births, deaths, and rates of natural increase and decrease that result from patterns of births and deaths. The dynamics of fertility and population aging are reported in the boxes at the bottom of the figure. The chart presents a picture of the general pattern of economic change that most countries undergo as they move from stage 1 to stage 5 of population growth. These generally "expected" patterns

The demographic transition in 5 stages

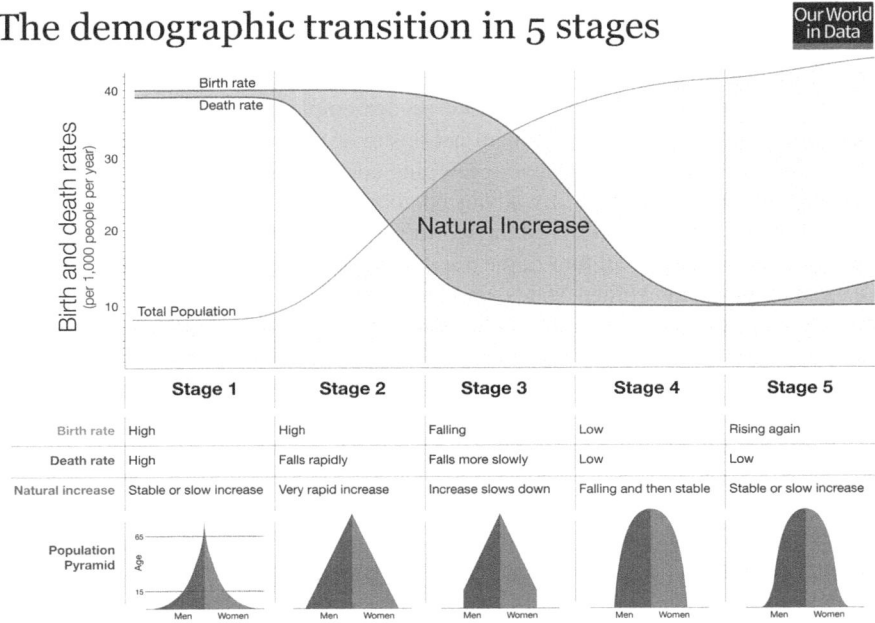

Fig. 2.3 Expected rate of population increase for the world by stage of development, birth rate, death rate, and rates of natural increase and decrease. (Roser, M., & Ortiz-Ospina, E., 2013/2017; Creative Commons Attribution-ShareAlike 4.0 International License)

are useful for comparing the population trends occurring within and between various groups of nations. In applying this framework, we can easily see variations that may prevent countries from moving from one developmental stage to another.

The differences that exist in population distribution patterns are apparent in charts such as that portrayed in Fig. 2.4, which summarizes the important age and gender distributions that take place in countries. This situation exists in many countries of the world and is illustrated in the various images of the "population pyramid[1]" of Mexico in 2018 located online at https://www.indexmundi.com/mexico/age_structure.html, which aggregates national populations by gender and age. The economically ideal pattern, of course, is to have many economically active persons (ages 15–64) who generate the resources needed to provide for age-dependent family members (< 15 years, > 60–65 years) to be able to financially support the overall development of these individuals and larger communities within which they reside.

---

[1]A population pyramid, also called an "age-sex pyramid," is a graphical illustration that shows the distribution of various age groups in a population (typically that of a country or region of the world), which forms the shape of a pyramid when the population is growing. This tool can be used to visualize the age of a particular population. It is also used in ecology to determine the overall age distribution of a population, an indication of the reproductive capabilities and likelihood of the continuation of a species (Wikipedia, 2018).

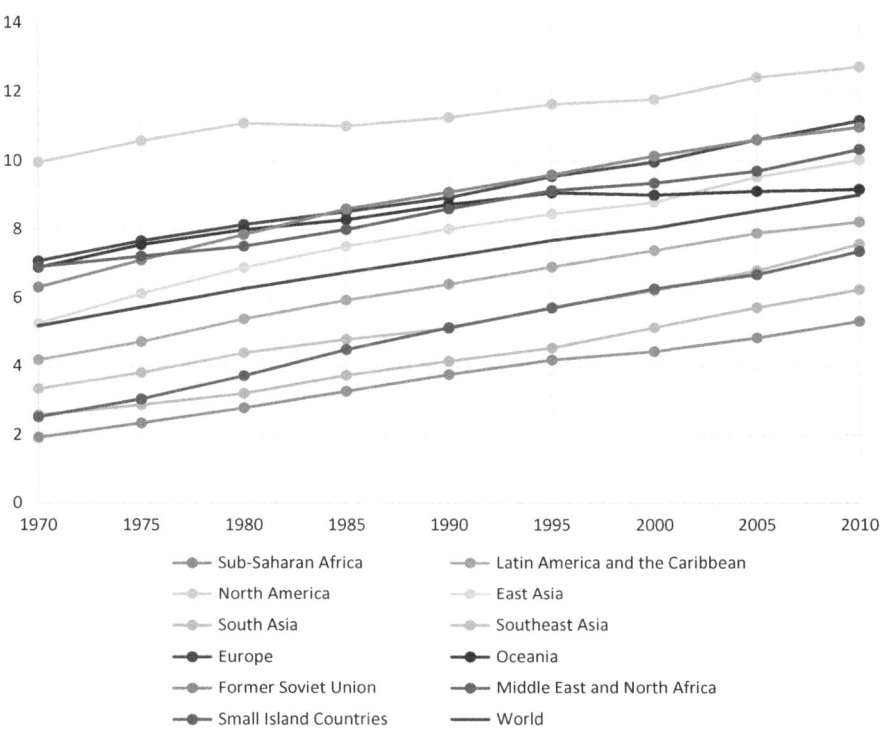

Fig. 2.4 Average years of total schooling among persons aged 15 years and older. (Data from World Bank, 2017; figure © *Advances in Well-Being: Towards a Better World*, by Richard J. Estes and M. Joseph Sirgy, published by Rowman & Littlefield International, 2018; reprinted with permission)

Mexico's population pyramid reflects the imbalance that exists between the numbers of noneconomically productive children, youth, and older persons vis-à-vis the numbers of persons in the economically active age group. In Mexico, the percentage is much lower than that of most postindustrial societies because of the large numbers of children in most Mexican families. The growing number of older persons, though still small, also makes large demands on the financial resources of the family and of the country. Taken as a percentage of Mexico's total population, the volume of demand for support placed on Mexican families by their children and their elders is large. At the same time, the proportion of economically active age groups in Mexico is steadily shrinking, which imposes yet another set of policy demands on a mid-level developing country.

What does this all mean? The economic burden placed on Mexico's economically active workforce is high as it struggles to meet the needs of so many children and a steadily increasing population of elderly persons. The demographic challenges for Mexico represented by these trends are substantial and have major well-being implications not only for Mexico but also for the world. Moreover, increased gender inequality, a lingering problem in Mexico, in combination with moderate to high rates of economic growth, has caused families to voluntarily reduce their birth rate and invest more in their elders (Ghose, 2013). Despite the complexity of these trends as well as the underlying drivers that support them, there is little determinism or fatalism that may be applied to these dynamics. Rather, these decisions are made by families themselves, and they, as with nearly all families, hold in their own hands the power to enhance their overall quality of life, standard of living, and well-being.

Private decision making and public policies formulated by policy makers in support of families play a vitally important role in enhancing the quality of life in society across the board. Evidence-based decisions of this kind provide the foundations upon which individuals, families, and societies achieve their collective progress. This is one of the many results of adopting a *positivist* approach to understanding and acting on the challenges that confront all sectors of personal and communal life.

Declining Rates of Infectious and Communicable Diseases

Perhaps most exciting and least appreciated in terms of making headlines has been the impact of modern medicine on the preponderance of infectious and communicable diseases such as diphtheria, pertussis, tetanus, polio, cholera, malaria, and tuberculosis. Each has declined to its historically lowest levels in response to aggressive health outreach services to large numbers of urban and rural dwellers. Vaccinations against crippling childhood diseases—diphtheria, pertussis, tetanus, and polio—now reach nearly 80% of the world's infants and children. If we think about this, this level of achievement in human progress is nothing short of a modern miracle. These diseases are entirely preventable, especially in their early stages, and the cost of vaccines has dropped to historically low levels. The recently launched United Nations Sustainable Development Goals initiative has been designed to reach the remaining 20% of unvaccinated, difficult to reach children. Every expectation exists for believing that this goal will be achieved by no later than 2025. Progress in treating drug-resistant tuberculosis likely will proceed more slowly, given the complexities of both the disease and the health delivery systems needed to treat the disease at its earliest stage.

The global sanitation movement, which is inextricably tied to the spread of communicable diseases, has fully taken hold. From the World Toilet Organization (http://worldtoilet.org/) down to the most dogged social enterprise working on the ground teaching people about the dangers to their health of exposure to open defecation, progress has been achieved to move the needle. Local communities around the world have developed highly effective approaches for processing liquid and solid wastes that previously littered their streets and even their homes.

The world's most environmentally aggressive communities formulate carefully thought through plans for disposing of solid and liquid wastes with an emphasis on waste reduction, waste reuse, and waste recycling. Less emphasis is placed on waste disposal and waste recovery, given the expense of these approaches and their often-negative impact on the poor into whose communities these wastes are often dumped. Rather, the most effective and, on balance, the least expensive approach to waste management has been to carefully "mine" the wastes to extract anything of value and then to use the remaining solid wastes as fuel in the production of low-cost energy delivered to communities with little or no previous access to the electric "grid."

Thanks to these rapidly spreading approaches for the effective and efficient management of waste, a larger share of the world's population need no longer depend on a single light bulb (or candle) to light their homes after dark. Instead, even low-income urban dwellers can have multiple outlets for receiving and using electrical services. This innovation, along with the significant advances that have occurred in the health, education, and economic sectors, have added measurably to the quality of life and well-being of many poor and low-income communities. The remaining challenge, of course, is to bring low-cost energy to the many hundreds of millions of rural dwellers who do not yet possess the ability to convert waste into low-cost energy. But this challenge is expected to be met in the decade just ahead.

Education and Well-Being

Housing and neighborhood living conditions also have improved significantly since 1950. Clean water is a new reality for the rich and the poor, one of the primary drivers of improved health conditions worldwide. The availability of clean piped water in developing countries has significantly improved the social situation of women and girls, who previously spent most of their time carrying heavy buckets of unsafe water from distant streams to their homes. At the same time, illiteracy is rapidly becoming a problem of the past, given that increasing numbers of children and adults (Fig. 2.4) have access to at least literacy education. The reduction of drudgery for the fulfillment of basic needs has created more space for other activities, not least of which include learning and the application of other basic productive skills in even the most deprived areas.

The global literacy rate for all men is 90.0% and the rate for all women is 82.7%. The rate varies throughout the world, with developed nations having a rate of 99.2% (2013); Oceania, 71.3%; South and West Asia, 70.2% (2015); and sub-Saharan Africa, 64.0% (United Nations, 2018).

Never in human history have we seen the major fundamental improvements in day-to-day living conditions and quality of life that have occurred during the decades following the end of World War II. Today, women and men and their school-age children can read newspapers or visit electronic sites using computers, do homework, write to others, and correctly read and interpret treatments prescribed by health service professionals, including pharmacists. Until now, the number of children who died because they or their illiterate parents were unable to read or understand labels on bottles of medicines prescribed by health care providers was very high (Estes & Sirgy, 2018a).

None of the preceding advances in human well-being would have been possible without the gains made in basic health, education, social welfare, engineering, and technology. Nor would they have been possible without the significant advances in community literacy levels, access to primary and secondary school education, and access to postsecondary education (colleges, universities, qualified evening schools, and continuing education programs designed to reach populations to which basic and advanced education were previously inaccessible). Major advances in vocational and technical training programs also have contributed to our century-long advances in health and education that serve as the cornerstone for improved quality of life everywhere in the world.

All the preceding efforts at advancing human well-being were supported by central and local governments and by an extraordinarily large number of generous private philanthropies. They also have been built on the foundation of economic growth and the foresight of informed business leaders and their enterprises that contributed to significant increases in per capita and household income levels—another of the critical drivers of advances in well-being (Gopal & Tikhvinsky, 2008).

Women and Girls

Significant gains in social progress since 1900, but especially since 1950, have been made in bringing historically disadvantaged population groups into the mainstream of society. These gains have been especially significant for women and girls who, increasingly, are achieving equity with men and boys. Most of the world's women are now able to vote and can participate fully as members of representative parliaments and congresses nearly everywhere in the world. Women and other members of historically disadvantaged population groups (e.g., children and youths, the elderly, sexual minorities, racial and ethnic minorities, migrants) also are receiving increasing levels of legal protection against occupational discrimination with the result that many are employed in the same types of positions as men, although the incomes of most women have not yet achieved full parity with those paid to men performing the same jobs. That situation, too, is changing rapidly as the so-called glass ceiling has more and more cracks. The contemporary achievements of women and other previously disenfranchised population groups in the sciences, business, education, health care, the performing arts, and competitive sports are especially noteworthy and have resulted in an entirely new cognitive "reframing" of their role in and rich contribution to male-dominated societies (UN Women, 2015).

It is truly notable that poverty rates throughout the world have declined dramatically. The rate of extreme poverty has been cut in half since 2000 and is expected to be cut in half again by 2030 in response to the ambitious poverty alleviation priorities embodied in the United Nations Sustainable Development Goals initiative with its thousands of local, national, and international private and public partners.

Average income levels of previously poor families have increased appreciably since 2000, and these averages are expected to continue to increase as the poor acquire new job skills and pursue training opportunities that previously were not available to them. These gains in poverty reduction have affected the rural poor most dramatically, especially in the poorest nations of East (China) and South Asia (India, Bangladesh, Pakistan), where hundreds of millions of the extreme poor have been lifted out of poverty. Every expectation exists for believing that this significant advance in human well-being will continue over at least the near term, during which time hundreds of millions of additional previously poor people will gain secure employment and stable incomes that exceed national and global poverty thresholds (World Bank, 2018).

The Drivers of Social Progress, Technological Innovation, and Well-Being

In addition to the dramatic social advances in human well-being just identified, major advances also have been made in improving worldwide access to science and technology. These advances in the collective scientific, technological, and engineering accomplishments are responsible for the impressive achievements that have been made since 1960 across all sectors of society. Some of these transformational innovations are described in the *Foreword* to this book and elsewhere (Estes & Sirgy, 2017, 2018a, 2018b; Estes & Tiliouine, 2014) and warrant a brief restatement, namely, completion of the sequencing of the human genome, gene-based treatment of cancers and other life-threatening diseases, phenomenal advances in the neurological sciences, and heretofore unimagined advances in the miniaturization of electronic devices along with the use of these devices for unparalleled ease of interpersonal communication and access to the sum total of all human knowledge using these devices to connect to supercomputers housed elsewhere ("cloud" computing). Technological advances in the medical sciences (including medical imaging systems such as computed tomography and magnetic resonance imaging), bioengineering approaches to aid physically disabled persons, the expansion of minimally invasive surgical techniques, and more effective medications for treating persons with serious mental and behavioral illnesses have emerged at a pace never previously experienced.

Additional major innovations across all sectors of human development are expected to continue to be achieved at an even more rapid pace as this still young century continues to unfold. The increasing pace of technological and broad-based social development will build on past achievements that provide the foundation for ever newer and more dramatic accomplishments…including the ability of humanity to travel to distance planets within our own solar system. At the same time, new possibilities for promoting a deepening sense of personal and collective well-being are expected to be within our grasp as well.

References

Estes, R. J., & Sirgy, M. J. (Eds.). (2017). *The pursuit of human well-being: The untold global history*. Cham, Switzerland: Springer.

Estes, R. J., & Sirgy, M. J. (2018a). *Advances in well-being: Towards a better world*. London: Rowman & Littlefield.

Estes, R. J., & Sirgy, M. J. (2018b). Advances in well-being in the MENA region: Accentuating the Positive. In L. Lambert & N. Pasha-Zaidi (Eds.), *Advances in well-being in the Middle East and North Africa (MENA) Region: Historical background and contemporary challenges*. Dordrecht, The Netherlands: Springer International Publishers. in press.

Estes, R. J., & Tiliouine, H. (2014). Islamic development trends: From collective wishes to concerted actions. *Social Indicators Research, 116*(1), 67–114.

Estes, R. J., & Zhou, H. M. (2014). A conceptual approach to the creation of public–private partnerships in social welfare. *International Journal of Social Welfare, 24*(4), 348–363.

Ghose, T. (2013, April 29). The secret to curbing population growth. *Live Science*. Retrieved August 19, 2018 from https://www.livescience.com/29131-economics-drives-birth-rate-declines.html

Gopal, S., & Tikhvinsky, S. L. (Eds.). (2008). *History of humanity: The Twentieth Century* (Vol. VII). Paris: United Nations Educational, Scientific, and Cultural Organization.

International Social Security Association. (2018). *Social security programs throughout the world, 2018*. Geneva, Switzerland: International Social Security Administration.

Roser, M., & Ortiz-Ospina, E. (2018). World Population Growth. [Online resource]. Retrieved September 1, 2018 from https://ourworldindata.org/world-population-growth

Tiliouine, H., & Estes, R. J. (2016). *The state of social progress of Islamic societies: Social, political, economic, and ideological challenges*. Dordrecht, The Netherlands: Springer International Publishers.

UN Women. (2015). *Progress of the world's women 2015–2016: Transforming economies, realizing rights*. New York: UN Women. Retrieved August 19, 2018 from http://www.unwomen.org/en/digital-library/publications/2015/4/progress-of-the-worlds-women-2015.

United Nations. (2018). *Least developed countries at a glance*. New York: UN Department of Economics and Social Affairs. Retrieved August 19, 2018 from https://www.un.org/development/desa/dpad/least-developed-country-category/ldcs-at-a-glance.html.

United Nations Children's Fund. (2018). *Research and reports [Web site]*. New York: UNICEF. Retrieved August 19, 2018 from https://www.unicef.org/research-and-reports.

United Nations Population Division (UNPOP). (2018). *Population trends*. Retrieved September 10 from http://www.un.org/en/development/desa/population/theme/trends/index.shtml

Van Soest, A., & Saha, U. (2012). *Birth spacing, child survival and fertility decisions: Analysis of causal mechanisms*. Center Discussion Chapter Series No. 2012–018. Retrieved June 13, 2017 from https://chapters.ssrn.com/sol3/chapters.cfm?abstract_id=2009852

Wikipedia. (2018). *Population pyramid*. Retrieved September 15, 2018 from https://en.wikipedia.org/wiki/Population_pyramid

World Bank. (2017). *Education statistics*. [Databank]. Retrieved September 13, 2018 from http://data.worldbank.org/data-catalog/ed-stats

World Bank. (2018). *World Development Report 2018: Learning to realize education's promise*. Washington, DC: World Bank. Retrieved August 19, 2018 from http://www.worldbank.org/en/publication/wdr2018.

World Health Organization. (2018). *Global health observatory (GHO): World health statistics 2018: Monitoring health for the SDGs*. Geneva: World Health Organization. Retrieved August 19, 2018 from http://www.who.int/gho/publications/world_health_statistics/2018/en/.

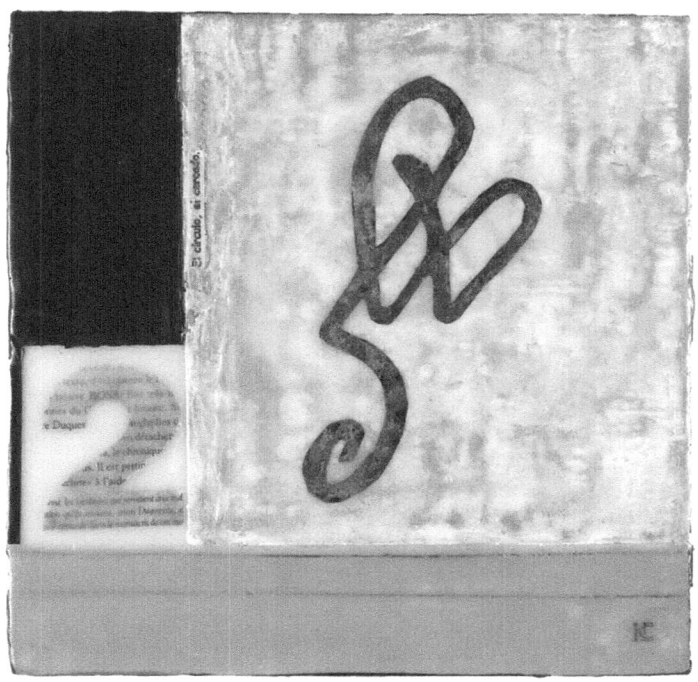

Part II

Image 2: © Lylia Ferero Carr: Muysca, BOSA

Chapter 3
Methodology

Comparative research using the world as the focus of analysis is very complex and requires multiple levels of conceptual and methodological decisions to implement correctly. The study reported in this volume is one of more than 40 such studies that have been conducted by this author at the global, regional, subregional, and national levels of analysis. The majority of these studies have been identified in the reference sections of the book's various chapters. The references identify the complexities of international comparative analysis and, at the same time, offer insights into the varied methodological solutions that other scholars may wish to consider.

This Study

The present study has been carried out in the tradition of the earlier inquiries into comparative analysis and examines global and national challenges and progress experienced by nations in providing for both the basic and enhanced needs of their growing populations. The methods used in implementing the study are discussed here and more fully in Appendix A, which focuses in greater detail on the study's statistical decisions.

The purpose of the present study and those that preceded it has been (1) to identify significant changes in the "adequacy of social provision"[1] occurring throughout the world and within specific continental and geopolitical regions; (2) to assess national progress in providing more adequately for the basic social and material needs of the world's growing population; and (3) to contribute to the creation of a comprehensive

---

[1] "Adequacy of social provision" refers to the changing capacity of governments to provide for the basic social, material, and other needs of the people living within their borders, e.g., for food, clothing, shelter, and access to at least basic health, education, and social services (Estes, 1988: 199–209).

© Springer Nature Switzerland AG 2019
R. J. Estes, *The Social Progress of Nations Revisited, 1970–2020*, Social
Indicators Research Series 78, https://doi.org/10.1007/978-3-030-15907-8_3

policy framework designed for use by governments, nongovernmental organizations, and people themselves for improving their material needs and subjective well-being.

Countries and Regions

This book reports a time-series analysis of the social development performances of 162 nations over the nearly 50-year period since 1970. Particular attention is given to human well-being at four levels of analysis: (1) selected countries; (2) major geopolitical subregions and regions including North America (N = 2), Oceania (N = 4), Europe (N = 35), Latin America (N = 26), Asia (N = 45), and Africa (N = 50); (3) well-being trends for the world as a whole; and (4) countries organized by the World Bank's major economic-political groupings of nations, i.e., developed market economies (N = 34), member states of the Commonwealth of Independent States (N = 21), developing countries (N = 67), and countries officially designated by the United Nations as least developed countries (N = 40). Countries grouped by these international geographic and sociopolitical levels of development are listed in Table 3.1.

Index of Social Progress

The primary instrument used in this study is the author's extensively pretested *Index of Social Progress* (ISP) and its statistically weighted version, the *Weighted Index of Social Progress* (WISP) (Table 3.2). In its present form, the ISP comprises 40 social indicators that are divided among 10 subindexes: *Education* (N = 4)*; Health Status* (N = 7)*; Women Status* (N = 4)*; Defense Effort* (N = 1)*; Economic* (N = 5)*; Demographic* (N = 3)*; Environmental* (N = 3)*; Social Chaos* (N = 5)*; Cultural Diversity* (N = 3); and *Welfare Effort* (N = 5). All 40 of the ISP's indicators in 2018 have been established to be valid indicators of social development and are used regularly in a broad range of development-focused studies conducted by other well-being policy-focused scholars.

Weighted Index of Social Progress

Owing to the volume of data gathered for the analysis, only statistically weighted index (WISP) (WISP70, WISP80, WISP90, WISP00, WISP10/11, WISP17/18) and subindex scores are reported in this book. The study's statistical weights were derived through a multistage principal component and varimax factor analysis in which indicator and subindex scores were analyzed separately for their relative contributions toward explaining the variance associated with changes in social progress over time (Table 3.3).

Table 3.1 Weighted index of social progress-18: Countries organized by continent and subregion (N = 162)

Africa (N = 50)	Asia (N = 45)	Latin America (N = 26)	Europe (N = 35)
East Africa (N = 15)	**East Asia (N = 7)**	**Caribbean (N = 7)**	**East Europe (N = 10)**
Burundi (LDC)	China (DC)	Bahamas (DC)	Belarus (CIS)
Comoros (LDC)	Hong Kong SAR (DME)	Belize (DC)	Bulgaria (CIS)
Djibouti (LDC)	Japan (DME)	Cuba (DC)	Czech Republic (DME)
Eritrea (LDC)	Korea, North (DC)	Dominican Republic (DC)	Hungary (DME)
Ethiopia (LDC)	Korea, South (DME)	Haiti (LDC)	Moldova (CIS)
Kenya (DC)	Mongolia (DC)	Jamaica (DC)	Poland (DME)
Madagascar (LDC)	Taiwan (DME)	Trinidad &Tobago (DC)	Romania (CIS)
Malawi (LDC)			Russian Federation (CIS)
Mauritius (DC)	**South Central Asia (N = 13)**	**Central America (N = 7)**	Slovak Republic (DME)
Mozambique (LDC)	Afghanistan (LDC)	Costa Rica (DC)	Ukraine (CIS)
Rwanda (LDC)	Bangladesh (LDC)	El Salvador (DC)	
Somalia (LDC)	Bhutan (LDC)	Guatemala (DC)	**North Europe (N = 10)**
Tanzania (LDC)	India (DC)	Honduras (DC)	Denmark (DME)
Uganda (LDC)	Iran (DC)	Mexico (DME)	Estonia (CIS)
Zambia (LDC)	Kazakhstan (CIS)	Nicaragua (DC)	Finland (DME)
	Kyrgyzstan (CIS)	Panama (DC)	Iceland (DME)
Middle Africa (N = 7)	Nepal (LDC)		Ireland (DME)
Angola (LDC)	Pakistan (DC)	**South America (N = 12)**	Latvia (CIS)
Cameroon (DC)	Sri Lanka (DC)	Argentina (DC)	Lithuania (CIS)
Central African Rep (LDC)	Tajikistan (CIS)	Bolivia (DC)	Norway (DME)
Chad (LDC)	Turkmenistan (CIS)	Brazil (DC)	Sweden (DME)
Congo, Rep (DC)	Uzbekistan (CIS)	Chile (DC)	United Kingdom (DME)
Congo, DR (LDC)		Colombia (DC)	
Gabon (DC)	**South East Asia (N = 9)**	Ecuador (DC)	**South Europe (N = 8)**
	Cambodia (LDC)	Guyana (DC)	Albania (CIS)
North Africa (N = 6)	Indonesia (DC)	Paraguay (DC)	Croatia (CIS)
Algeria (DC)	Lao, PDR (LDC)	Peru (DC)	Greece (DME)
Egypt, UAR (DC)	Malaysia (DC)	Suriname (DC)	Italy (DME)
Libya (DC)	Myanmar (LDC)	Uruguay (DC)	Macedonia, TFYR (CIS)

(continued)

Table 3.1 (continued)

Africa (N = 50)	Asia (N = 45)	Latin America (N = 26)	Europe (N = 35)
Morocco (DC)	Philippines (DC)	Venezuela (DC)	Portugal (DME)
Sudan (LDC)	Singapore (DME)		Slovenia (CIS)
Tunisia (DC)	Thailand (DC)		Spain (DME)
	Viet Nam (DC)		
Southern Africa (N = 6)		**North America (N = 2)**	**West Europe (N = 7)**
Botswana (DC)	**West Asia (N = 16)**	Canada (DME)	Austria (DME)
Lesotho (LDC)	Armenia (CIS)	United States (DME)	Belgium (DME)
Namibia (DC)	Azerbaijan (CIS)		France (DME)
South Africa (DC)	Bahrain (DC)		Germany (DME)
Swaziland (DC)	Cyprus (DC)		Luxembourg (DME)
Zimbabwe (DC)	Georgia (CIS)		Netherlands (DME)
	Iraq (DC)	**OCEANIA (N = 4)**	Switzerland (DME)
West Africa (N = 16)	Israel (DME)	**Australia-New Zealand (N = 2)**	
Benin (LDC)	Jordan (DC)	Australia (DME)	
Burkina-Faso (LDC)	Kuwait (DC)	New Zealand (DME)	
Cape Verde (LDC)	Lebanon (DC)		
Cote d'Ivoire (DC)	Oman (DC)	**Melanesia (N = 2)**	
Gambia (LDC)	Qatar (DC)	Fiji (DC)	
Ghana (DC)	Saudi Arabia (DC)	Papua-New Guinea (DC)	
Guinea-Bissau (LDC)	Syria (DC)		
Guinea (LDC)	Turkey (DME)		
Liberia (LDC)	Yemen (LDC)		
Mali (LDC)			
Mauritania (LDC)			
Nigeria (DC)			
Niger (LDC)			
Senegal Leone (LDC)			
Sierra (LDC)			
Togo (LDC)			

CIS Commonwealth of Independent States, *DC* developing countries, *DME* developed market economies, *LDC* least developed countries

Standardized indicator scores (N = 40) were multiplied by their respective factor loadings and averaged within their subindex. The average subindex scores (N = 10), in turn, were subjected to a second statistical weighting. A constant value of +50 was added to the formula to eliminate the many negative values that resulted for the world's socially least developed countries. The resulting values from this two-stage statistical weighting process formed the basis for computing the composite WISP scores summarized in Table 3.4.

Table 3.2 Indicators on the Weighted Index of Social Progress-18 by subindex (40 indicators and 10 subindexes)

Index of Social Progress, 2018 (ISP2018, WISP2018) (40 Indicators, 10 Subindexes)
Education Subindex (N = 4)
Public expenditure on education as percentage of gross domestic product, 2015–2017 (+)
Primary school completion rate, 2015–2017 (+)
Secondary school net enrollment rate, 2015–2017 (+)
Adult literacy rate, 2015–2017 (+)
Health Status Subindex (N = 6)
Life expectation at birth, 2015–2017 (+)
Infant mortality rate, 2015–2017 (−)
Under-five child mortality rate, 2015–2017 (−)
Physicians per 100,000 population, 2015–2017 (+)
Percent of population undernourished, 2015–2017 (−)
Public expenditure on health as percentage of gross domestic product, 2015–2017 (+)
Women Status Subindex (N = 4)
Female adult literacy as percentage of male literacy, 2015–2017 (+)
Maternal mortality ratio, 2015–2017 (−)
Female secondary school enrollment as percentage of male enrollment, 2015–2017 (+)
Seats in parliament held by women as percentage of total, 2015–2017 (+)
Defense Effort Subindex (N = 1)
Military expenditures as percentage of gross domestic product, 2015–2017 (−)
Economic Subindex (N = 5)
Per capita gross national income (as measured by purchasing power parity), 2015–2017 (+)
Percent growth in gross domestic product, 2015–2017 (+)
Unemployment rate, 2015–2017 (−)
Total external debt as percentage of gross domestic product, 2015–2017 (−)
Gini Index score [most recent year (most available year available)] (−)
Demography Subindex (N = 3)
Average annual rate of population growth, 2015–2017 (−)
Percent of population aged <15 years, 2015–2017 (−)
Percent of population aged >64 years, 2015–2017 (+)
Environmental Subindex (N=3)
Percentage of nationally protected area, 2015–2017 (+)
Average annual number of disaster-related deaths, 2015–2017 (−)
Per capita metric tons of carbon dioxide emissions, 2015–2017 (−)
Social Chaos Subindex (N=6)
Strength of political rights, 2015–2017 (−)
Strength of civil liberties, 2015–2017 (−)
Number of internally displaced persons per 100,000 population, 2015–2017 (−)
Number of externally displaced persons per 100,000 population, 2015–2017 (−)
Estimated number of deaths from armed conflicts (low estimate), 2015–2017 (−)
Perceived Corruption Index, 2015–2017 (+)
Cultural Diversity Subindex (N=3)

(continued)

Table 3.2 (continued)

Index of Social Progress, 2018 (ISP2018, WISP2018) (40 Indicators, 10 Subindexes)
Largest percentage of population sharing the same or similar racial/ethnic origins, 2015–2017 (+)
Largest percentage of population sharing the same or similar religious beliefs, 2015–2017 (+)
Largest share of population sharing the same mother tongue, 2015–2017 (+)
Welfare Effort Subindex (N=5)
Age First National Law—old age, invalidity & death, 2015–2017 (+)
Age First National Law—sickness & maternity, 2015–2017 (+)
Age First National Law—work injury, 2015–2017 (+)
Age First National Law—unemployment, 2015–2017 (+)
Age First National Law—family allowance, 2015–2017 (+)

Table 3.3 Weighted Index of Social Progress-18 factors and factor loadings (N = 162)

Factor 1 Adequacy of Social Provision (N = 5)
.90 * STN Health Status 2018 Subindex
.90* STN Women's Status 2018 Subindex
.89 * STN Demographic Status 2018 Subindex
.73 * STN Education 2018 Subindex
.55 * STN Welfare Effort 2018 Subindex
Factor 2 National Environment and Diversity Resources (N = 2)
.84 * STN Environmental Status 2018 Subindex
.81 * STN Cultural Diversity 2018 Subindex
Factor 3 Defense and Military Expenditures (N = 1)
.97 * STN Defense Effort 2018 Subindex
Factor 4 Economic Resources and Stress (N = 2)
.92 * STN Social Chaos 2018 Subindex
.75 * STN Economic Status 2018 Subindex

Data Sources

The majority of the data used in the analysis were obtained from the annual reports supplied by individual countries to specialized agencies of the United Nations, the United Nations Development Programme (2018), the World Bank (2018), the Organization for Economic Cooperation and Development (2018), the International Social Security Association (2018), the International Labour Organization (2018), the International Monetary Fund (2018a, 2018b), and other major international data collection and reporting organizations. Data for the *Environmental* subindex were obtained from the World Resources Institute (2018) and the United Nations Commission on Sustainable Development (2018). Data for the *Social Chaos* subindex were obtained from Amnesty International (2018), Freedom House (2018), the International Federation of Red Cross and Red Crescent Societies (2018), the

Table 3.4 Application of factor loadings to create the Weighted Index of Social Progress-18 (N = 162)

Final statistical weights used in constructing the Weighted Index of Social Progress-18
WISP2018 = {[(.456 * Factor 1) + (.169 * Factor 2) + (.128 * Factor 3) + (.245 * Factor 4)]} + 50
where:
Factor 1 = {[(Health18 * .90) + (Woman18 * .90) + (Demographic18 * .89) + (Education18 * .73) + (Welfare19 * .55)] +
Factor 2 = [(Cultural Diversity18 * .81) – (Environmental18 * .84)] +
Factor 3 = [(Defense Effort18 * .97)] +
Factor 4 = [(Social Chaos18 * .92) + (Economic19 * .75)]} + 50

Stockholm International Peace and Research Institute (2018), and Transparency International (2018). Data for the *Cultural Diversity* subindex were gathered from the Central Intelligence Agency's *World Factbook* (2018) and from the work of independent scholars in the fields of comparative language, religion, and ethnology. Data sources for the individual demographic, economic, and political indicators are reported in relevant tables.

Country Selection

The 162 countries selected for inclusion in the study satisfied at least three of the following four criteria: (1) a population size either approaching or exceeding one million people; (2) a reasonable degree of political stability such that timely and reliable data collection could be undertaken by governmental or nongovernmental bodies, or both; (3) the availability of comprehensive, reliable, and time-series social indicator data; and (4) the country's inclusion in the author's earlier studies of international comparative social development and well-being. Countries with missing, inadequate, incomplete, or distorted data on three or more of the ISP's 40 indicators and for which reasonable estimates for the missing data could not be calculated, were excluded from the analysis. This latter group of countries consist primarily of the ocean-locked island nations situated in the Pacific Ocean with their substantially fewer than one million people (United Nations Office of the High Representative for the Least Developed Countries, Landlocked Developing Countries and Small Island Developing States, 2017).

Levels of Analysis

Throughout the book, data are reported for four levels of analysis: (1) development trends occurring for the world as a whole (N = 1); (2) development trends occurring at the continental (N = 6) and subcontinental levels (N = 19); (3) development trends occurring within socioeconomic-political groupings (i.e., developed market economies, the Commonwealth of Independent States, developing countries, least developed countries (N = 4); and (4) development trends occurring within each of the 162 countries, including the study's 40 socially least developed countries.

Time Frame

Index and subindex findings are reported separately for each of the study's six time periods, i.e., 1970, 1980, 1990, 2000, 2010/2011, and 2017/2018. Thus, this analysis reports both archival and original cross-sectional analyses of the "state of well-being" reflective of development trends for approximately 95% of the world's population over a 50-year period (1970–2017/18).

References

Amnesty International. (2018). *Research*. [Web site Homepage]. Retrieved July 10, 2018 from https://www.amnesty.org/en/latest/research/?contentType=2564&issue=1253&sort=date
Central Intelligence Agency. (2018). *World factbook* (p. 2018). Washington, DC: U.S. Department of State.
Estes, R. J. (1988). *Trends in world social development: The social progress of nations, 1970–1987*. New York: Praeger.
House, F. (2018). *Freedom throughout the world, 2018*. New York: Freedom House.
International Federation of Red Cross and Red Crescent Societies. (2018). *Annual report, 2018*. Retrieved July 10, 2018 from https://media.ifrc.org/ifrc-pages/
International Labour Organization. (2018). *Statistics and databases*. [Database]. Retrieved July 10, 2018 from http://www.ilo.org/global/statistics-and-databases/lang%2D%2Den/index.htm
International Monetary Fund. (2018a). *IMF data*. [Database]. Retrieved July 8, 2018 from http://www.imf.org/en/Data
International Monetary Fund. (2018b) *World economic outlook, 2018*. April. Retrieved July 8, 2018 from https://www.imf.org/en/Publications/WEO/Issues/2018/03/20/world-economic-outlook-april-2018
International Social Security Association. (2018). *Social security programs throughout the world*. [Database]. Geneva: International Social Security Association. Retrieved August 24 from https://www.ssa.gov/policy/docs/progdesc/ssptw/
Organization for Economic Cooperation and Development. (2018). *OECD data*. [Database]. Retrieved September 4, 2018 from https://data.oecd.org/
Stockholm International Peace Research Institute. (2018). *SIPRI yearbook 2018: Armaments, disarmament and international security*. Stockholm, Sweden: Stockholm International Peace Research Institute.
Transparency International. (2018). *Corruptions perception index*. [Organization Web site.] Berlin: Transparency International. Retrieved August 24, 2018 from https://www.transparency.org/research/cpi/overview
United Nations Commission on Sustainable Development. (2018). *Knowledge platform*. [Organization Web site]. Retrieved July 10, 2018 from https://sustainabledevelopment.un.org/frameworks

United Nations Development Programme. (2018). *Human development report. 2018.* New York: United Nations Development Programme.

United Nations Office of the High Representative for the Least Developed Countries, Landlocked Developing Countries and Small Island Developing States. (2017). *Enhancing the participation of the landlocked states in the implementation of Sustainable Development Goal (SDG) 14.* Retrieved July 1, 2018 from http://unohrlls.org/event/enhancing-participation-landlocked-states-implementation-sustainable-development-goal-sdg-14/

World Bank. (2018). *World development report* (p. 2018). Washington, DC: World Bank Group.

World Resources Institute. (2018). *Maps and data.* [Institution Web site]. Retrieved August 24, 2018 from http://www.wri.org/resources/maps

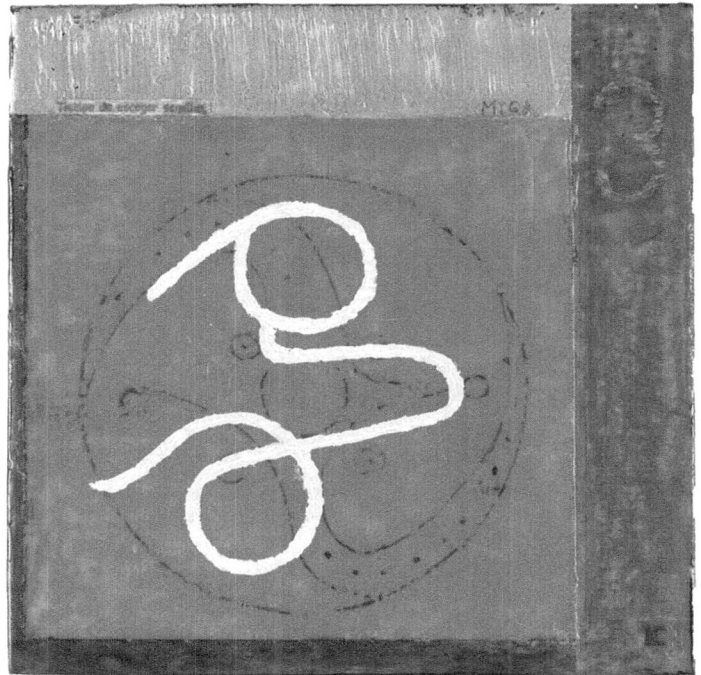

Part III

Image 3: © Lylia Ferero Carr: Muysca, Miqa

Chapter 4
World Social Development and Well-Being Trends

The most dramatic findings on the *Weighted Index of Social Progress* (WISP) over the entire 50-year period reported in this study are summarized in Fig. 4.1 (renumbered Fig. 1.1 in Chap. 1) and Fig. 4.2 (renumbered Fig. 1.2 in Chap. 1). These 2 figures show the average WISP scores and percent change in WISP scores for each decade over the 50-year period between 1970 and 2020 (est.). These two figures summarize changes in world social development by major world region for the entire 50-year period reported on in this study. The patterns reported in these figures are significant and offer a vivid picture of the changes that have taken place over the extended period reported in this chapter. They are consistent with the focus of this chapter, whose central concern is progress at the global level in advancing quality of life and well-being of all of the world's nations, the latter of which reflects changing social patterns within 95% of the world's current total population.

1. The world's *two most socially developed regions* are Europe (N = 35, WISP18 = 90.7) and North America (N = 2, WISP18 = 88.6). This pattern has existed since 1970 and reflects the extraordinarily high level of education, quality health care, technological innovation, and social provision that characterizes the countries of these regions. This pattern also reflects national and regional attention focused on the complex social needs of especially vulnerable population groups that exist along the periphery of each of the societies that form these regions, i.e., children and youth, the elderly, the poor, and persons with severe physical or emotional disabilities or both, and military veterans and their widows, among others. These social trends also indicate a strong and increasing commitment to environmental protection, including the creation of green spaces, public parks, and protected lands (Estes & Sirgy, 2018a, 2018b).

© Springer Nature Switzerland AG 2019
R. J. Estes, *The Social Progress of Nations Revisited, 1970–2020*, Social Indicators Research Series 78, https://doi.org/10.1007/978-3-030-15907-8_4

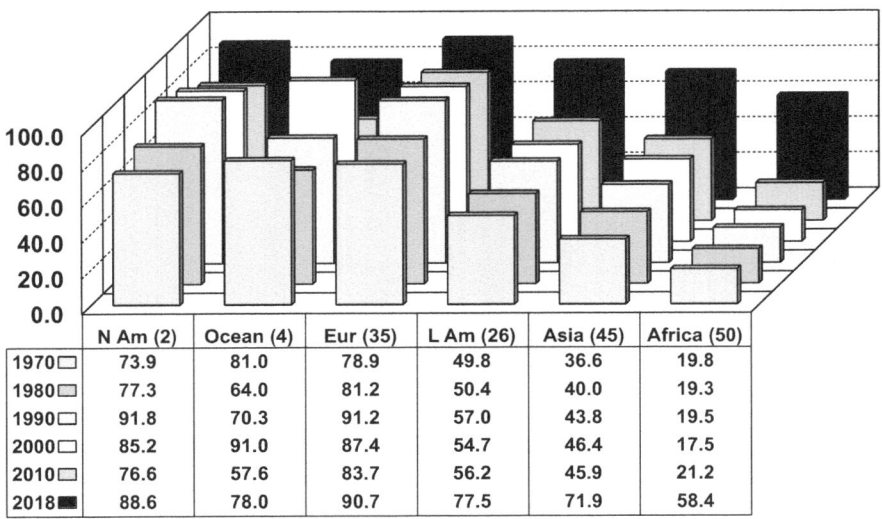

	N Am (2)	Ocean (4)	Eur (35)	L Am (26)	Asia (45)	Africa (50)
1970☐	73.9	81.0	78.9	49.8	36.6	19.8
1980☐	77.3	64.0	81.2	50.4	40.0	19.3
1990☐	91.8	70.3	91.2	57.0	43.8	19.5
2000☐	85.2	91.0	87.4	54.7	46.4	17.5
2010☐	76.6	57.6	83.7	56.2	45.9	21.2
2018■	88.6	78.0	90.7	77.5	71.9	58.4

Fig. 4.1 Average Weighted Index of Social Progress scores by continent, 1970–2018 (N = 162)

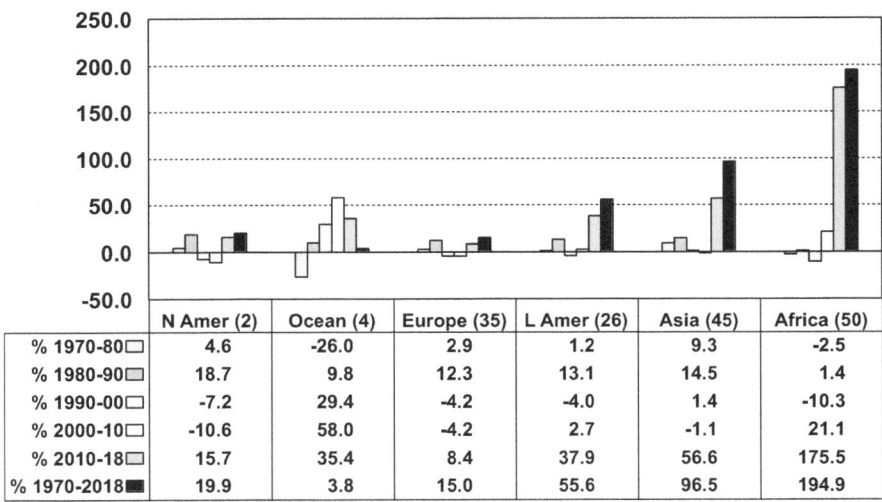

	N Amer (2)	Ocean (4)	Europe (35)	L Amer (26)	Asia (45)	Africa (50)
% 1970-80☐	4.6	-26.0	2.9	1.2	9.3	-2.5
% 1980-90☐	18.7	9.8	12.3	13.1	14.5	1.4
% 1990-00☐	-7.2	29.4	-4.2	-4.0	1.4	-10.3
% 2000-10☐	-10.6	58.0	-4.2	2.7	-1.1	21.1
% 2010-18☐	15.7	35.4	8.4	37.9	56.6	175.5
% 1970-2018■	19.9	3.8	15.0	55.6	96.5	194.9

Fig. 4.2 Percent change in average Weighted Index of Social Progress scores by continent, 1970–2018 (N = 162)

(a) They also reflect the high levels of national and foreign direct investments (FDI) and regional development assistance to less developed countries and regions, including preferential trade arrangements (Investopedia, 2018).[1]

---

[1] A preferential trade area (also referred to as a "preferential trade agreement" or "PTA," is a trading bloc that gives preferential access to certain products from the participating countries. This is

(b) Of some interest, too, is the fact that many of the populations of these countries tend to be culturally more homogeneous (often Protestant) and to engage in levels of international development assistance more than the United Nation's requested contribution of 0.07% of a donor country's national income. Aid provided by the Scandinavian countries, for example, currently averages 1.2% of the gross national income (Estes, 2010a; Organization for Economic Cooperation and Development, 2018).

(c) These countries also tend to be characterized by comparatively low levels of diversity-related conflict, albeit the growing presence of large numbers of immigrants since the 1980s, many of whom are people of color and Muslim, has created unexpected levels of racial, religious, and ethnic stress vis-à-vis their traditional population majority (CIA, 2018).

(d) Economic and labor shortfalls are driving immigration into these countries, especially in response to their low birth rates relative to concentrations of people who did, indeed, share genetic links with one another (IOM, 2018).

2. The world's *two least socially developed regions* are Africa (N = 50, WISP18 = 58.4) and Asia (N = 45, WISP18 = 71.9). These regions have consistently been the least socially developed since 1970, but in 2018, they reflect tremendous social achievements as a result of the laser-sharp activities associated with the United Nations' *Millennium Development Campaign* (2000–2016) and, in the case of Asia, a combination of the *Millennium Development Campaign* and dramatically increased financial investments in the region, but especially in the People's Republic of China and India. More than 100 million people have been lifted out of abject poverty in China since 2000, especially in rural areas in the Peoples Republic of China (Wu, 2016). The expectation is that this number, perhaps even more, given the rapid rate of the country's economic growth, again will be lifted out of extreme poverty by 2025, especially if the People's Republic of China is able to retain its position as "manufacturer to the world" (Weingast & Wittman, 2006; World Bank, 2018).[2]

3. The positive enhancements in well-being in another major world region, South Asia (e.g., Bangladesh, India, Pakistan), have resulted from high levels of FDI, impressive advances in technological development and innovation, and their early-stage advances in the health, education, and social welfare sectors. Other countries in the region are benefitting from these advances as well and, together, are contributing to the rapid pace of social and economic development in the larger region.

Significant environmental challenges remain for South Asia, including much needed improvements in the availability of fresh water and the disposal of solid

---

done by reducing tariffs but not by abolishing them completely. A PTA can be established through a trade pact. It is the first stage of economic integration (Investopedia, 2018).

[2] The reader need only examine the origin of many of the items on her/his desk to determine how many of those items originated in China (or other economically emerging East Asian economies) including the cell phone, tablet, computer(s), and other electronics on which many of us now depend.

waste. These areas remain significant challenges for South Asia and contribute to its chronic problems with infectious and communicable diseases. This reality is further compounded by the fact that at least 65% of South Asia's total population of more than 1901 million people reside in rural communities where a comparatively low level of public expenditures is allocated, even though the United Nations and other international development assistance organizations invest heavily in the region.

The large number of sub-Saharan African *and* Asian nations, including those of South Asia, share with more economically advanced nations critical challenges associated with diversity-related social conflict, high levels of financial poverty among these groups, limited opportunities for well-paying jobs, and, in general, the goal of participating as co-equal members in the social, political, and economic systems of society (International Monetary Fund, 2018; World Bank, 2018).

(a) The above situation is especially evident among the more than a handful of sub-Saharan nations located in middle Africa where the combination of recurrent warfare and high levels of financial poverty has proven to be especially intractable (International Monetary Fund, 2018).

(b) Nearly all the nations of Middle Africa are landlocked, which greatly impedes their ability to engage in significantly increased levels of international commerce with nations that are located nearby and those that can be reached via rivers and trains over great distances that separate producers and foreign purchasers of these usually handmade goods and services. This situation exists despite the rich network of underutilized waterways and other traditional transportation systems (well-established land pathways) that cross-cut throughout the region and that often are blocked due to recurrent intra- and interregional warfare and violence and intergroup ethnic conflicts (African River Networks, 2018; Stockholm International Peace Research Institute, 2018).

(c) Asian countries struggle both with the size of their populations, which account for more than 40% of the world's total population, and with the great distances that separate large Asian nations from one another (United Nations Population Division, 2018).

(d) There also exists a long history of comparative tolerance for issues such as extreme poverty in combination with low-wage labor in many Asian nations whose religions and cultures promote self-sacrifice, personal denial, and the minimization of needs and wants to their lowest possible levels, e.g., as reflected in the daily lives of the region's many monks and nuns as well as the pursuit of nirvana, which only can be achieved through self-denial of even the most basic needs (World Bank, 2018).

(e) Not infrequently, the large pool of inexpensive labor available in the Asian region, especially in South and Southeast Asia, is needed for the large numbers of countries who economies are based on large-scale agrobusinesses, machine-made clothing, electronic factories, and labor-intensive assembly plants (World Bank, 2018).

(f) Often low-skilled assembly jobs in Asia are carried out in the homes of workers themselves, which, in turn, frequently impinge on the physical space, time, and missed hours of sleep of the wives and children of the primary wage earners and, in extreme cases, that of elderly persons living in the same household (International Labour Organization, 2018).

4. Though the countries of **Latin America** currently are in a major "take off" phase, as in the past, social development and level of well-being are progressing more slowly in comparison with the rates of social development taking place within the developing countries of Africa and Asia. Even so, the decades of social stagnation that characterized the region's development in the past, the often referred to "lost decades" (Hayes, 1989) of development, are now in the past, with the result that accelerated rates of social progress have become major features of the region's social progress since 2000. In time, development trends in Latin America are expected to more closely approximate those of the nations located in North America.

(a) Latin America's average WISP18 scores approach those of its neighbors to the north (N = 26, WISP18 = 77.6 vs. 49.8 in 1970).

(b) Ironically, and despite the impoverished conditions under which many of the people of Latin America reside, their reported levels of subjective "happiness" are among the highest in the world (Helliwell, Layard, & Sachs, 2018). These latter measures depend primarily on polling data and, in the main, reflect people's views of their own quality of life at specific moments in time. Missing are the much-needed in-depth analyses of changing levels of happiness and well-being of the same individuals, families, and households over an extended period (a single year would work just fine initially). Graciela Tonon (2016) and Mario Rojas-Herrera (2016) and the teams of scholars associated with them are beginning to fill in this critical data gap, the outcomes of which likely will emerge over the next several years. The data and methods that these investigators are providing for a seriously misunderstood population (and region) will aid considerably in national, regional, and international planning on the part of both intergovernmental and not-for-profit organizations that promote national, regional, and world-wide well-being.

(c) The large combined populations of Mexico, Central America, and South America are experiencing significant increases in their objective conditions of life, which, in turn, are adding to increases in years of average life expectancy; enhanced rates of infant, child, and maternal survival; and significant advances in income security and protection of economically vulnerable population groups; they have also made impressive gains in protection of their forests, air, water, and other critical environmental resources. These gains have been highly successful in improving the quality of life and well-being of the peoples of this region.

5. **Oceania** is a vast region of the world. Although it has only a comparatively small population, it contains literally hundreds of islands on which people live, some of which already have emerged as independent nation-states. Most of this latter

group of nations are doing well economically but their land is threatened by global warming and repeated flooding. Some are in danger of sinking below the seas entirely.

(a) Because these small island nations are surrounded entirely by water, trade within and between most of them is sparse and is even more so among nations that are separated by thousands of miles of water. The major improvements in the region's development have resulted primarily from FDI. As has been the situation for many centuries, the international financial and human capital assistance has come from more affluent nations—many of which were former colonizing powers within the region—and from major international nongovernmental aid organizations.

(b) The social situations of the four nations of Oceania included in this study (Australia, New Zealand, Papua New Guinea, and Fiji) differ appreciably from those reported for the other groups of nations.

(c) These differences are reflected in the fact that, for the first 30 years of data reporting, the WISP values focused on the well-being status of just two of the region's largest economies, i.e., Australia and New Zealand. WISP data for Fiji and Papua New Guinea were added after 1990, given two realities: (a) Australia and New Zealand invested heavily and with success in the development of Fiji and Papua New Guinea; and (b) reliable data are now available from both governmental and nongovernmental sources for Fiji and Papua New Guinea, who now meet all four of the criteria needed for their inclusion in the analysis.

(d) Further, and only in recent years, WISP scores for Fiji and Papua New Guinea have begun to approximate those of the region's more economically advanced countries (N = 4, WISP18 = 78.0 versus 81.0 for Australia and New Zealand alone in 1970). This represents a dramatic leap forward for the smaller island nations of Oceania and, in time, a larger number of Pacific Ocean island groups of nations are expected to join Fiji and Papua New Guinea as social leaders in the region. This is especially expected to be the case for the Pacific nations that are already on their way to becoming more economically advanced developing countries.

(e) Viewed from a well-being perspective, all four countries of Oceania included in this study are moving forward toward progressively higher levels of objective quality of life and well-being. The economies of all four countries are vibrant albeit their products differ appreciably, i.e., the economy of Papua New Guinea depends on agriculture, fishing, and mineral extraction; that of Fiji, on both the preceding plus light manufacturing; and those of New Zealand and Australia are postindustrial societies whose economies are dominated by a wide range of human and related services.

(f) Unfortunately, the most basic needs of many of the region's aboriginal peoples are satisfied imperfectly. One critical indicator of this reality is the extraordinarily disproportionate numbers of indigenous men and women who are either incarcerated or functioning under direct court supervision

(Wikipedia, 2018a). This highly negative pattern of human well-being has greatly interrupted the family lives of the thousands of men and women who have only marginal access to their families in addition to having poor educations, weak job skills, and high dependencies on welfare services that came into being to serve the income security needs of entirely different populations—children and youth, the sick and elderly, persons with severe disabilities, unemployed and injured workers and, in some cases, families with large numbers of children (International Social Security Association, 2018).

(g) There is, however, no indication that the prevailing pattern of social marginalization of Oceania's large number of poor and socially disenfranchised people will be significantly altered over the near term, despite the fact that the majority of the ancestors of the region's nonindigenous people settled there either as former prisoners of the British Crown or as political refugees, but most often as economic migrants in search of new job and other financial opportunities.

(h) Further, due to global warming, many of Oceania's nations are experiencing serious flooding (Flood List News, 2018) and, in time, some are expected to succumb to the rising seas and disappear entirely as nation-states with defined geographic territories (Guardian, 2016). If they are to survive, the populations (and cultures) of these nations will need to migrate entirely to neighboring countries whose land masses are significantly above sea level. This process is already happening (UN Office of the High Representative for the Least Developed Countries, Landlocked Developing Countries and Small Island Developing States, 2018).

Overview of Regional Social Development and Well-Being

In all, the data and trends just reported, and the percentage changes in WISP70 through WISP18/20 scores summarized in Fig. 4.2 (see Fig. 1.2 in Chap. 1), reflect an optimistic view of advances that have taken place among 95% of the world's population between 1970 and the present. The trends often are dramatic and emphasize the high levels of national, regional, and world investments that have taken place during this period of human history, especially among the devastatingly poor nations of developing sub-Saharan Africa and Asia for which significant social gains have been realized since 1970 to the present. These gains are to be applauded, and every effort must be made to sustain them into the future, even if to do so is to require progressively higher levels of government or intergovernmental intervention (Estes, 2010b). The decline in global poverty rates has been especially significant in East, South, and Southeast Asia, where nearly 70% of the world's absolute poor lived prior to 2000. Gains in alleviating world poverty have been significant in these areas. At the same time, years of average life expectancy increased appreciably between 2000 and 2018, whereas rates of infant, child, and maternal mortality declined in every region worldwide and did so at a steady pace with substantial

accomplishments. Welfare, health, education, income security, and improved housing, more available and affordable public transportation as well as environmental
protection initiatives reached unparalleled levels in human well-being (Estes &
Sirgy, 2018a, 2018b). These gains in social development reversed centuries-long
disparities in health, education, housing, and sanitation that have kept the poor and
other socially disadvantaged groups trapped in constricted socioeconomic
environments.

Diversity-related social conflict within and between the nations of the Middle
East and North Africa (the frequently referred to as the "MENA region"), however,
has continued to persist well after 2000 CE. As of the writing of this chapter, there
is no reason to believe that these centuries-old animosities will end any time soon—
instead, we have only the promise of more death, more permanently incapacitating
injuries, and more destruction of important historical urban sites and monuments.
Further, elements of these conflicts have now taken the form of jihadist terrorism,[3]
suicide bombings, and other organized and independent acts of aggression directed
at Western cities and major centers of financial activity. The author, along with a
group of eminent social scientists, is at work attempting to understand more fully
the root causes of the devastating acts and, where possible, to reduce their numbers
(Rahtz & Estes, 2019; Sirgy & Estes, 2018; Sirgy, Estes, & Rahtz, 2018; Sirgy,
Joshanloo, & Estes, 2018).

Performance of Development Groups on the Weighted Index of Social Progress

In addition to summarizing changes over time in the WISP scores for countries
organized by major continental groupings, this chapter also provides data that summarize shifts over time in the well-being of countries organized by major geo-
economic and geopolitical groupings. These countries were considered "developed
market economies" (DME; N = 34) and were classified as such by the United
Nations (2018) and the World Bank (2018). The 34 nations that form the DME are
located primarily in Europe and North America with additional nations located in
Asia (Japan, Korea, Singapore, Taiwan) and Oceania (Australia, New Zealand). The
three other major socio-geographic-political groupings are the countries that comprise the successor states of the former Soviet Union and that now are member
states of the Commonwealth of Independent States (CIS, N = 21); developing countries (DC; N = 67); and least developed countries (N = 40).

---

[3] Jihadi, or jihadist, refers to a person who believes that an Islamic state governing the entire community of Muslims must be created and that this necessity justifies violent conflict with those who
stand in its way (Estes & Sirgy, 2016; Tiliouine & Estes, 2016).

Table 4.1 Selected social, political, economic, and other characteristics for nations grouped by socio-geographic-political groupings (4 groups, N = 162 countries)

	DMEs (N = 34)	CISs (N = 21)	DCs (N = 67)	LDCs (N = 40)	World (N = 162)
Population—Total	1,303,189,798	333,113,907	4,789,592,619	964,213,360	7,390,109,684
Avg country pop size	38,329,112	15,862,567	71,486,457	24,105,334	45,617,961
Percent pop <14 years old	16.9	16.8	28.6	41.0	27.7
Percent pop >64 years old	16.8	12.8	6.1	3.3	8.5
Percent pop growth rate	2.8	0.3	3.3	2.3	2.5
Mortality rates					
Infants per 1000	3.1	12.5	21.0	50.3	23.4
Children <age 5	6.0	14.5	26.8	71.7	31.9
Maternal	18.2	23.5	133.4	469.4	177.9
Selected health investments and outcomes					
Physicians per 100,000	3.6	3.0	1.5	0.3	1.8
Avg years life expectancy	79.6	73.6	71.5	62.1	71.2
Per capita gross domestic product	47.4	18.5	17.0	2.8	20.1
Economic growth rate	2.8	4.0	3.3	4.1	3.5
Unemployment rate	6.4	8.2	13.1	13.8	11.2
Political freedoms	1.5	4.0	3.9	4.9	3.7
Civil liberties	1.5	3.7	3.8	4.7	3.5

Countries with Developed Market Economies

The world's nations with DME have retained their advanced social, political, and economic status throughout the entire period covered by this study. This pattern, along with that of the world's other developing groups of nations, is confirmed in the data reported in Table 4.1 and Figs. 4.3 and 4.4. These 34 countries, for example, remain the world's leaders in civil liberties and political freedoms (Freedom House, 2018). The countries have the lowest rates of infant and child mortality and of maternal deaths (World Health Organization, 2018). By 2040, these already remarkably low levels of deaths associated with pregnancy are expected to decline another 50%, especially within the social democratic nations of Northern and Western Europe (Glatzer, Camfield, Møller & Rojas, 2015).

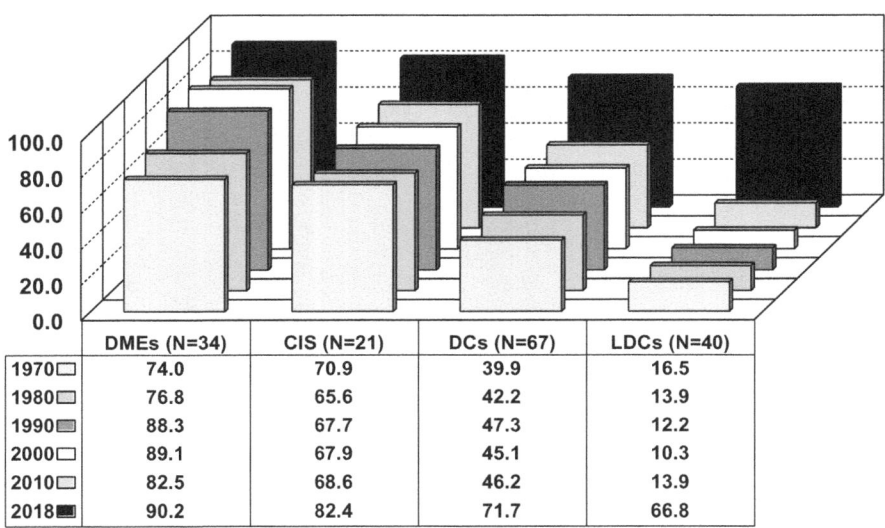

Fig. 4.3 Average Weighted Index of Social Progress scores by major geopolitical groupings, 1970–2018 (N = 162) (*CIS* Commonwealth of Independent States, *DC* developing country, *DME* developed market economy, *LDC* least developed country)

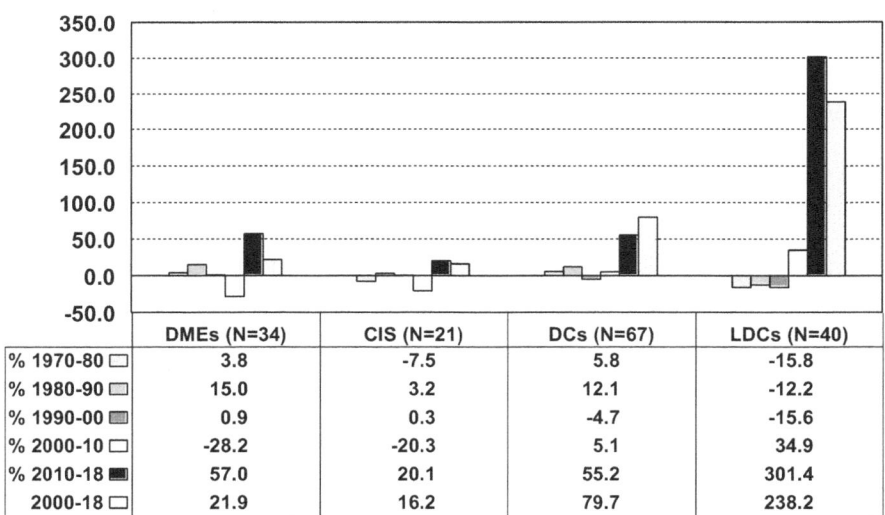

Fig. 4.4 Average percent changes in Weighted Index of Social Progress scores by major geopolitical groupings, 1970–2018 (N = 162) (*CIS* Commonwealth of Independent States, *DC* developing country, *DME* developed market economy, *LDC* least developed country)

The United States is a comparative "social laggard" among this group of nations on most of the social elements of well-being even as it continues to lead the world with the largest and most influential economic drivers and to be a military and political leader (United Nations Development Programme, 2018; Weingast & Wittman, 2006). Even a cursory examination of the nation's long and painful history of poverty, including 20% of her children, make clear the dual and contradictory forces at work within the United States that prevent the country from achieving a level of social and economic parity commensurate with its political achievements—this despite the country's historical political leadership role among DME nations (North American Treaty Organization, 2018) (Figs. 4.5a, 4.5b, 4.5c, 4.5d, 4.5e and 4.5f).

DMEs serve as the models against which other nations compare their own developmental gains and frequently serve as the basis for less developed countries to set their own development goals and objectives. As a group, the DMEs have developed the world's most sophisticated social welfare systems that reach the largest possible population of their most economically vulnerable citizens. High levels of political and civil rights freedom characterize these countries, as do moderate to high levels of press and religious freedom. In summary "these countries have it all"—vigorous systems of participatory political participation, high levels of press and religious freedom, and comparatively comprehensive and strong social welfare systems that provide for the income security needs of the most vulnerable populations living within their borders.

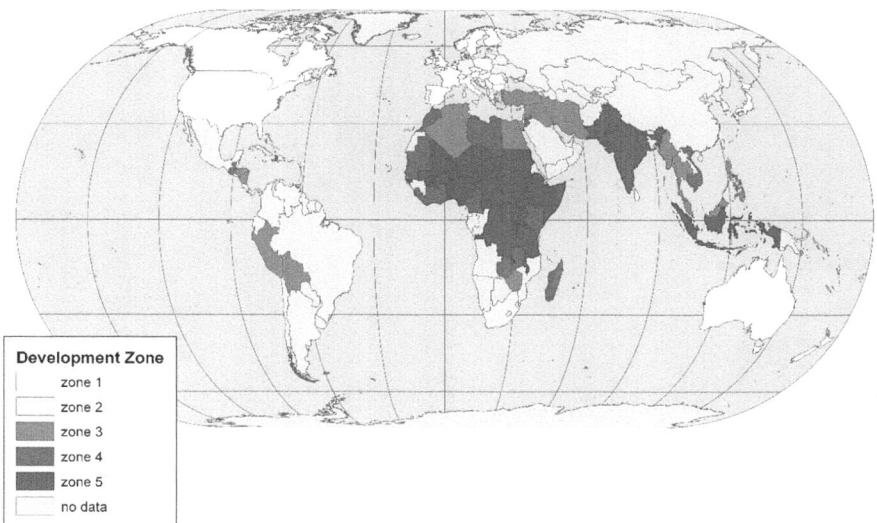

Fig. 4.5a Distribution of Weighted Index of Social Progress scores by country and development zone, 1970. (Map created by Amy Hillier)

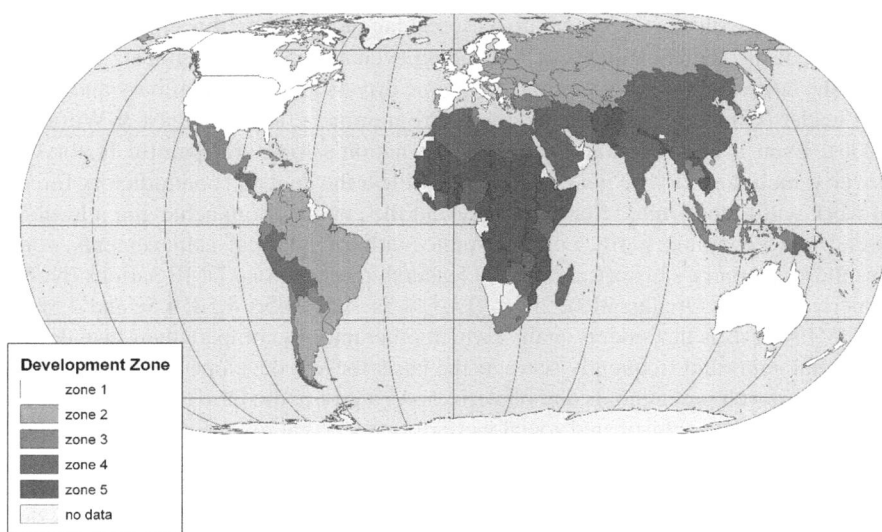

Fig. 4.5b Distribution of Weighted Index of Social Progress scores by country and development zone, 1980. (Map created by Amy Hillier)

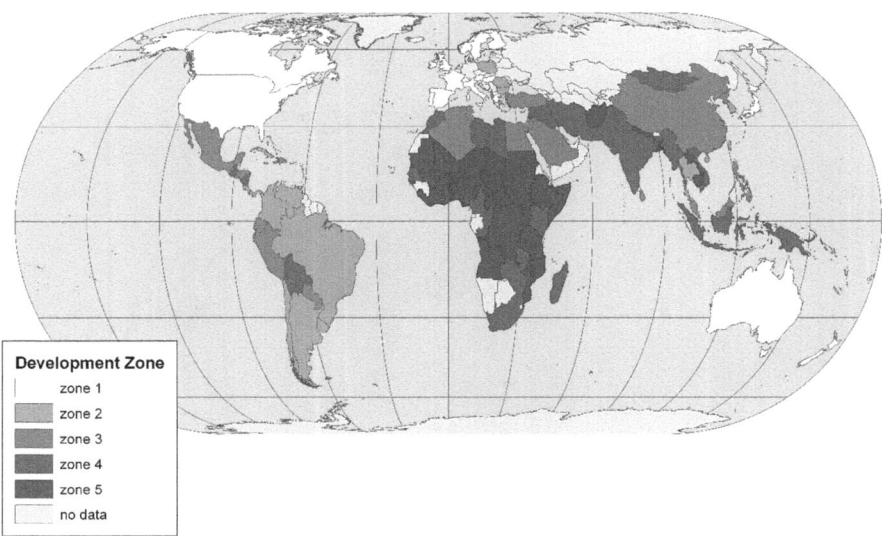

Fig. 4.5c Distribution of Weighted Index of Social Progress scores by country and development zone, 1990. (Map created by Amy Hillier)

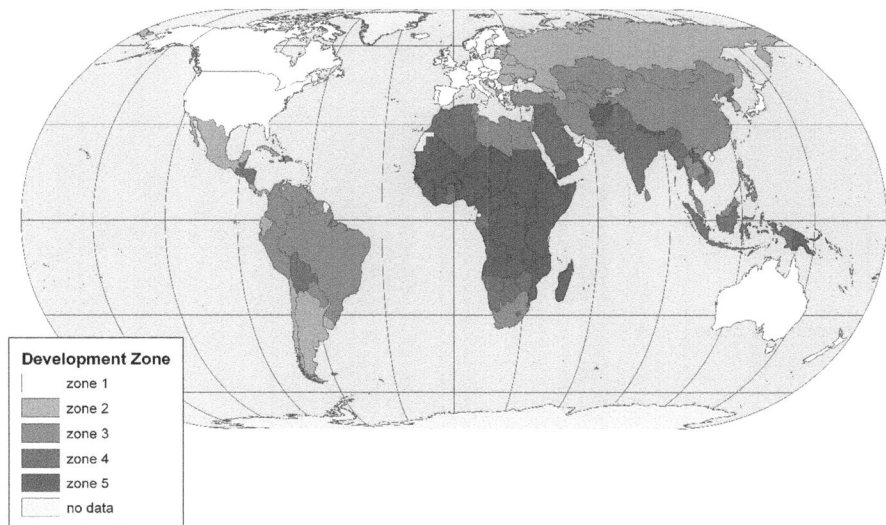

Fig. 4.5d Distribution of Weighted Index of Social Progress scores by country and development zone, 2000. (Map created by Amy Hillier)

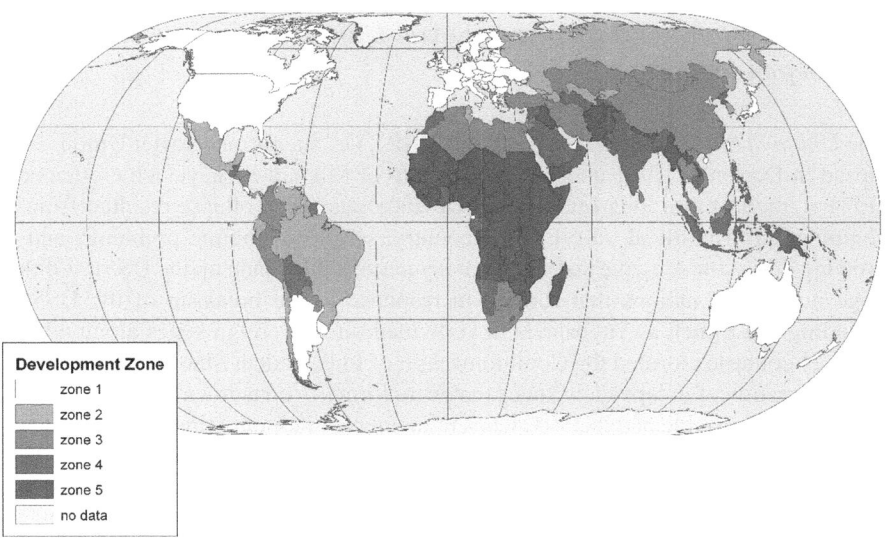

Fig. 4.5e Distribution of Weighted Index of Social Progress scores by country and development zone, 2009. (Map created by Amy Hillier)

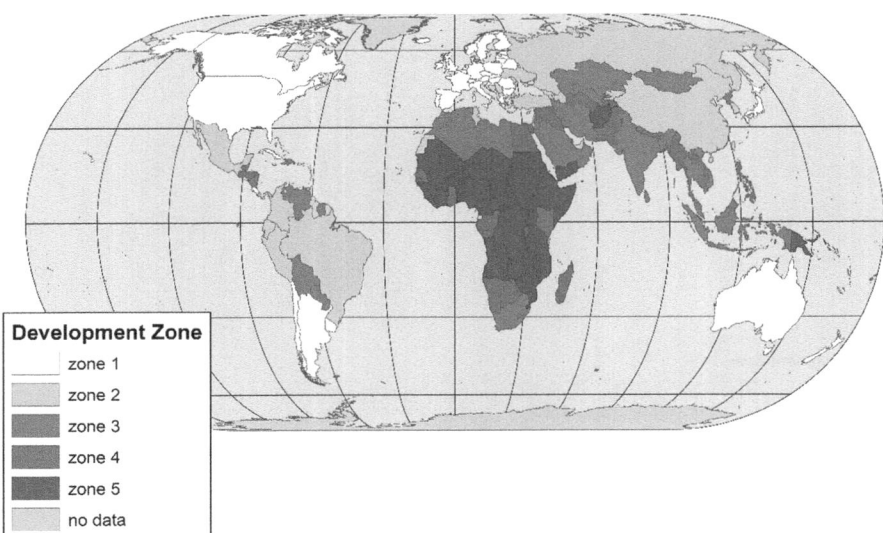

Fig. 4.5f Distribution of Weighted Index of Social Progress scores by country and development zone, 2018. (Map created by Amy Hillier, 2018)

Successor States to the Former Soviet Union/(Commonwealth of Independent States)

The *Union of Soviet Socialist Republics* (USSR), i.e., the former Soviet Union, collapsed in December 1991 under the leadership of Mikhail Sergeyevich Gorbachev (1931–), the last in a long line of political autocrats. The collapse resulted from a combination of political unrest in the country, serious economic problems, and a growing desire for self-rule among the many nations that made up the USSR. Of the large number of nations that formed in response to the break-up of the USSR, including those such as Yugoslavia, that divided into sovereign states along ethnic lines, 21 countries formed the Commonwealth of Independent States (CIS; N = 21), a confederation of independent states that were formerly constituent republics of the Soviet Union, established in 1991. Current member states are Armenia, Azerbaijan, Belarus, Kazakhstan, Kyrgyzstan, Moldova, the Russian Federation, Tajikistan, and Uzbekistan. Turkmenistan and Ukraine are associate members.

The members of the CIS comprise the second most socially developed group of nations. Though the population of these countries is small relative to the other three groups of nations under discussion, their land mass is substantial and their human capital and natural resource reserves are extraordinarily high. Indeed, the country with the largest land mass, the Russian Federation, has produced many of the world's most preeminent scholars and scientists and, today, is the largest exporter of natural gas and petroleum products on which the nations of Europe heavily depend. Even so, the economies of most of these countries are highly vulnerable, and their linkages to nations outside of the CIS have not been fully realized even though extensive trade relationships exist among these other more economically and politically developed nations.

Well-being among most member nations of the CIS is highly advanced as reflected in their higher than average years of life expectancy, low rates of infant and child deaths, and the significant leadership roles that women perform in politics, the sciences, academic life, and, as in the past, the performing arts. Population growth rates are favorable and slow, and per capita gross domestic product and other critical economic variables are stable and increasing at a steady pace. Considerable evenness, however, exists among these nations with respect to advances in quality of life post-transition compared to DME; nonetheless, they are making substantial progress toward achieving the goals of their five-year plans and are providing more adequately for the basic and enhanced needs of their growing populations (Estes, 2012b; Graham & Werman, 2017)

Unlike other highly and moderately economically advanced nations and despite their relative affluence, however, most member states of the CIS contribute sparingly to the total financial and technical assistance needs of their countries. This is an unfortunate pattern given the critical role these sectors play in helping the region's countries become more economically related sectors. Spending on official development assistance among these nations is higher only for the Russian Federation, albeit the percentage share of their gross domestic product represented by these investments in poorer countries has not been consistent or adequate compared to that needed by poorer countries (Library of Congress, 2018). The reasons for this trend are associated with the lack of a history of humane assistance to member states outside their direct sphere of influence and, even within their sphere of influence, aid is limited to mostly military and police actions. Most of these countries also must draw on their own resources to finance their own national development. Not now, but in the future, as these countries become more affluent, they likely will develop robust programs of international development assistance to less developed countries in Asia, Africa and, perhaps, Latin America, depending on their trade relationships.

In any case, the countries of the CIS are building on the social philosophy, practices, and administrative legacies that existed while all these nations were part of the social system of the former USSR, thus their designations as "successor states to the former Soviet Union." They learned many critical lessons from this multilayered socio-political-economic-military relationship, and these lessons continue to inform much of their contemporary approaches to social provision (both within their countries and those with which they have developed critical multilateral trade and other types of relationships). The approaches taken by the member states of the modern CIS to political and economic development, however, are new and are now bringing them into the mainstream of economically advanced nations. This process of entering the mainstream of global relations almost certainly will continue well into the decades just ahead (Estes, 2012a, 2012b). In time, the nations of the CIS almost certainly will become world leaders in economic and technological development—positions for which they are well suited historically and in the global economy.

Developing Countries

The largest group of countries discussed in this section is that classified by the World Bank as developing countries (DCs; N = 67). Consisting of a population of more than 4.8 thousand million people, or approximately 64% of the world's total, the countries in which these persons reside are in developing Africa, Asia, and Latin America. Although they are more advanced than nearly all lessor developed states, the populations of the DCs experience high levels of infant and child deaths and, tragically, of many women of child-bearing age (ca. 14–50 years old). Mothers most often die from complications of childbirth associated with inadequate access to skilled prenatal care and, following delivery, the unavailability of adequate levels of continuing postnatal care. Unclean water is a leading cause of both child and maternal deaths, but especially of the death of the children who are bathed in contaminated water, which is also used by women to prepare infant formula and other child "nourishment" food products. However, *poverty*, with all the limitations that it places on the health choices available to pregnant women and their families, is the true cause of death (and epidemic levels of neonatal "failure to thrive").

The data summarized in Table 3.1 also reflect lower years of average life expectancy for people living in DCs as well as painfully slow rates of economic growth and per capita income levels and, not surprisingly, compromised systems of political freedom and civil liberties. Many of these countries produce comparatively low levels of goods and services that can be sold in international markets; hence, they tend to be far more dependent on domestic productivity for their consumer goods and services. This pattern will likely change in the decades ahead, especially for the top half of the DCs whose human capital reserves are increasing rapidly and, in time, will provide the leadership needed to accelerate the pace of social development in their respective countries. Of interest, too, is the fact that several of the most economically vigorous DCs trade regularly with neighboring states and countries who may further process the goods and services they import from neighboring countries for resale on international markets.

Unemployment levels in DCs considered as a group are remarkably high (13.1%) as is the population younger than 14 years of age (28.6%). In effect, these patterns reflect progressively high levels of joblessness for countries where growth in employment is critical to their development, especially in export-oriented industries. The current situation represents disproportionately low levels of technology and technological innovation in the economic and scientific sectors. These innovations are of critical importance to the overall well-being of societies. An overdependence on agricultural and low to moderately skilled manufacturing work accounts for the preceding factors along with high drop-out rates at the postsecondary level. All these patterns need to be reversed rather dramatically if the DCs are to gain an important place in the global market and internal trade. International nongovernmental organizations may be able to provide substantial assistance to the economically impoverished DCs, but this assistance must be guided by the carefully formulated goals and objectives of the United Nations *Sustainable Goals Campaign*, which has successfully involved governmental, nongovernmental, and private philanthropists in the execution of its goals. The critical partners in driving development, however, must be highly selective with respect to the goals on which they work and the criteria that are to be used to carefully evaluate national and regional progress in attaining these goals. The absence of thoughtful attention to all the preceding will simply sustain the low levels of social, political, and economic development that already afflict too many of the DCs.

Least Developing Countries

The world's economically least developed countries (LDCs) and socially (and economically) least developed countries (N = 40) are the poorest, most socially disadvantaged nations in the world. They lack adequate food supplies, skilled health care personnel, transportation, and communications infrastructure and have little to no publicly organized social welfare infrastructure designed to meet the needs of their most vulnerable populations, but especially those of children and youth who represent the future of these nations. The countries also are characterized by low levels of quality housing, high levels of environmental pollution, and little in the way of occupational health and safety protections. Unionized or other types of protected work is virtually unknown to most workers in the LDCs and socially least developed countries, even in the small "mom and pop" shops and light industry factories in which nonagricultural workers seek employment.

The average years of life expectancy among the 964 thousand million residents of the LDCs have improved dramatically since 1970 but, as of 2020, continue to lag substantially behind those of the DCs, CIS, and DME (United Nations Commission on Trade and Development [UNCTAD], 2018). This pattern is not likely to change appreciably in the years ahead, even if the actual number of years of average life expectancy in the LDCs increases. Similarly, infant and child rates of mortality remain high, as do the number of maternal deaths both prior to and following the delivery of newborns.

Rates of economic growth in the LDCs also are low relative to those in other clusters of nations worldwide, whereas unemployment rates and inflation trends continue to increase. Technological innovation in many of these countries remains virtually nonexistent and, to the extent that contemporary technology exists in these countries, comprises "out of box" technologies purchased from either the DME where they are developed or from the DME where they are produced, e.g., iPhones, iPads, Macs, and the like (with the exception of Samsung products, which are designed, promoted, and exported worldwide from Korea).

Graphic Illustration of Global Data

Professor Amy Hillier, director of the Master of Science in Social Policy program at the University of Pennsylvania School of Social Policy & Practice, was kind enough to prepare a series of geographic information system figures for me that use the concept of "development zones" and color shadings ranging from white (most favorable) to bright red (least favorable) to illustrate the major changes that have taken place in WISP scores between 1970 and 2018. In each figure, the world is divided into five "development zones" and the countries associated with each zone are shaded on a scale of white (zone 1) to bright red (zone 5). The world's 40 most socially progressive nations are grouped together in zone 1 and the remaining 122 countries are distributed equally across the remaining four remaining development zones. The geographic information system maps that result from this approach to data aggregations of nations are powerful and vividly present the study's major findings in a simplified, easily understandable manner.

The data presented using the format of *Geographic Information System Mapping*[4] (GIS) are quite rich and present a definitive picture of the changes over time in the level of social development and, hence, well-being of all the world's nations. Indeed, simply examining the changes in these charts that have taken place over 1970–2018 (2020) are quite distinct and offer a vivid graphical presentation of net gains and losses in development over the entire 50-year period beginning 1970. These GIS images, however, do not take the place of the detailed analyses summarized throughout the volume, including the nation-specific data for each nation by the WISP's 10 subindexes. For a more detailed understanding the major drivers of development as well as the outcomes associated with these drivers one must read the entirety of the book and only then will the richness of the data summarized in the GIS figures be fully interpretable.

Discussion

This chapter has provided a wide range of data that confirms that significant positive advances in human well-being and broad-based social development have occurred since 1970. Progress in these areas has been particularly impressive in the health, education, social welfare, technological, environmental, and economic sectors.

---

[4] A geographic information system (GIS) is a framework for gathering, managing, and analyzing data. Rooted in the science of geography, GIS integrates many types of data. It analyzes spatial location and organizes layers of information into visualizations using maps and 3D scenes. With this unique capability, GIS reveals deeper insights into data, such as patterns, relationships, and situations—helping users make smarter decisions. A GIS is a framework for gathering, managing, and analyzing data. Rooted in the science of geography, GIS integrates many types of data. It analyzes spatial location and organizes layers of information into visualizations using maps and 3-dimensional scenes. With this unique capability, a GIS provides deeper insights into data, such as patterns, relationships, and situations—helping users make smarter decisions (ESRI, 2018).

Women and girls also have made unparalleled levels of social progress with the result that they are more literature than at any other time in history, have greater control over their reproductive cycles, are able to be part of the paid workforce and are able to maintain greater control over their earnings. Women also can hold land in their own name, take out personal or commercial loans, receive and retain control over inheritances gifted to them in their name and can, when appropriate, initiate divorce in response to failed marriages (United Nations Development Programme, 2018; World Bank, 2018).

Social welfare systems are better funded and are reaching larger numbers of economically vulnerable children and youth, the aged, persons with severe emotional and physical disabilities, and others who live on the margins of society (International Social Security Association, 2018). These improvements strengthen all societies and make available fiscal and human capital resources needed to sustain robust economic activities for decades to come. Social welfare income support services also make possible opportunities for the poor and other disadvantaged population groups to promote their own well-being and, with considerable personal and collective effort, to become fully functioning members of society. These processes also certainly will continue well into the future and will strengthen the social, political, and economic capacity of nations, regions, and the world as a whole (Weingast & Wittman, 2006).

International Trade Agreements

The world's economies also are strengthening and expanding at a rapid pace (International Monetary Fund, 2018; World Bank, 2018). Economic expansion rates are especially impressive among the very large group of developing countries who, overall, are the major drivers of global economic growth, low levels of inflation, and strong intraregional and international trade agreements in the form of social, political, military, and economic "trade pacts." Among many others the most significant international trading pacts include those identified in Box 4.1.

> **Box 4.1 Partial listing of major international trade agreements by year of establishment and listed alphabetically (Wikipedia, 2018b)**
> - Andean Community – 1969
> - ASEAN Free Trade Area (AFTA) – 1992
> - ASEAN–Australia–New Zealand Free Trade Area (AANZFTA) – 2010
> - Asia-Pacific Trade Agreement (APTA) – 1975
> - Central American Integration System (SICA) – 1993
> - Central European Free Trade Agreement (CEFTA) – 1992
> - Commonwealth of Independent States Free Trade Area (CISFTA) – 2011
> - Common Market for Eastern and Southern Africa (COMESA) – 1994
> - G-3 Free Trade Agreement (G-3) – 1995

(continued)

Box 4.1 (continued)

- Greater Arab Free Trade Area (GAFTA) – 1997
- Dominican Republic–Central America Free Trade Agreement (DR-CAFTA) – 2004
- East African Community (EAC) – 2005
- Eurasian Economic Union (EAEU) –2015
- European Economic Area (EEA; European Union–Norway–Iceland–Liechtenstein) – 1994
- European Union Customs Union (EUCU; European Union–Turkey–Monaco–San Marino–Andorra) – 1958
- European Free Trade Association (EFTA) – 1960
- Gulf Cooperation Council (GCC) – 1981
- International Grains Agreement – 1995 Comprising a Grains Trade Convention (GTC) and a Food Aid Convention (FAC)
- North American Free Trade Agreement (NAFTA) (Pending replacement by USMCA) - 1994
- Pacific Alliance Free Trade Area (PAFTA) – 2012
- South Asian Free Trade Area (SAFTA) – 2004
- Southern African Development Community Free Trade Area (SADCFTA) – 1980
- Southern Common Market (MERCOSUR) – 1991

These trade agreements have fostered not only economic development but social and political development as well. They also have helped to lift tens of millions of people out of extreme poverty by providing a secure and stable income and, with it, at least the beginnings of social benefits associated with employment, e.g., unemployment, health insurance, at least the beginnings of a retirement income security system and, in many countries, family support systems as well as programs that serve persons who are severely injured on the job. These agreements have fostered international travel on the part of at least company managers who, without the support of their companies, would never have the opportunity to experience international travel and sometimes the dramatic cultural exchanges that take place between themselves and their counterparts in other countries (not infrequently with persons employed by the same multinational corporation). All these social innovations have added measurably to the well-being of nations and people themselves through the significant levels of economic benefits associated with these newly created jobs and other previously nonexistent employment opportunities (Manyika, 2017) (Box 4.2).

Box 4.2 Stockholm International Peace Research Institute Databases (SIPRI, 2018)
SIPRI Databases
SIPRI Arms Transfers Database

The Stockholm International Peace Research Institute (SIPRI) Arms Transfers Database shows all international transfers of major conventional arms since 1950 and is the most comprehensive publicly available source of information on international arms transfers.

SIPRI Arms Industry Database

The SIPRI Arms Industry Database contains information on the 100 largest arms-producing and military services companies.

SIPRI Multilateral Peace Operations Database

The SIPRI Multilateral Peace Operations Database offers information on all peace operations conducted since 2000, including location, dates of deployment and operation, mandate, participating countries, number of personnel, costs, and fatalities.

SIPRI Military Expenditure Database

The SIPRI Military Expenditure Database gives the annual military spending of countries since 1949, allowing comparison of countries' military spending in local currency at current prices; in US dollars at constant prices and exchange rates; and as a share of gross domestic product.

Other resources

SIPRI keeps comprehensive collections of material covering arms control and disarmament.

Arms Embargoes

SIPRI provides information on all arms embargoes that have been implemented by an international organization, such as the European Union or the United Nations, or by a group of nations. All embargoes that are in force, or have been in force since 1998, are included.

National Reports on Arms Exports

SIPRI provides links to all publicly accessible national reports on arms exports. These are constantly updated to include links to newly published national reports on arms exports.

Financial Value of the Global Arms Trade

Using reports from the National Reports Archive, SIPRI estimates the financial value of arms exports.

The Government of Peru provided a financial donation to SIPRI's databases in 2016.

Nations also have engaged in more efforts to promote environmental protection of their most precious national and international resources. These efforts have contributed to cleaner air, the setting aside of protected land and other green spaces, and protection of endangered animals, flora and, yes, people themselves. The latter group of living beings have been protected through improved systems for the safe disposal of solid and liquid wastes, the use of recycled materials to generate electricity (particularly for use by the poor), clean water, and national protection of forests, open lands, streams, seas and, increasingly, of oceans on a more extensive level. These global efforts at environmental protection have been highly effective and, today, continue to be reflected as major targets of the recently launched *17 Sustainable Development Goals* (SDG) initiative of the specialized agencies of the United Nations in collaboration with governments and hundreds of private sector partners at all levels of corporate enterprises, charitable foundations, and nongovernmental development assistance organizations, and individual philanthropists. People themselves also are substantially involved in this initiative and, most importantly, as full and equal partners in the implementation of the SDG initiative. Together, these are the stakeholders needed to make the SDG campaign a success.

Thus, major actions are taking place at the global level to reverse centuries of social discrimination with the result that previously persecuted groups are now moving forward at a substantial pace…as is the world itself. These significant gains are not to be minimized but, instead, reflect even more broad-based changes that have occurred throughout the world since at least 1970 and beyond.

Trade Agreements and Expenditures for Defense

Regional trade pacts have proven to be highly effective in promoting job development within participating companies and corporations. These pacts also have added to increased levels of political and economic stability among participating nations and are adding dramatically to the human resources and capacities of all these nations. Better educated, more competitive persons with experience in the new types of jobs created through advanced technologies also are a major outcome of these important regional and international trade arrangements.

However, one of the major challenges confronting regional trade pact agreements is that many also contain paragraphs that pledge mutual military support to members of the pact from external threats from nations either in the region or outside that are not members of the trade pact. Where implemented, these secondary mutual defense agreements add considerable additional expense to the administration of these pacts. These agreements also have added to national and regional expenditures for military hard- and software, e.g., for both conventional (high-powered rifles, tanks) and specialized nonconventional weapons (mostly small missiles with nuclear tips, stealth jets), or both. The cost of these expenditures for regional defense are substantial and typically range between 5 and 8% of national and regional GDP. Often, these were unanticipated expenses associated with international trade agreements, but they are perceived by member states of the agreements to be essential to their success, especially in countries with recurrent civil unrest or with protracted histories of diversity-related social conflict (Freedom House, 2018; Stockholm International Peace Research Institute, 2018).

The above costs are incurred in the production, marketing, sales, and purchases of both aggressive and defensive weapons of war. The costs to nations and the world are extraordinary and significantly reduce the resources that are available for critical social programs that are needed for income vulnerable population groups. The money used for military expenditures also adds comparatively little to the economies of nations but exposes them to major conflicts with neighboring states. Further, spending for national defense significantly reduces the resources that are available for improvements in education, health, housing, sanitation, road and communications infrastructure development, and so on. In all cases, countries with high levels of defense expenditures frequently are left poorer and remain so if such expenditures continue to increase in response to actual or perceived existential threats.

Next Chapters

All the data reported thus far provide the foundation on which the following data-driven chapters (Chaps. 5 and 6) add additional understanding to the global data reported in this chapter, i.e., *regional* development trends (Chap. 5) and *national* development trends (Chap. 6). These chapters are more analytical in nature and report a rich set of disaggregated data using the global database as their point of reference. Similarly, the chapters in Part 6 focus not on geopolitical regions but, instead, on at-risk population groups that are vulnerable to high levels of repeated income insecurity based on racial or ethnic discrimination (Chap. 7), gender (Chap. 8), or recurrent poverty status (Chap. 9). *A reading of all these chapters is needed to fully understand the global patterns and trends summarized in this chapter.*

References

African River Networks (ARN). (2018). *About ARN*. Kampala, Uganda: ARN. Retrieved December 9, 2018 from https://sites.google.com/site/africanriversnetwork/Home/about-us

ESRI. (2018). *What is graphic information imaging systems?* Retrieved December 11, 2018 from https://www.esri.com/en-us/what-is-gis/overview.

Estes, R. J. (2010a). The world social situation: Development challenges at the outset of a new century. *Social Indicators Research, 98*, 363–402.

Estes, R. J. (2010b). Toward sustainable development: From theory to praxis. *Social Development Issues, 15*(3), 1–29.

Estes, R. J. (2012a). Economies in transition: Continuing challenges to quality of life. In K. Land, A. C. Michalos, & M. Joseph Sirgy (Eds.), *Handbook of quality of life research* (pp. 433–457). Dordrecht, The Netherlands: Springer.

Estes, R. J. (2012b). Failed and failing states: Is quality of life possible? In K. Land, A. C. Michalos, & M. J. Sirgy (Eds.), *Handbook of quality of life research* (pp. 555–580). Dordrecht, The Netherlands: Springer.

Estes, R. J., & Sirgy, M. J. (2016). Is quality of life related to radical Islamic militancy and acts of terrorism? In H. Tiliouine & R. J. Estes (Eds.), *The state of social progress of Islamic societies: Social, political, economic, and ideological challenges* (pp. 575–606). Dordrecht, The Netherlands: Springer.

Estes, R. J., & Sirgy, M. J. (2018a). *Advances in well-being: Towards a better world.* London: Rowman and Littlefield.

Estes, R. J., & Sirgy, M. J. (2018b). Global advances in quality of life and well-being: Past, present, and future. *Social Indicators Research*, [First Online: 01 March 20] 18, in press. https://doi.org/10.1007/s11205-018-1869-4.

Flood List. (2018). *Australia – Ex-tropical cyclone Owen dumps record rain in Queensland.* December 17. Retrieved December 22, 2018 from http://floodlist.com/australia/australia-ex-tropical-cyclone-owen-dumps-record-rain-in-queensland

Freedom House. (2018). *Freedom throughout the world.* New York: Freedom House.

Glatzer, W., Camfield, L., Møller, V., & Rojas, M. (Eds.). (2015). *Global handbook of quality of life: Exploration of well-being of nations and continents.* Dordrecht, The Netherlands: Springer.

Graham, C., & Werman, A. (2017). Well-being in the transition economies of the successor states of the former Soviet Union: the challenges of change. In R. J. Estes & M. J. Sirgy (Eds.), *The pursuit of human well-being: The untold global history* (pp. 493–521). Dordrecht, The Netherlands: Springer.

The Guardian (2016). *Five Pacific islands lost to rising seas as climate change hits.* Retrieved December 22, 2018 from https://www.theguardian.com/environment/2016/may/10/five-pacific-islands-lost-rising-seas-climate-change.

Hayes, M. D. (1989). *The U.S. and Latin America: A lost decade?* Washington, DC: Inter-American Development Bank.

Helliwell, J. F., Layard, R., & Sachs, J. D. (2018). *World happiness report, 2018.* New York: Sustainable Development Solutions Network. Retrieved August 1, 2018 from http://worldhappiness.report/ed/2018/

Hillier, A. (2018). *Graphics illustrator.* University of Pennsylvania School of Social Policy & Practice (SP2).

International Labour Organization (ILO). (2018). *Future of work.* Geneva, Switzerland: ILO Global Commission on Work. Retrieved December 8, 2018 from https://www.ilo.org/global/topics/future-of-work/WCMS_569528/lang–en/index.htm.

International Monetary Fund (IMF). (2018). *Sub Saharan regional economic outlook, 2018: Capital flows and the future of work.* Washington, DC: IMF.

International Organization for Migration (IOM). (2018). *Global migration indicators* (p. 2018). Geneva: IOM.

International Social Security Association. (2018). *Social security programs throughout the world, 2018.* Geneva, Switzerland: International Social Security Administration.

Investopedia. (2018). Economic integration. *Investopedia.* Retrieved December 9, 2018 from https://www.investopedia.com/terms/e/economic-integration.asp.

Library of Congress. (2018). *Regulation of foreign aid: Russian Federation.* Washington, DC: Library of Congress. Retrieved August 1, 2018 from https://www.loc.gov/law/help/foreign-aid/russia.php.

Manyika, J. (2017). Technology, jobs, and the future of work. *McKinsey Global Institute: Executive summary.* Retrieved December 14, 2018 from https://www.mckinsey.com/featured-insights/employment-and-growth/technology-jobs-and-the-future-of-work.

North American Treaty Organization. (2018). *NATO summit guide: Brussels.* Brussels: North American Treaty Organization.

Organization for Economic Cooperation and Development. (2018). *Net official development assistance.* [Database]. Paris: Organization for Economic Cooperation and Development,

Development Assistance Committee. Retrieved August 1, 2018 from https://data.oecd.org/oda/net-oda.htm

Rhatz, D., & Estes, R. J. (2019). *The universal soldier: The dynamics of gang formation among Jihadist terrorists*. (in preparation).

Rojas-Herrera, M. (Ed.). (2016). *Handbook of happiness research in Latin America*. Dordrecht, The Netherlands: Springer.

Sirgy, M. J., & Estes, R. J. (2018). Understanding jihadist terrorism in the MENA and Gulf States region: Quality-of-life implications for counterterrorism. In L. Lambert (Ed.), *Positive psychology in the Middle East and North Africa: Research, policy, and practice*. Dordrecht, The Netherlands: Springer. In press.

Sirgy, M. J., Estes, R. J., & Rahtz, D. R. (2018). Combatting jihadist terrorism: A quality-of-life perspective. [On line]. *Journal of Applied Research in Quality of Life*. https://doi.org/10.1007/s11482-017-9574-z

Sirgy, M. J., Joshanloo, M., & Estes, R. J. (2018). The global challenge of jihadist terrorism: A quality-of-life model. [On line]. *Social Indicators Research*. https://doi.org/10.1007/s11205-017-1831-x

Stockholm International Peace Research Institute (SIPRI). (2018). *SIPRI yearbook, 2018: Armaments, disarmaments, and international security*. Stockholm: SPIRI.

Tiliouine, H., & Estes, R. J. (Eds.). (2016). *The state of social progress of Islamic societies: Social, political, economic, and ideological challenges*. Dordrecht, The Netherlands: Springer.

Tonon, G. (Ed.). (2016). *Indicators of quality of life in Latin America*. Dordrecht, The Netherlands: Springer International.

United Nations. (2018). *UN country classification system*. Retrieved July 30, 2018 from http://www.un.org/en/development/desa/policy/wesp/wesp_current/2014wesp_country_classification.pdf

United Nations Conference on Trade and Development. (2018). *List of least developed countries*. Geneva, Switzerland: United Nations Conference on Trade and Development. Retrieved July 1, 2018 from http://unctad.org/en/pages/ALDC/Least%20Developed%20Countries/UN-list-of-Least-Developed-Countries.aspx.

United Nations Development Programme. (2018). *Human development reports 2018*. New York: United Nations Development Programme. Retrieved August 26, 2018 from http://hdr.undp.org/en/year/2018.

United Nations High Representative for Small Island and Land-Locked Nations (UN-OHRLLS). (2018). *Sustainable development goals*. Retrieved December 17, 2018 from https://www.un.org/sustainabledevelopment/blog/2018/10/small-island-developing-states-from-around-the-world-to-assess-progress-on-sustainable-development/.

United Nations Population Division (UNPOP). (2018). World population prospects. 2018. New York: UNPOP.

Weingast, B. R., & Wittman, D. (2006). *The Oxford handbook of political economy*. New York/Oxford UK: Oxford University Press.

Wikipedia. (2018a). *List of countries by incarceration rate*. Retrieved September 19, 2018 from https://en.wikipedia.org/wiki/List_of_countries_by_incarceration_rate.

Wikipedia. (2018b). *Operational (trade) agreements*. Retried December 10, 2018 from https://en.wikipedia.org/wiki/List_of_multilateral_free-trade_agreements.

World Bank. (2018). *World development report 2018: Learning to realize education's promise*. Washington, DC: World Bank.

World Health Organization. (2018). *Annual statistical report* (p. 2018). Geneva: World Health Organization.

Wu, G. (2016). *Four factors that have driven poverty reduction in China*. Geneva, Switzerland: World Economic Forum. Retrieved August 1, 2018 from https://www.weforum.org/agenda/2016/10/four-factors-that-have-driven-poverty-reduction-in-china.

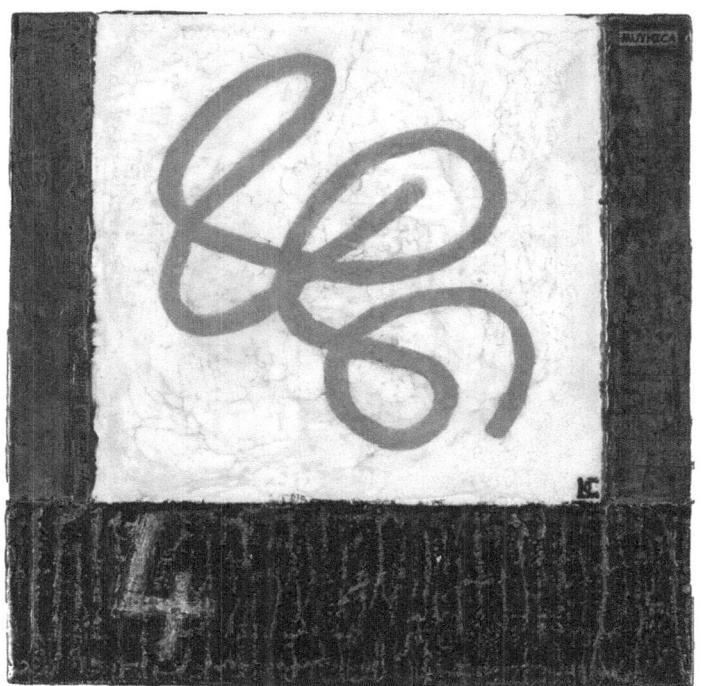

Part IV

Image 4: © Lylia Ferero Carr: Muysca, Muyhica

Chapter 5
Regional and Subregional Variations on the Weighted Index of Social Progress, 1970–2020

This chapter reports an analysis of the development and well-being trends of the 162 countries included in the comprehensive analysis. These 162 countries, as previously reported, represent a total of 95% of the world's population. The only exceptions to this total are the small island developing and, in some cases, land-locked nations of developing Africa, Asia, Latin America, and the Caribbean (UN Office of the High Representative for the Least Developed Countries, Landlocked Developing Countries and Small Island Developing States, 2018). These countries account for only a small percentage of the world's total population but, due to rapid global warming, are among the most vulnerable global populations worldwide, especially with respect to massive flooding, tsunamis, and the like. In any case, the special conditions and unique conditions confronting this important block of 5% of the world's countries are not discussed at length here.

The focus of this chapter is the 19 regions/subregions into which the world's seven continental groupings are divided. The regions are separated by discrete socio-political-economic history and are identified in Fig. 5.1. In addition to identifying the regions, Fig. 5.1 reports scores for the *Weighted Index of Social Progress* (WISP18) for each of the 19 subregions as well as the percentage changes in WISP scores between 2000 (WISP00) and 2018 (WISP18).

Figure 5.1 reports the WISP18 scores over the 20-year period beginning 1990. The figure is easy to understand and summarizes a wealth of data not readily available when presented in tabular form alone. Further, the figure reports these scores and ranks group nations by overall level of social performance since 1990. Thus, Fig. 5.1 and the other figures contained in this chapter offer an often-vivid portrait of changes in well-being at the global, regional, and subregional levels over at least a minimum of a 20-year period, often for the full 50-year period of the study. In their order of presentation in the chapter, the figures show data for the 162 nations of Europe (N = 35), Africa (N = 50), Asia (N = 35), and Latin America (N = 25) as well as for the four nations of Oceania (Australia, Fiji, Papua New Guinea, and New Zealand) and the two nations of North America (Canada and the United States).

© Springer Nature Switzerland AG 2019   69
R. J. Estes, *The Social Progress of Nations Revisited, 1970–2020*, Social
Indicators Research Series 78, https://doi.org/10.1007/978-3-030-15907-8_5

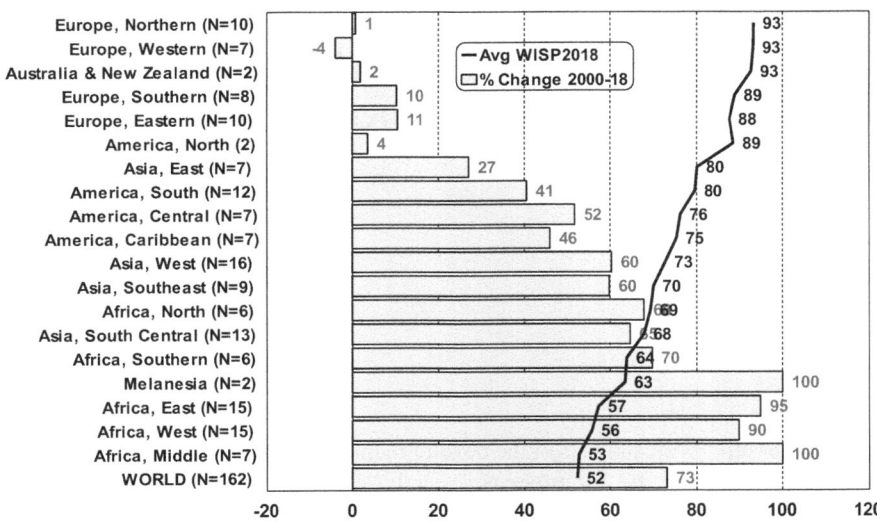

Fig. 5.1 Ranked ordered regional average Weighted Index of Social Progress-18 scores by subregion and percent change, 2000–2018 (N = 162). *WISP*, Weighted Index of Social Progress

Only the small island developing nations of the South Pacific and elsewhere with populations well below 50,000 and with limited social indicator sources are not included in the present analyses (UN Office of the High Representative for the Least Developed Countries, Landlocked Developing Countries and Small Island Developing States, 2018). These countries are identified in Box 5.1 by major geographic location.

Chapter Focus

The chapter provides a summary of social development and well-being accomplishments for all 162 countries included in the study group organized by the world's 19 major geographic regions and subregions. The purpose of the chapter is to identify the world's regions that are making the most and least progress in attaining their quality of life objectives. The data presented are primarily quantitative, albeit many inferences also are made concerning changes in people's subjective assessment of their own well-being.

Thus, the chapter contains a comprehensive picture of changes in the historical objective and subjective well-being over the most recent two decades. These patterns suggest the directions that future regional development is likely to assume (Aslam & Corrado, 2012; Morrison, 2017; Schyns, 2002).

Box 5.1 Small Island Developing Countries (UN Office of the High Representative for the Least Developed Countries, Landlocked Developing Countries and Small Island Developing States, 2018)

Caribbean	Pacific	Africa, Indian Ocean, Mediterranean and South China Sea
Anguilla	American Samoa	Bahrain
Antigua and Barbuda	Cook Islands	Cape Verde
Aruba	Federated States of Micronesia	Comoros
Bahamas	Fiji	Guinea-Bissau
Barbados	French Polynesia	Maldives
Belize	Guam	Mauritius
British Virgin Islands	Kiribati	São Tomé and Príncipe
Cuba	Marshall Islands	Seychelles
Dominica	Nauru	Singapore
Dominican Republic	New Caledonia	
Grenada	Niue	
Guyana	Northern Mariana Islands	
Haiti	Palau	
Jamaica	Papua New Guinea	
Montserrat	Samoa	
Netherlands Antilles	Solomon Islands	
Puerto Rico	Timor-Leste	
Saint Kitts and Nevis	Tonga	
Saint Lucia	Tuvalu	
Saint Vincent and the Grenadines	Vanuatu	
Suriname		
Trinidad and Tobago		
US Virgin Islands		

Ranked Ordered Regional Performances on the Weighted Index of Social Progress

Geopolitical regions and subregions are represented in two ways in this chapter, i.e., by Weighted Index of Social Progress (WISP) scores accrued for each of the world's 19 major regions as identified in Fig. 5.1 and WISP development zones (ranging from 1 to 5 with the most favorable rating closest to "1"). As summarized in Fig. 5.1, the regions with the most favorable WISP scores are concentrated among the nations of Europe, North America, and selected countries in Oceana. Conversely, the least favorable WISP scores and average WISP score regional averages are associated with the nations of Africa and the poorer nations (and subregions) of Asia, especially those of South and Southeast Asia, and selected subregions in Latin America and the Caribbean. The very well-off and the poorest nations of these subregions are discussed more fully in Chap. 6, which lists countries by socio-development level and period. Of critical importance in this section, however, is to appreciate the often subtle, but important, differences that exist between the subregions of each continental grouping. The reader is also encouraged to consult Appendix B, which reports WISP and WISP subindex scores for the entire 50 years covered by the study.

The following sections of this chapter discuss the major WISP subregional/sub-continental findings reported for each continent since 1970. Country data trends by index (Index of Social Progress [ISP], WISP) and subindex scores (N = 10 subindexes per country) over the 50-year period are, as already indicated, reported in Appendix B for all 162 nations by major development grouping. The table reprinted in Appendix B includes baseline data that can be used by other scholars to monitor future changes in development and well-being that will have taken place during future decades, including assigning their own system of statistical weights.

European Social Development Trends

The WISP data reported in Figs. 5.2 and 5.3 summarize scores for each decade from 1970 to the present. These figures report innovative well-being objective data for the European region and its four subregions of 35 nations divided among four major subregions, i.e., northern (N = 10), eastern (N = 10), southern (N = 8), and Western (N = 7) Europe. Countries that make up each of the subregions are identified by name and locale in Chap. 3. All 35 of the European countries have been included in the WISP database since 1970; hence, the chart reflects a rich set of data for a full 50 years for one of the world's most socially advanced regions and four subregions. (Note, too, that the author has published many articles and book chapters on a variety of aspects of European social development for the entire 50-year period, a period that captures the maturation of Europe into a region characterized by comprehensive welfare states that are the envy of many non-European societies [Estes, 2004, 2010, 2012, 2015]).

Thus, the data reported in this section of the chapter summarize the steady pace of social gains made by the region over a full half century. These gains have been remarkable given the political turbulence that occurred in the Eastern European subregion following the dissolution of the former Soviet Union. Today, this region is at the same level of social development as the other subregions in Europe. Not surprisingly, European nations from all four subregions are among the most socially developed and happiest nations in the world (Helliwell, Layard & Sachs, 2018). We shall see the complete WISP18 listing of nations for each of Europe's subregions, as

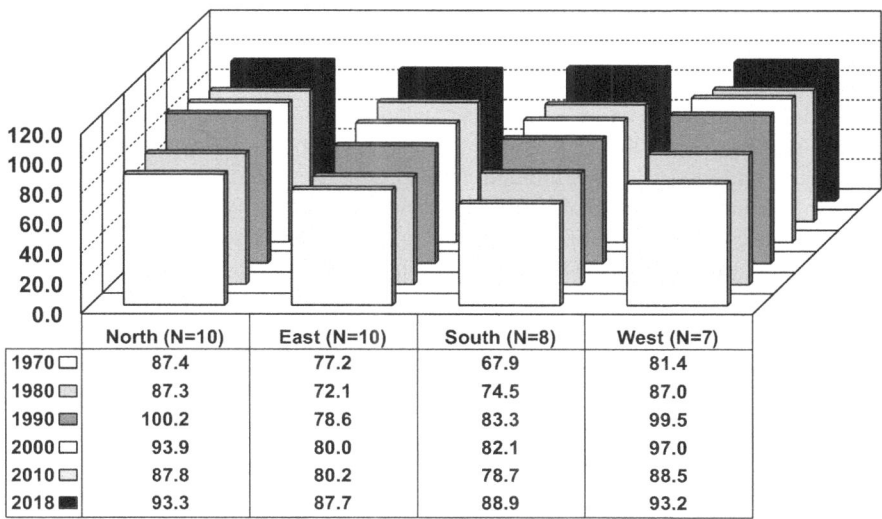

	North (N=10)	East (N=10)	South (N=8)	West (N=7)
1970 ☐	87.4	77.2	67.9	81.4
1980 ☐	87.3	72.1	74.5	87.0
1990 ▥	100.2	78.6	83.3	99.5
2000 ☐	93.9	80.0	82.1	97.0
2010 ☐	87.8	80.2	78.7	88.5
2018 ■	93.3	87.7	88.9	93.2

Fig. 5.2 Average Weighted Index of Social Progress scores for the European region by subregion, 1970–2018 (N = 35)

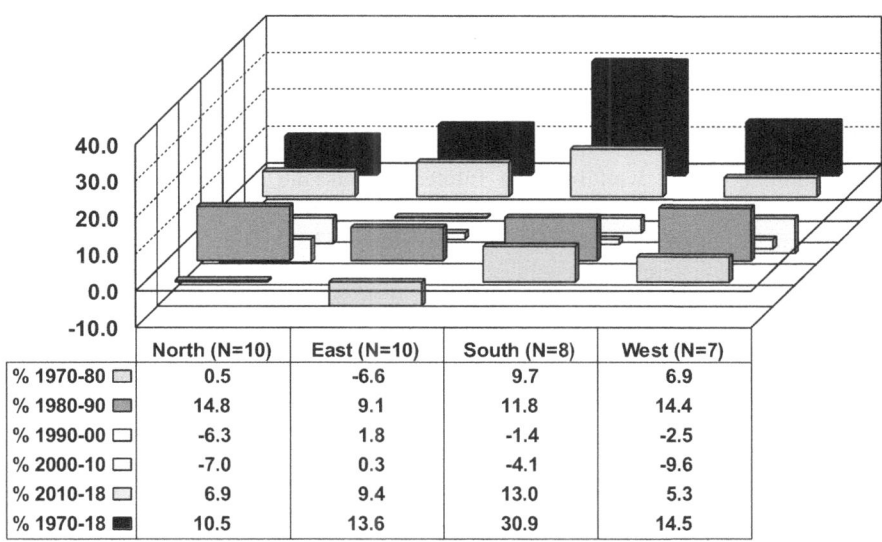

	North (N=10)	East (N=10)	South (N=8)	West (N=7)
% 1970-80 ☐	0.5	-6.6	9.7	6.9
% 1980-90 ▥	14.8	9.1	11.8	14.4
% 1990-00 ☐	-6.3	1.8	-1.4	-2.5
% 2000-10 ☐	-7.0	0.3	-4.1	-9.6
% 2010-18 ☐	6.9	9.4	13.0	5.3
% 1970-18 ■	10.5	13.6	30.9	14.5

Fig. 5.3 Percentage changes in average Weighted Index of Social Progress scores for the European region by subregion, 1970–2018 (N = 35)

well as those of other major geopolitical regions and subregions, in the next chapter. Appendix B provides even more comprehensive data for each nation in the two WISP indexes and 10 subindexes for the period 1970–2020. In effect, 72 scores are presented for each country over this time span except for the Eastern European countries who gained their independence from the former Soviet Union in 1991.

Europe, as reported previously in this chapter, is the most socially developed of the world's regions and enjoys one of the highest levels of quality of life (Fig. 5.2). Twenty-one of the world's three most socially developed regions are the socially progressive nations of Europe, including the 17 countries that make up northern and Western Europe. Rates of infant, child, and maternal mortality are remarkably low in the countries as are years of average life expectancy (only selected economically advanced nations of East Asia have a slightly higher average life expectancy). Years of age-appropriate primary and secondary school education are just slightly short of reaching 100% enrollment, whereas postsecondary education is available to all qualified students at virtually no cost to themselves. Technological innovations by individuals in the European states compete favorably with the patentable accomplishments of North Americans, who, indeed, have developed technologies rooted in European science and technology, e.g., the theoretical and applied science of innovations first created by French, German, and other northern European scientists, e.g., the contributions made by Louis Pasteur (France, 1822–1895), Marie and Pierre Curie (France, 1864–1934, 1859–1906), Albert Einstein (Germany, 1877–1955), Niels Bohr (Denmark, 1885–1962), and Wernher von Braun (Germany, 1912–1977), among many others who contributed to the North American spirit of scientific exploration and innovation that, in time, took, humanity to the stars (Selian and McKnight, 2017).

The social status of women during the modern area reached a zenith in Europe (Roth, 2008). The social, economic, corporate, and political status of European women equals or exceeds that of men and women everywhere in the world and it is expected to continue well into the future. Indeed, the status of contemporary European women has become the standard by which the social, political, and economic progress of women throughout the world is judged. Today, in Europe, many women are enrolled in higher education, own and operate complex social enterprises, engage in highly profitable businesses of their own, enjoy universal suffrage, are represented in substantial numbers as elected officials in national parliaments and in critical intergovernmental bodies, and, in some cases have been empowered to a level equal to that of men. The region's women are fully aware that they are the successors of the remarkable women in each country who have preceded them—a lesson that men frequently have minimized or forgotten altogether but would do well to refresh their memory of the revolutionary progressive social history that followed the beginning of the Industrial Revolution in Germany, the United Kingdom, and other parts of Europe before moving on to North America (European Commission, 2009).

Europeans also enjoy access to a full spectrum of publicly financed social welfare schemes that commence well before birth and continue throughout their entire lives to the point that personal savings levels among working class Europeans are among the lowest of the economically advanced societies (Estes & Zhou, 2015; Trading Economics, 2018). The origins of the "welfare state," for example, are attributed to the German Otto von Bismarck (1815–1898), then chancellor of the German Empire (1871–1890), who sought to use the "give them bread" function of welfare to control the high levels of social conflict in the country resulting from long-term unemployment and hunger. The approach adopted succeeded in achieving its goals and, subsequently, served as a model for the rest of Europe confronting the same types of income insecurity problems with their populations. Today, commonly referred to as "social security," the programs that resulted from these social innovations have proven to be among the most successful publicly adopted approaches to income security for vulnerable populations worldwide. Indeed, these wide expanses of income security programs for highly vulnerable populations have been adopted by virtually all nations worldwide even as the richness of the benefits they provide has increased to cover an increasing number of income vulnerable populations in nearly all countries (International Social Security Association, 2018).

Finally, the European region also is known for its careful attention to environmental protection. This attention comprises complex interventions intended to conserve water and energy, efficient recycling and repurposing of liquid and solid waste, a rich array of policies that prevent the use of nonbiodegradable products including the mandatory separation by consumers of waste into designated household or public containers. The region's nations also are known for their willingness to set aside large expanses of forests, rivers, and streams as well as urban green spaces for use by the public. The city streets of most European cities also are relatively free of litter. The use of tobacco products in most public spaces also is strictly prohibited, albeit some local taverns and bars permit the use of these products in their public spaces. Extensive research is being undertaken to identify more efficient ways to produce energy (including the repurposing of waste materials) including the production of nuclear-generated energy in most European nations. Within Europe, as elsewhere, however, the disposal of nuclear waste materials used in the production of energy remains problematic and is not yet resolved. Very likely, European nuclear-dependent nations will need to find more effective and efficient approaches to fissionable materials or, possibly, to refrain from depending entirely on nuclear sources (World Nuclear Association, 2018).

Within Europe as a region, its northern and western subregions are the most developed (Fig. 5.2) and have high rates of sociopolitical development (Fig. 5.3). Even so, Europe's southern and eastern subregions have attained WISP scores closely approximating those of the other two regions but are also achieving improvements in overall well-being as measured by the WISP that are comparable with those reported for northern and western Europe, especially when one examines the net social gains achieved by all four subregions from 1970 to the present. Almost certainly, the WISP scores for the entire European region will reach full parity on all the WISP's 40 social indicators and 10 subindexes in the decades just ahead.

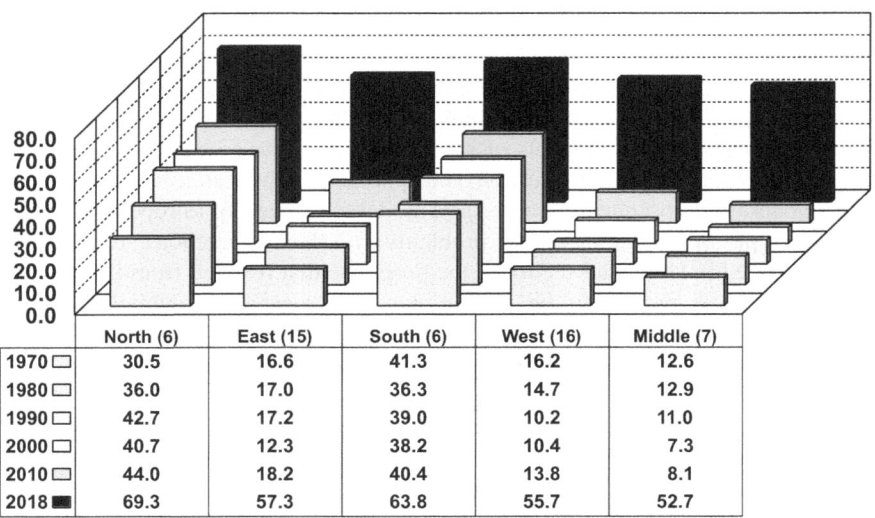

	North (6)	East (15)	South (6)	West (16)	Middle (7)
1970 □	30.5	16.6	41.3	16.2	12.6
1980 □	36.0	17.0	36.3	14.7	12.9
1990 □	42.7	17.2	39.0	10.2	11.0
2000 □	40.7	12.3	38.2	10.4	7.3
2010 □	44.0	18.2	40.4	13.8	8.1
2018 ■	69.3	57.3	63.8	55.7	52.7

Fig. 5.4 Average Weighted Index of Social Progress scores for Africa by subregion, 1970–2018 (N = 50)

African Social Development Trends

The African region (N = 50) is home to approximately 1400 million people, or 18.4% of the world's total. The 50 nations are divided among five subregions and are among the world's most rapidly developing countries (Figs. 5.4 and 5.5). The rapid rates of social development and well-being have been occurring for the past 20 years and are expected to continue well into the future, especially as the United Nations 17 Sustainable Development Goals (SDG) are realized. The 17 SDG build directly on the accomplishments associated with the goals of the 10-year Millennium Development Campaign (MDC) that was launched by the United Nations General Assembly in 2000. One of the unique features of the MDC was that, for the first time in history, government, intergovernmental bodies, nongovernmental bodies, and families and households created a working partnership to reduce poverty and, at the same time, to promote the general well-being of societies themselves. Substantial sums of money were invested in the launching of the MDC with the promise that even more money would be made available from both governments and nongovernmental organizations, on an as needed basis.

The eight goals of the MDC were:

Goal 1: To eradicate extreme poverty and hunger, but especially income poverty among the poorest persons (mostly women, children, youth, and the aged) in rural communities of the world's socially least developed countries.
Goal 2: To achieve universal primary education with special attention assigned to the education of women and illiterate adults.

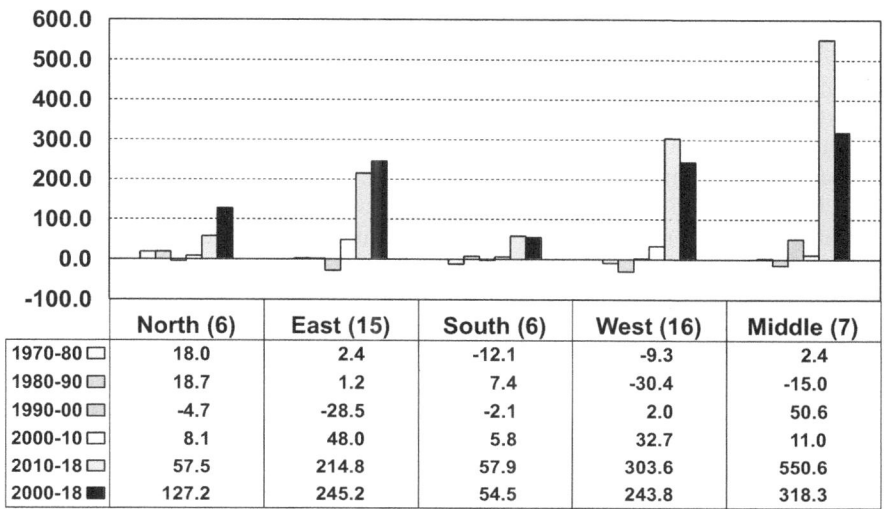

	North (6)	East (15)	South (6)	West (16)	Middle (7)
1970-80 ☐	18.0	2.4	-12.1	-9.3	2.4
1980-90 ☐	18.7	1.2	7.4	-30.4	-15.0
1990-00 ☐	-4.7	-28.5	-2.1	2.0	50.6
2000-10 ☐	8.1	48.0	5.8	32.7	11.0
2010-18 ☐	57.5	214.8	57.9	303.6	550.6
2000-18 ■	127.2	245.2	54.5	243.8	318.3

Fig. 5.5 Percentage change in average Weighted Index of Social Progress scores for Africa by subregion, 1970–2018 (N = 50)

Goal 3: To promote gender equality and empower women with a special focus on women in the poorest countries of developing Africa, Asia, and Latin America.

Goal 4: To reduce child mortality in developing Africa, Asia, and Latin America.

Goal 5: To improve maternal health for women everywhere in the world through enhanced preventive and primary health care.

Goal 6: To combat HIV/AIDS, malaria and other diseases in all regions of the world.

Goal 7: To ensure environmental sustainability including the creation of major protected forest other flora, fauna, and the seas.

Goal 8: To develop a global partnership for development but especially with economically advanced and developing nations. Intergovernmental and major international nongovernmental organization partnerships also are a priority.

Other goals were specified as "objectives" in the detailed body of the MDC's foundational documents but were of no less importance than these formally identified goals (United Nations Development Programme, 2016).

The MDC was a major success as reflected in the extraordinary social gains attained by many of Africa's poorest nations, which could not fund the complex, expensive human service and technological programs that the MDC made possible. Following the completion of the first campaign and building on the remarkable success attained by the MDC, the United Nations authorized a successor initiative intended to continue and deepen the critical successes achieved by the MDC, i.e., what is now referred to as the SDG or *Social Development Campaign*. This SDG campaign was launched in 2015 and, once again, identified as the primary beneficiaries the poorest of the poor nations located in developing Africa, Asia, and Latin

America (Hanson, Puplampu, & Shaw, 2017; UNCTAD, 2018). The initial successes of this campaign are reflected in the WISP scores reported for the majority of Africa's subregions (Figs. 5.4 and 5.5), especially among the desperately poor nations of Central, Southern, and Western Africa. The predominately Islamic nations of North Africa, most of which have direct access to the Mediterranean Sea, were already comparatively advantaged African nations at the time the series of studies began, as were the countries of East Africa, which had direct access to other trade routes.

The SDGs reflect 17 closely intertwined goals (actually "aspirations"), all of which impact directly advancing development and well-being in Africa: **Goal 1:** no poverty; **Goal 2:** zero hunger; **Goal 3:** good health and well-being; **Goal 4:** quality education; **Goal 5:** gender equality; **Goal 6:** clean water and sanitation; **Goal 7:** affordable and clean energy; **Goal 8:** decent work and economic growth; **Goal 9:** industry, innovation and infrastructure; **Goal 10:** reduced inequalities; **Goal 11:** sustainable cities and communities; **Goal 13:** climate action; **Goal 14:** life below water; **Goal 15:** life on land; **Goal 16:** peace, justice, and strong institutions; and, **Goal 17:** partnerships for the goals.

Asian Social Development Trends

Asia is the world's largest and most culturally diverse region. Asia is made up of four distinct subregions in which its population of 4500 million people reside (vs. 2120 million people in 1970). The region contains three of the world's "population super giants": China (1400 million people), India (1300 million people), and Indonesia (275 million people). The United States, because its Western coastline of more than 1500 land miles along the Pacific Ocean, also is a "Pacific power" but is not part of Asia (population in 2018 = ca. 330 million people).

Advancements in Asia in the objective conditions of life and well-being have been among the most rapid and impressive worldwide (Figs. 5.6 and 5.7). Life expectancy in the region ranges from the mid-70 years on average to that of the world's longest living nation, Japan (average years of life expectancy = 84.2 years for both genders). Infant, child, and maternal mortality rates have dropped dramatically in the region's countries since 2000 and, today, exceed world average gains. Social gains in these critical areas of well-being are especially impressive and represent one of the central goals of social development over time (Estes & Sirgy, 2018a; World Bank, 2018).

The region's gains in primary and secondary school education since 2000 also are impressive—sectors that require the investment of significant national resources to achieve notable goals. Most of the "social laggards" along these dimensions are the small island nations of the South Pacific (UN Office of the High Representative for the Least Developed Countries, Landlocked Developing Countries and Small Island Developing States, 2018). These countries are identified in Box 5.1. The same pattern also prevails among the poorest countries of South and Southeast Asia, including Bangladesh, India, and Indonesia. Asia also is one of the world's major

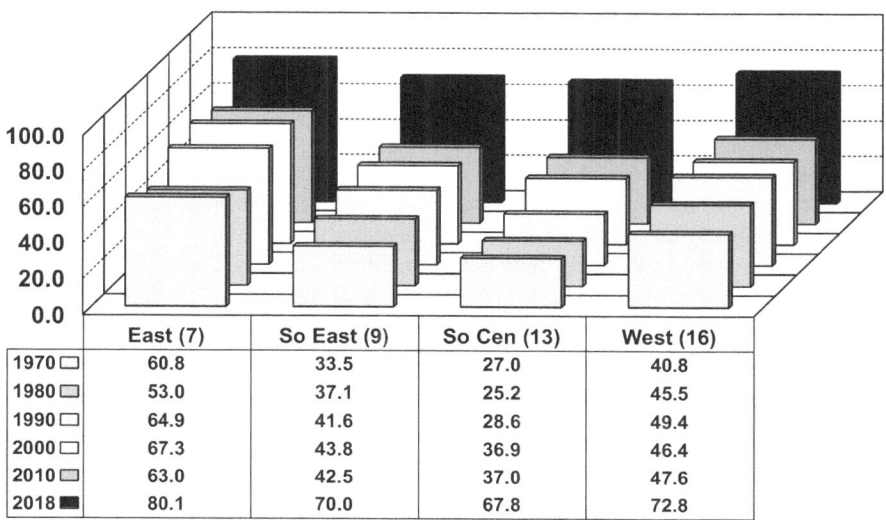

Fig. 5.6 Average Weighted Index of Social Progress scores for Asia by subregion, 1970–2018 (N = 45). (So, south)

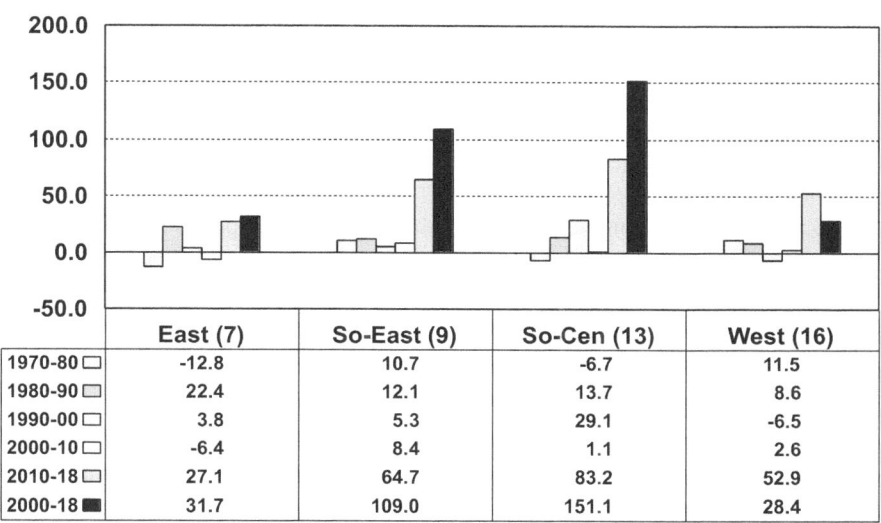

Fig. 5.7 Percent change in average Weighted Index of Social Progress scores for Asia by subregion, 1970–2018 (N = 45). (So, south)

centers of higher learning (United Nations Development Programme, 2016, 2018) and, increasingly, is a region of designation for higher education and training in automated technologies, but especially in software and hardware development. Costs, though, prohibit many young people from availing themselves of the services of these institutions, which, as a result, seek to attract increasing numbers of foreign students. Nearly everywhere in East and Southeast Asia, families spend inordinate sums of money on informal tutoring for their children, especially in the physical sciences, mathematics, and at least colloquial English. These latter forms of education are very expensive for the families and result in these students allocating as much as 10–12 h daily on education alone.

The granting of full social, political, and economic parity to the girls and women of these regions has been slow. This pattern is especially surprising among Asia's most economically advanced countries, which recognize the importance of the contributions made by women to their development but overtly discriminate against women of child-bearing age and those 40 years of age and older. Indeed, Asia's social profile would be significantly enhanced were full equity and administrative power granted to that half of their extraordinarily well-educated population.

The Asian region also is making steady gains in technology, environmental protection, and the safe and efficient disposal of liquid and solid wastes. Significant gains also are being made in the elimination of Asia's long-standing slums and temporary housing and, in their place, cleaner, more spacious, family-friendly housing is becoming increasingly available. The region's social safety nets are more secure than those of the past, but, still, large numbers of the poor, self-employed, and independent merchants continue to be left out of these systems. Income security services for chronically poor families, individuals, and communities remain weak, especially among those persons and communities located in Asia's extensive rural areas. Progress is being made in this sector, if only gradually (Estes, 2015).

Poverty alleviation has become a major hallmark of the Asian region and its subregions (United Nations Development Programme, 2018). In China alone, for example, since 1990 more than 100 million chronically poor individuals and households have been lifted out of poverty due to a wide range of government investments and international development assistance. This initiative has been nothing short of remarkable given the complex dynamics that contribute to policy formation. The fact that these persons are now part of China's tax-paying working class is a significant net social gain for the country. China's new *Five-Year Plan* (2015–2020) calls for the lifting of yet another 100 million people out of extreme poverty during the current era. Comparable, but somewhat less far-reaching initiatives in reducing national and regional poverty, have been adopted by India and Indonesia, and every reason exists for believing that these countries, too, will achieve the complex goals associated with the alleviation of poverty. All three of these nations must be acknowledged for their substantial investments in working to bring about such a dramatic level of social and economic development among people who are typically left out of major national and regional development initiatives.

Asia is one of world's leaders in technology, especially in the miniaturization of electronic devices developed elsewhere. This accomplishment is especially notable in China and India and selected countries of Southeast Asia. Further, many of the software programs on which most of the world's corporations, scholars, and others depend are written in Asia. Book production, apart from the actual printing, including this book, also is a major Asian export owing to the availability of accomplished coders, related software, and high levels of human capital found within the region.

Unfortunately, though, some Asian nations also are major violators of intellectual property agreements, especially China and India, and have been the subjects over decades of dozens of international lawsuits by many international businesses that license the use of their software, e.g., Adobe, Microsoft Corporation. In the main, however, these lawsuits have not prevented the continued illegal copying and sale of much of the software for use by individual consumers (Clark & Hagan, 2018; Rapoza, 2012).

Unfortunately, the Asian region also is besieged by chronic levels of diversity-related social conflict. The emergence of jihadism in West Asia and, with it, terrorism both home and abroad, has become a major negative feature of the region despite its many successes (Estes & Sirgy, 2018a, 2018b, 2018c; Sirgy, Estes, & Rahtz, 2018; Sirgy, Joshanloo, Estes, & Rahtz, 2018). Though occurring with less frequency (START, 2018) in some subregions, the problem of West Asia-originated global terrorism still has not been resolved, especially the acts of terrorism directed at global financial, political, and military centers in Europe, North America, and selected countries of Oceania (Global Terrorism Database, 2018). Economically developed nations are spending hundreds of millions of dollars annually to prevent the flow of terrorism into their nations.

Latin American Social Development Trends

Social progress in the Latin America region (N = 26) is best characterized as "start and stop," given the slow to negative changes in development and well-being that characterized the region for the first 30 years of this analysis (Estes, 2004; Rojas-Herrera, 2016; Tonon, 2016). This pattern is reflected in Figs. 5.8 and 5.9, which summarize the region's subregional performances on the WISP since 1970. Many of these negligible changes are concentrated across all three regions in which people have struggled under difficult circumstances to meet their basic needs but especially those associated with access to quality housing, continuity of health care, basic literacy, and a modicum of income security during periods of serious illness or injuries. Meeting the income and social security needs of children and youth, the aged and disabled, and those of other historically disadvantaged population groups has proven to impose difficult challenges for the highly unstable governments and administrative bureaus through which these services typically are provided (International Social Security Association, 2018).

The education of children at both the primary and secondary school levels has, however, been a consistent priority of the region's 25 national and 75 subregional governments. These critical investments in the future of children and young people and, in turn, the larger society have had a highly positive impact on the region's development as has the creation of a broad spectrum of specialized programs of postsecondary higher education and vocational and professional training. Among the results of these investments has been the formation of appreciably high levels of human capital reserves that, in turn, have contributed to the region's development of

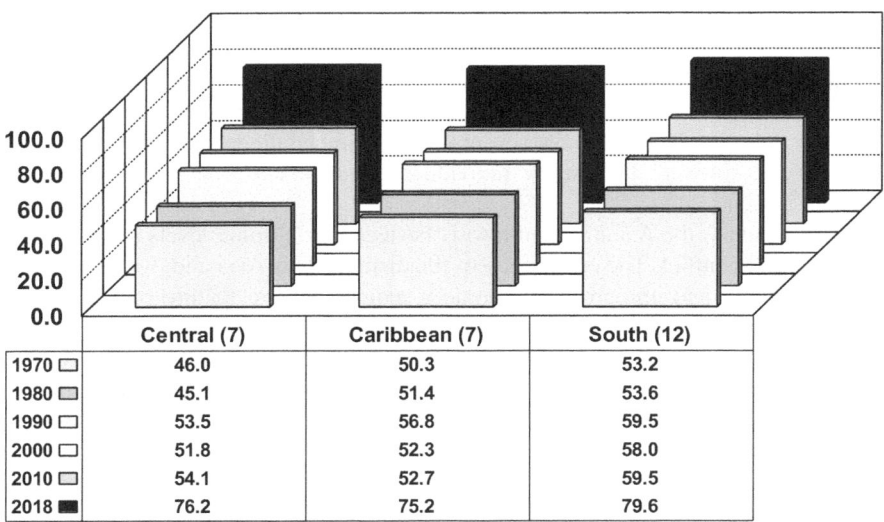

	Central (7)	Caribbean (7)	South (12)
1970 ☐	46.0	50.3	53.2
1980 ☐	45.1	51.4	53.6
1990 ☐	53.5	56.8	59.5
2000 ☐	51.8	52.3	58.0
2010 ☐	54.1	52.7	59.5
2018 ■	76.2	75.2	79.6

Fig. 5.8 Average Weighted Index of Social Progress scores for Latin America by subregion, 1970–2018 (N = 26)

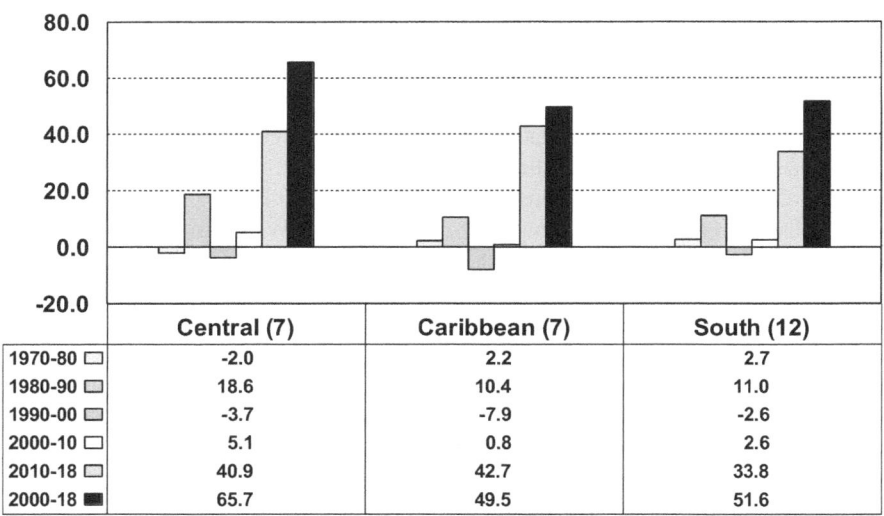

	Central (7)	Caribbean (7)	South (12)
1970-80 ☐	-2.0	2.2	2.7
1980-90 ☐	18.6	10.4	11.0
1990-00 ☐	-3.7	-7.9	-2.6
2000-10 ☐	5.1	0.8	2.6
2010-18 ☐	40.9	42.7	33.8
2000-18 ■	65.7	49.5	51.6

Fig. 5.9 Percent change in average Weighted Index of Social Progress scores for Latin America by subregion, 1970–2018 (N = 26)

a technologically prepared workforce, greater gender equality for women, increased opportunities for geographic and social mobility, and significantly improved systems of social provision that each year reach a progressively greater number of previously unqualified people.

Since the year 2000, the Latin American region and each of its three major subregions have experienced significant advances in (a) years of average life expectancy; (b) dramatically reduced rates of infant, child, and maternal mortality; (c) significantly higher numbers of age appropriate children attending government-financed and private schools; (d) improved housing, sanitation, and solid and liquid waste disposal; (e) improved occupational and health standards; and (f) improved pension and publicly managed fiduciary arrangements focused on helping retired workers enjoy postemployment lives of dignity. Development progress in these sectors has added significantly to the region's quality of life and well-being. Nearly all specialists in this area of research agree that the positive momentum of these forces will continue over the long term—certainly for at least the next two decades (Rojas-Herrera, 2016; Tonon, 2016).

Families, the quality of family life, and family solidarity have been the rocks on which all other advances in the social well-being of the region's residents have depended. In recognition of the importance of these three of four legs of social policy, people, working through their governments, are gradually weaving more secure social safety nets that focus on the aged and families with large numbers of children—many of which go unsupervised for long periods given that both parents must work to support and enrich the socioeconomic status of the whole family. Thus, governments and private nongovernmental organizations carry increasing responsibility for developing programs of child social, emotional, and recreational support for increasingly larger numbers of the region's children and their families (especially in situations in which members of the region's multilayered extended kinship systems are not available to perform these functions).

In short, Latin America is a major world region that is "on the move" toward progressively higher levels of happiness, life satisfaction, quality of life, and well-being (Helliwell, Layard, & Sachs, 2018; United Nations Development Programme, 2018). This forward-looking trajectory is the result of the removal of major obstacles to personal, collective, and community development that characterized the region during its earlier three decades of competitive development stagnation in providing more completely for the needs of its rapidly expanding population (Bates, Coatsworth, Williamson, 2006). Today, the future of Latin America is one in which people themselves have been placed at the center of development. The world community supports this priority and is providing substantial levels of financial and technical aid in support of helping the 26 nations of Latin America achieve the ambitious development objectives that they have established for themselves.

Regional and National Quality of Life and Well-Being and the Prognosis for the Future

The next chapter shifts from a discussion of global (N = 1) and regional analyses (N = 19) of quality of life and well-being to a discussion of well-being trends since 1970 and shifts to a discussion of those trends at the national level for the period 1970–2020 (est.) (N = 162). The discussion in the next chapter provides an intraregional perspective on the major social development gains and losses that have occurred within all these countries for the full 50-year period covered. Where necessary and appropriate, however, estimated data for the period 2018–2020 are reported as well, though in most cases the data summarized are comprehensive for the period. The chapter should be read with reference to Appendix B, which reports detailed data for each nation for the WISP's two composite indexes (ISP, WISP) and the ten component subindexes that are used to form the composite index scores, e.g., *health, education, social welfare provision, national expenditures for defense, changes in the status of women, levels of internal and intraregional social chaos, demographic trends, efforts to enhance the income security of financially vulnerable population groups, and advances in environmental protection.* In all, more than 72 data points are reported for the largest number of nations. Data are less complete for the recently independent nations of Eastern Europe following the collapse of the former Soviet Union in 1991, but their social comparability to other subregions of Europe is without parallel. WISP scores for the newly independent nations of the former Soviet Union almost certainly will be comparable to those of Western Europe by 2030. The WISP scores of other geopolitical regions can be expected to improve over the same period, and some will likely exceed the social gains they achieved during even earlier decades with far fewer national and international resources available to them than during earlier decades. All the world's major regions and subregions will achieve higher standards of living and quality of life than those which already exist today. This expectation for steady and increasing levels of global progress exists for the small island developing countries of the South Pacific, Caribbean, and coastal areas of sub-Saharan Africa already identified in the chapter and for the currently poor and socially least developed countries of Africa, Asia, and Latin America.

References

Aslam, A., & Corrado, L. (2012). The geography of well-being. *Journal of Economic Geography, 12*(3), 627–649.

Bates, R. H., Coatsworth, J. H., Williamson, J. G. (2006). Lost Decades: Lessons from Post-Independence Latin America for Today's Africa. *NBER Working Paper No. 12610.* Retrieved December 18, 2018 from https://www.nber.org/papers/w12610

Clark, G., & Hagan. (2018). Quicktake: What's intellectual property and does China steal it? *Bloomberg,* March 22. Retrieved July 1, 2018 from https://www.bloomberg.com/news/articles/2018-03-22/what-s-intellectual-property-and-does-china-steal-it-quicktake

Estes, R. J. (2004). Development challenges of the 'New' Europe. *Social Indicators Research, 69*(2), 123–166.

Estes, R. J. (2010). Toward sustainable development: From theory to praxis. *Social Development Issues, 15*(3), 1–29.

Estes, R. J. (2012). Economies in transition: Continuing challenges to quality of life. In K. Land, A. C. Michalos, & M. Joseph Sirgy (Eds.), *Handbook of quality of life research* (pp. 433–457). Dordrecht, The Netherlands: Springer International Publishers.

Estes, R. J. (2015). Development trends among the world's socially least developed countries: Reasons for cautious optimism. In B. Spooner (Ed.), *Globalization: The crucial phase* (pp. 23–70). Philadelphia: University of Pennsylvania Museum Press.

Estes, R. J., & Sirgy, M. J. (2018a). *Advances in well-being: Towards a better world*. London/New York: Rowman & Littlefield Ltd..

Estes, R. J., & Sirgy, M. J. (2018b). Advances in well-being in the MENA region: Accentuating the positive. In L. Lambert & N. Pasha-Zaidi (Eds.), *Advances in well-being in the Middle East and North Africa (MENA) region: Historical background and contemporary challenges*. Dordrecht, The Netherlands: Springer. (in press).

Estes, R. J., & Sirgy, M. J. (2018c). Is quality of life related to radical Islamic militancy and acts of terrorism? In H. Tiliouine & R. J. Estes (Eds.), *The state of social progress of Islamic societies: Social, political, economic, and ideological challenges* (pp. 575–606). Dordrecht, The Netherlands: Springer.

Estes, R. J., & Zhou, H. (2015). A conceptual approach to the creation of public–private partnerships in social welfare. *International Journal of Social Welfare, 24*(4), 348–363.

European Commission. (2009). *Women in European politics—Time for action*. Office for Official Publications of the European Communities.

Global Terrorism Database. (2018). *START Program*. College Park MD: University of Maryland. Retrieved December 18, 2018 from https://www.start.umd.edu/gtd/

Hanson, K. T., Puplampu, K. P., & Shaw, T. M. (Eds.). (2017). *From millennium development goals to sustainable development goals*. London/New York: Routledge.

Helliwell, J. F., Layard, R., & Sachs, J. D. (2018). *World happiness report, 2018*. New York: Sustainable Development Solutions Network. Retrieved August 28, 2018 from http://world-happiness.report/ed/2018/

International Social Security Association. (2018). *Social security programs throughout the world, 2018*. Geneva: International Social Security Association. Also available for 2017 at https://www.ssa.gov/policy/docs/progdesc/ssptw/

Morrison, P. S. (2017). *Subjective wellbeing and the region: multilevel approaches (draft)*. Victoria University of Wellington, New Zealand, Departmental Working Paper. Retrieved December 18, 2018 from https://az659834.vo.msecnd.net/eventsairwesteuprod/production-ersa-public/d9bec9dda2bd4dfca013a6cb2d349187

Rapoza, K. (2012). In China, why piracy is here to stay. *Forbes, July 22*.

Rojas-Herrera, M. (Ed.). (2016). *Handbook of happiness research in Latin America*. Dordrecht, The Netherlands: Springer International.

Roth, S. (2008). *Gender politics in the expanding European Union: Mobilization, inclusion, exclusion*. New York/Oxford: Berghahn Books.

Schyns, P. (2002). Wealth of nations, individual income and life satisfaction in 42 countries: A multilevel approach. *Social Indicators Research, 60*, 5–40.

Selian, A. N., & McKnight, L. (2017). The role of technology in the history of well-being: Transformative market phenomena over time. In R. J. Estes & M. J. Sirgy (Eds.), *The pursuit of human well-being: The untold global history* (pp. 639–687). Cham, Switzerland: Springer International.

Sirgy, M. J., Estes, R. J., & Rahtz, D. W. (2018). Combatting jihadist terrorism: A quality-of-life perspective. *Journal of Applied Research in Quality of Life, 13*(4), 813–837.

Sirgy, M. J., Joshanloo, M., Estes, R. J., & Rahtz, D. W. (2018). The global challenge of jihadist terrorism: A quality-of-life model. *Social Indicators Research*, in press. doi:https://doi.org/10.1007/s11205-017-1831-x.

Tonon, G. (Ed.). (2016). *Indicators of quality of life in Latin America*. Dordrecht, The Netherlands: Springer.

Trading Economics. (2018). *European Union gross household saving rates, 1999–2018*. Retrieved August 28, 2018 from https://tradingeconomics.com/european-union/personal-savings

United Nations Conference on Trade and Development (UNCTAD). (2018). *List of least developed countries*. Geneva, Switzerland: United Nations Conference on Trade and Development. Retrieved August 28, 2018 from http://unctad.org/en/pages/ALDC/Least%20Developed%20Countries/UN-list-of-Least-Developed-Countries.aspx.

United Nations Development Programme. (2016). *Ending poverty: The MDGs and beyond 2015*. New York: United Nations Development Programme. Retrieved August 28, 2018 from http://www.un.org/millenniumgoals/.

United Nations Development Programme. (2018). *Human development reports, 2018. [Web site]*. New York: United Nations Development Programme. Retrieved August 28, 2018 from http://hdr.undp.org/en/year/2018.

United Nations High Representative for Small Island and Land-Locked Nations (UN-OHRLLS). (2018). Sustainable development goals. Retrieved December 17, 2018 from https://www.un.org/sustainabledevelopment/blog/2018/10/small-island-developing-states-from-around-the-world-to-assess-progress-on-sustainable-development/.

World Bank. (2018). *World development report, 2018: Learning to realize education's promise*. Washington, DC: World Bank. Retrieved August 28, 2018 from http://www.worldbank.org/en/publication/wdr2018.

World Nuclear Association. (2018). *Nuclear power in the European Union*. Retrieved December 18, 2018 from http://www.world-nuclear.org/information-library/country-profiles/others/european-union.aspx

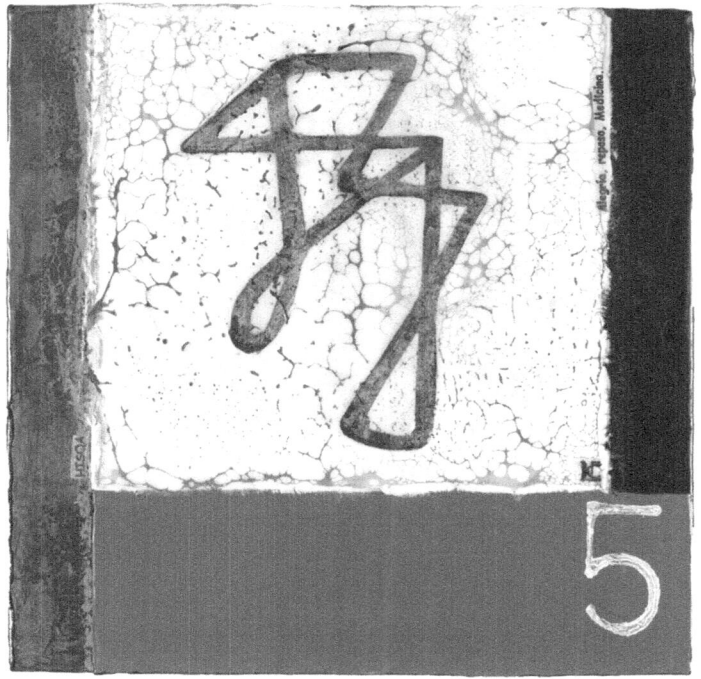

Part V

Image 5: © Lylia Ferero Carr: Muysca, Hisqa

Chapter 6
National Quality of Life and Well-Being: 50 Years of Development and Well-Being Challenges and Progress

Thus far, we have documented major shifts that have occurred in quality of life and well-being worldwide from 1970 to the present. Along with selected estimates for the next 2 years, these data illustrate national trends in well-being by decade over the most recent 50-year period. The author has previously reported on interim trends for the period 1970–2020. These trends have been strongly positive and forward-oriented over the entire period covered by the earlier reports (Estes, 1976, 1988, 1998a, 1998b, 2007, 2010, 2012a, 2012b, 2015b, 2018). In recent years, and with other scholars working on the same period, national studies also have been undertaken on countries characterized by extensive histories of diversity-related social conflict that, in the case of North Africa and West Asia, has taken the form of religiously inspired acts of terrorism in both their own and other nations (el-Aswad, 2019; Sirgy, Estes, & Rahtz, 2018). Targets of the latter have been primarily major population and financial centers in Western nations (of Europe and North America) as well as the national capitals and centers of national defense and defense intelligence within these countries (Central Intelligence Agency, 2018). Though the number of acts of international terrorism has successfully been reduced in the last several years, even so, horrific acts of terrorism continue to take place in the countries of origin and their nearby neighbors, e.g., Afghanistan, Iran, Iraq, and Syria, among others.

World Social Leaders and Socially Least Developing Countries

The world's social leaders (SL) and socially least developed countries (SLDC) are identified in Figs. 6.1 and 6.2 and in Tables 5.1 and 5.2. The two figures show Weighted Index of Social Progress (WISP) 2000 and WISP18 scores and percentage changes in WISP scores that occurred in the index over nearly two decades. The figures also identify the socially most and socially least developed countries, their

© Springer Nature Switzerland AG 2019

R. J. Estes, *The Social Progress of Nations Revisited, 1970–2020*, Social Indicators Research Series 78, https://doi.org/10.1007/978-3-030-15907-8_6

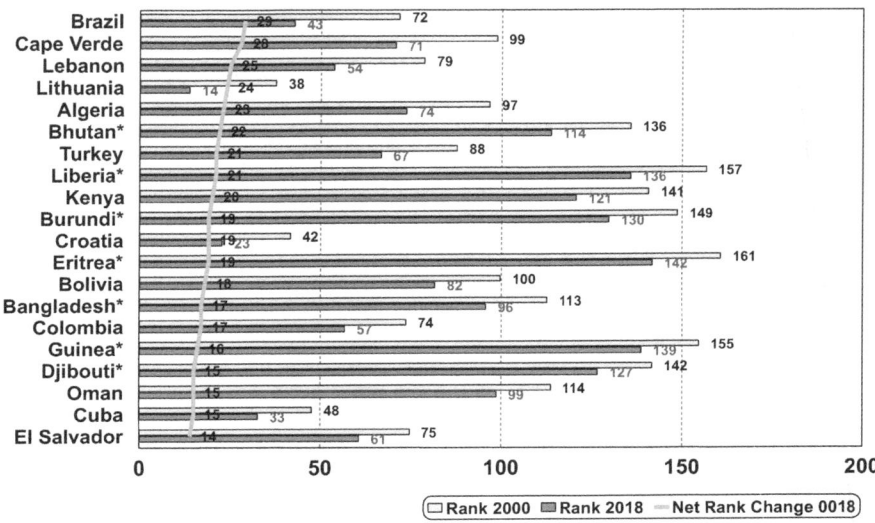

Fig. 6.1 Countries with the highest number of social rank gains on the Weighted Index of Social Progress between 2000 and 2018 (N = 20). (United Nations Commission on Trade and Development, 2018). *Officially designated "least developed country"

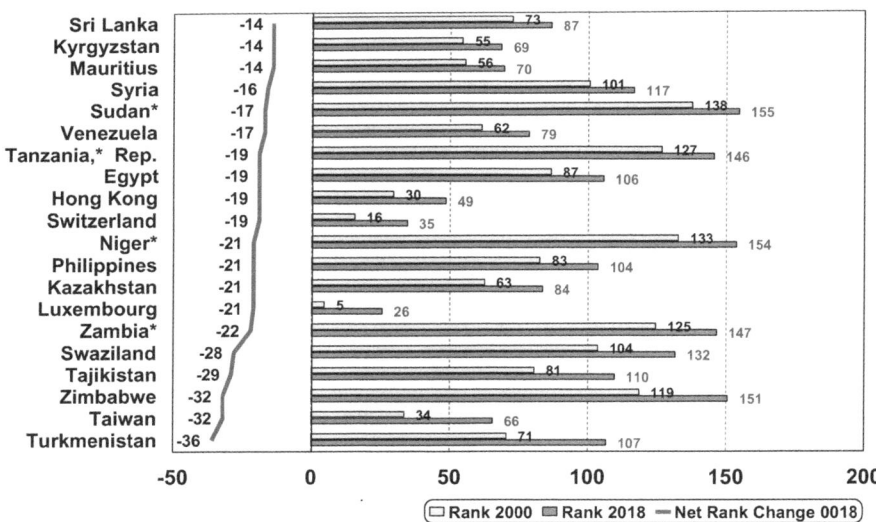

Fig. 6.2 Countries with the highest number of social rank losses on the Weighted Index of Social Progress 2018 between 2000 and 2017/18 (N = 20) (United Nations Commission on Trade and Development, 2018) *Officially designated "least developed country"

Table 6.1 Top 25 performing countries on the Weighted Index of Social Progress 2018 (WISP18), 1990–2017/18 (N = 25) (United Nations Commission on Trade and Development, 2018)

WISP 2000	WISP 2010/2011	WISP 2017/2018	COUNTRY	WISP RANK 2000	WISP RANK 2010/2011	WISP RANK 2017/2018
107	72	99	Denmark	2	1	1
100	71	98	Germany	6	4	2
100	70	97	Austria	7	5	3
91	65	97	Japan	18	17	4
107	71	95	Sweden	1	3	5
98	67	95	Italy	9	12	6
101	66	95	Finland	4	13	7
98	68	95	Iceland	8	8	8
97	68	94	Belgium	10	9	9
104	72	94	Norway	3	2	10
95	67	94	Netherlands	13	11	11
93	66	93	New Zealand	17	15	12
90	64	93	Portugal	20	21	13
74	59	93	Lithuania	38	37	14
96	65	92	United Kingdom	11	19	15
94	67	92	France	14	10	16
89	62	92	Bulgaria	23	28	17
94	65	92	Ireland	15	20	18
88	66	92	Czech Rep	24	14	19
89	68	92	Australia	22	7	20
81	57	91	Estonia	31	44	21
96	65	91	Spain	12	18	22
70	62	91	Croatia	42	27	23
90	65	91	Greece	21	16	24
86	64	90	Canada	26	24	25

WISP Weighted Index of Social Progress

ranked social performances for the year 2018 relative to all 162 countries included in the study and the baseline scores for 2000 vis-à-vis 2018. The data presented in these figures are instructive and clearly indicate that 20 nations in each group have been the most and least successful in providing for both the basic and the enhanced social, political, economic, and other well-being needs of their growing populations.

Tables 6.1 and 6.2, by comparison, summarize country-specific WISP scores for the world's SL and SLDC for 2000, 2010/2011, and 2017/2018 and the WISP score rank positions for all 50 of the countries included in these tables relative to all 162 countries included in the more comprehensive worldwide analysis of changes in the quality of life and well-being of the hundreds of thousands of people who reside in the 50 SL and SLDC (United Nations Commission on Trade and Development, 2018). The highest numbers of the world's SL are located in Europe, North America,

Table 6.2 Bottom 25 performing countries on the Weighted Index of Social Progress 18, 2000–2017/18 (N = 25) (United Nations Commission on Trade and Development, 2018)

WISP 2000	WISP 2010/2011	WISP 2017/2018	COUNTRY	WISP RANK 2000	WISP RANK 2010/2011	WISP RANK 2017/2018
2	32	41	Cen African Rep[a]	151	152	162
−4	26	47	Chad[a]	154	156	161
−10	25	48	Sierra Leone[a]	159	159	160
8	35	48	Yemen[a]	145	141	159
1	17	48	Somalia[a]	152	161	158
−4	37	48	Nigeria	156	137	157
7	37	49	Uganda[a]	146	135	156
13	35	49	Sudan[a]	138	142	155
14	35	50	Niger[a]	133	143	154
−19	17	51	Afghanistan[a]	162	162	153
−12	38	51	Ethiopia[a]	160	134	152
24	37	51	Zimbabwe	119	136	151
12	35	52	Cote D'Ivoire	143	145	150
−10	26	52	Angola[a]	158	158	149
13	39	52	Mali[a]	137	130	148
22	39	54	Zambia[a]	125	126	147
20	42	54	Rep. of Tanzania[a]	127	115	146
15	36	54	Cameroon	132	138	145
−2	26	54	Congo, DR[a]	153	157	144
3	40	54	Burkina Faso[a]	150	125	143
−15	29	55	Eritrea[a]	161	153	142
14	34	55	Togo[a]	135	147	141
4	33	55	Mozambique[a]	148	149	140
−4	32	56	Guinea[a]	155	151	139
13	34	56	The Gambia[a]	139	146	138

WISP Weighted Index of Social Progress.
[a]Officially designated "least developed country."

Australia, and New Zealand. The largest number of SLDC is concentrated in sub-Saharan Africa, especially among those nations that have been officially classified by the United Nations as least developed countries.[1]

The reader is referred to Appendix B, which includes indexes (N = 2) and subindexes (N = 10) for the six periods (1970, 1980, 1990, 2000, 2010, 2018). Appendix B also shows the net percentage change in WISP scores over the approximately 50-year period 1970–2018.

---

[1] The least developed countries are identified in the figures and charts with an (*) following their name (United Nations Commission on Trade and Development, 2018).

Zones of Quality of Life and Well-Being

Many nations share characteristics in common with one another, including overall level of quality of life and well-being. Figure 6.3a–e groups nations into related zones of well-being and social development. The cut-off points used to divide countries into zones of well-being are identified in the title of each subtable, as are the numbers of countries included in each zone, which, except for Zone 1, show little variation.

Following Figs. 6.3a–e is a graphical information system representation of these zones prepared by Amy Hillier of the University of Pennsylvania (Fig. 6.4), who also prepared the earlier versions from 1970 to the present reprinted in Chap. 4.

(a) Well-being development zone 1 (Weighted Index of Social Progress 18 score range: 99.5–87.5; N= 40)

Denmark	Netherlands	Estonia	Slovakia
Germany	New Zealand	Spain	Costa Rica
Austria	Portugal	Croatia	Cuba
Japan	Lithuania	Greece	Chile
Sweden	United Kingdom	Canada	Switzerland
Italy	France	Luxembourg	Belarus
Finland	Bulgaria	Slovenia	Uruguay
Iceland	Ireland	Hungary	Romania
Belgium	Czech Rep	Poland	United States
Norway	Australia	Argentina	Latvia

(b) Well-being development zone 2 (Weighted Index of Social Progress 18 score range: 85.5–76.5;N= 30)

Ukraine	Moldova	El Salvador
Korea, South	Albania	Azerbaijan
Brazil	Bahamas	Singapore
Cyprus	Lebanon	Tunisia
Armenia	Macedonia	China
Israel	Guyana	Taiwan
Georgia	Colombia	Turkey
Russia	Panama	Peru
Hong Kong SAR	Ecuador	Kyrgyzstan
Mexico	Jamaica	Mauritius

Fig. 6.3a, b, c, d and e Countries (N = 162) grouped by well-being and social development zones (N = 5) using Weighted Index of Social Progress 2018 scores. *Indicates countries officially classified by the United Nations and the World Bank as "least developed countries." Many of these countries are either land- or sea-locked and have recent histories of colonization by European powers, high levels of diversity-related social conflict, civil war, or wars with neighboring states (Central Intelligence Agency, 2018; Stockholm International Peace Research Institute, 2018)

(c) Well-being development zone 3 (Weighted Index of Social Progress 18 score range: 75.5–70.5; N= 30)

Cape Verde	Paraguay	Jordan
Dominican Rep	Bolivia	Bahrain
Viet Nam	Uzbekistan	Kuwait
Algeria	Kazakhstan	Indonesia
Thailand	Suriname	Saudi Arabia
Trinidad-Tobago	Nicaragua	Bangladesh*
Libya	Sri Lanka	Belize
Mongolia	Iran	India
Venezuela	Morocco	Oman
South Africa	Malaysia	Korea, Nor

(d) Well-being development zone 4 (Weighted Index of Social Progress 18 score range: 70.0–58.5;N= 30)

Qatar	Comoros*	Kenya
Botswana	Nepal*	Laos*
Fiji	Guatemala	Pakistan
Philippines	Bhutan*	Haiti*
Honduras	Myanmar*	Rwanda*
Egypt	Lesotho*	Madagascar*
Turkmenistan	Syria	Djibouti*
Namibia	Ghana	Congo, Rep
Cambodia *	Iraq	Senegal*
Tajikistan	Gabon	Burundi*

(e) Well-being development zone 5 (Weighted Index of Social Progress 18 score range: 58.0–41.5; N= 32)

Mauritania*	Togo*	Zimbabwe	Chad*
Swaziland	Eritrea*	Ethiopia*	Central African
Papua New Guinea	Burkina Faso*	Afghanistan*	Rep*
Malawi*	Congo, DR*	Niger*	
Guinea-Bissau*	Cameroon	Sudan*	
Liberia*	Tanzania, * Republic	Uganda*	
Benin*	Zambia*	Nigeria	
Gambia, * The	Mali*	Somalia*	
Guinea*	Angola*	Yemen*	
Mozambique*	Cote D'Ivoire	Sierra Leone*	

Fig. 6.3a, b, c, d and e (continued)

Country Scores on the Weighted Index of Social Progress

Table 6.3 shows the WISP scores for all 162 countries included in the study for the years 2000, 2010, and 2018 as well as the rank order position of these countries for each period. The data range from the strongest performing countries on the WISP to those that continue to struggle with meeting at least the basic social needs of their

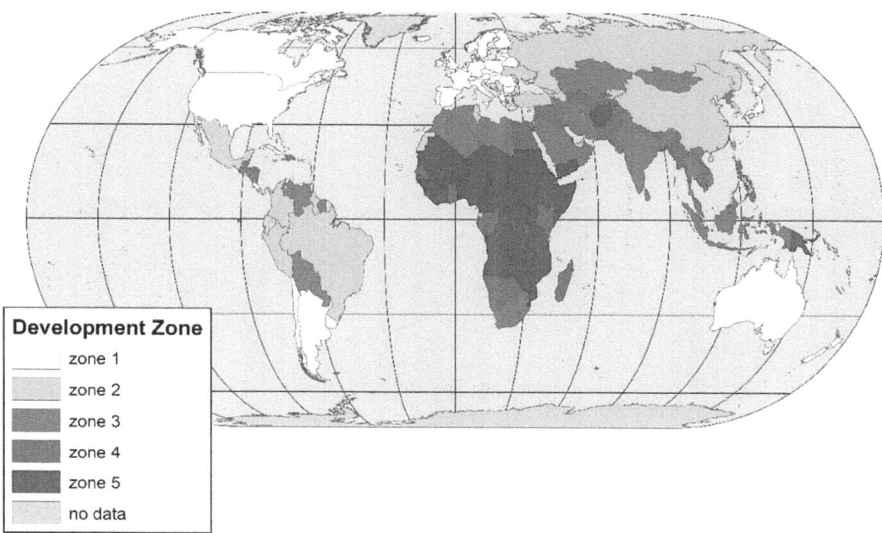

Fig. 6.4 Graphical information system distribution of Weighted Index of Social Progress 18 scores by country and development zone (Map by Amy Hillier)

rapidly increasing populations. The table, through the rank ordering of countries, identifies the major well-being challenges and accomplishments of 95% of the world's total population. The data reported in these tables and figures, however, are composite WISP scores *only* and *not* national performances on the 10 component subindexes of the WISP, i.e., the health, education, welfare, women, and six other sectors. These detailed data are reported in Appendix B of this book and elsewhere (Estes, 2019).

World Social Leaders

Not all of the world's nations that have been identified as leaders remain permanently in those positions. Indeed, the list of world development and well-being leaders identified in Table 6.1, as reported by this author, has changed over time—sometimes dramatically but always in response to social, political, and economic shifts occurring within their societies. That having been said, Table 6.1 identifies those countries that consistently have outperformed others with respect to their composite WISP scores over time. These changes, and the earlier rank order positions ascribed to these nations, are closely associated with their values, norms, and traditions. All three of these factors, in turn, are deeply steeped in the histories of these societies and in the contemporary political, economic, technological, and environmental pressures with which they are confronted.

Table 6.3 Scores and ranks on the Weighted Index of Social Progress by country, 1970–2018

WSPRNK18 (N = 162)	WSPRNK10 (N = 162)	WSPRNK00 (N = 162)	WSPRNK90 (N = 124)	WSPRNK80 (N = 124)	WSPRNK70 (N = 107)	COUNTRY (N = 162)	WISP18 (N = 162)	WISP10 (N = 162)	WISP00 (N = 162)	WISP90 (N = 124)	WISP80 (N = 124)	WISP70 (N = 107)
1	2	2	1	3	2	Denmark	99	72	107	108	92	91
2	4	6	.	.	.	Germany	98	71	100	.	.	.
3	6	7	4	5	8	Austria	97	70	100	101	90	83
4	11	18	14	10	22	Japan	97	65	91	95	86	73
5	1	1	3	4	1	Sweden	95	71	107	102	91	95
6	8	9	8	2	12	Italy	95	67	98	97	93	81
7	7	4	9	15	14	Finland	95	66	101	97	81	80
8	5	8	.	.	.	Iceland	95	68	98	.	.	.
9	15	10	10	8	11	Belgium	94	68	97	97	89	81
10	3	3	2	6	3	Norway	94	72	104	103	90	89
11	19	13	5	9	4	Netherlands	94	67	95	100	87	87
12	20	17	16	16	9	New Zealand	93	66	93	93	81	82
13	16	20	23	26	31	Portugal	93	64	90	87	70	62
14	21	38	.	.	.	Lithuania	93	59	74	.	.	.
15	13	11	12	12	5	United Kingdom	92	65	96	96	84	87
16	9	14	6	7	10	France	92	67	94	98	90	81
17	18	23	26	23	18	Bulgaria	92	62	89	79	72	77
18	35	15	13	11	7	Ireland	92	65	94	95	85	84
19	22	24	.	.	.	Czech Republic	92	66	88	.	.	.
20	27	22	17	14	13	Australia	92	68	89	91	82	80
21	34	31	.	.	.	Estonia	91	57	81	.	.	.
22	12	12	19	17	24	Spain	91	65	96	90	78	72
23	30	42	.	.	.	Croatia	91	62	70	.	.	.
24	23	21	21	20	29	Greece	91	65	90	87	76	64
25	33	26	15	18	19	Canada	90	64	86	93	78	76

						Country						Rank
			100	56	90	Luxembourg				5	10	26
	75		85	60	90	Slovenia	15			27	17	27
79	71	87	91	64	90	Hungary	17	22	22	19	14	28
78	60	80	85	63	89	Poland	33	25	25	29	28	29
61		73	69	59	89	Argentina		35	31	44	39	30
	69		87	64	89	Slovakia	34			25	24	31
60	59	75	68	58	89	Costa Rica	26	28	29	45	40	32
67	54	65	65	60	88	Cuba	30	37	41	48	41	33
62	83	69	75	57	88	Chile	20	49	36	37	44	34
75		96	93	68	87	Switzerland		13	11	16	25	35
	63		78	60	87	Belarus	27			33	29	36
66	70	78	79	63	87	Uruguay	21	31	27	32	32	37
74	77	69	77	59	87	Romania	23	27	37	35	31	38
72		90	85	61	87	United States		19	18	28	37	39
			77	55	87	Latvia				36	36	40
	55		71	57	85	Ukraine	49			41	26	41
49	57	74	71	58	85	Korea, South	35	46	30	40	49	42
56		63	53	54	85	Brazil		41	45	72	50	43
			70	59	84	Cyprus				43	45	44
	63		65	49	84	Armenia				49	43	45
55		73	72	58	84	Israel	37	32	32	39	47	46
			63	51	83	Georgia				53	51	47
	59		67	53	82	Russia	46			46	46	48
50	51	71	84	60	82	Hong Kong		38	34	30	38	49
		59	60	51	82	Mexico	32	54	48	57	57	50
			67	53	81	Moldova				47	48	51
61	54	55	65	53	81	Albania		48	54	50	53	52

(continued)

Table 6.3 (continued)

WISP70 (N = 107)	WISP80 (N = 124)	WISP90 (N = 124)	WISP00 (N = 162)	WISP10 (N = 162)	WISP18 (N = 162)	COUNTRY (N = 162)	WSPRNK70 (N = 107)	WSPRNK80 (N = 124)	WSPRNK90 (N = 124)	WSPRNK00 (N = 162)	WSPRNK10 (N = 162)	WSPRNK18 (N = 162)
.	.	.	58	53	80	Bahamas	.	.	.	64	55	53
53	64	45	52	52	80	Lebanon	41	30	68	79	79	54
.	.	.	63	47	80	Macedonia	.	.	.	52	69	55
.	.	.	55	51	79	Guyana	.	.	.	69	63	56
50	57	64	53	46	79	Colombia	44	40	43	74	74	57
56	56	63	62	52	79	Panama	36	43	46	54	60	58
49	53	57	60	51	79	Ecuador	47	51	52	58	66	59
55	62	67	59	51	78	Jamaica	38	34	38	61	58	60
48	43	53	53	50	78	El Salvador	50	58	56	75	78	61
.	.	.	60	52	78	Azerbaijan	.	.	.	59	54	62
50	60	70	64	55	78	Singapore	45	36	35	51	61	63
44	48	57	57	53	78	Tunisia	53	56	51	66	52	64
.	36	49	56	50	77	China	.	73	62	68	88	65
.	58	75	77	60	77	Taiwan	.	39	28	34	42	66
44	49	55	48	47	77	Turkey	54	55	53	88	72	67
38	37	48	53	50	76	Peru	58	69	64	76	70	68
.	.	.	61	53	76	Kyrgyzstan	.	.	.	55	64	69
.	56	67	61	52	75	Mauritius	.	45	39	56	56	70
.	.	.	40	49	75	Cape Verde	.	.	.	99	81	71
47	53	57	59	51	75	Dominican Republic	51	52	50	60	71	72
28	33	34	49	50	75	Viet Nam	73	77	82	84	80	73
36	36	50	42	49	75	Algeria	61	74	59	97	77	74
45	52	62	54	49	75	Thailand	52	53	47	70	75	75
54	57	66	58	51	74	Trinidad-Tobago	40	42	40	65	65	76

						Country						
21	40	44	46	46	74	Libya	84	62	70	89	90	77
.	37	43	57	48	74	Mongolia	.	70	72	67	67	78
55	63	63	59	52	74	Venezuela	39	33	44	62	59	79
51	43	44	52	47	74	South Africa	43	59	71	77	85	80
49	54	53	51	49	73	Paraguay	48	50	55	80	76	81
35	37	27	40	46	73	Bolivia	63	67	87	100	97	82
.	.	.	52	52	73	Uzbekistan	.	.	.	78	62	83
.	.	.	59	49	73	Kazakhstan	.	.	.	63	68	84
.	.	.	49	47	72	Suriname	.	.	.	86	94	85
38	33	39	43	50	72	Nicaragua	57	78	75	96	82	86
51	55	57	53	46	72	Sri Lanka	42	47	49	73	73	87
32	38	45	46	47	72	Iran	67	66	69	90	91	88
29	36	45	38	49	72	Morocco	71	72	67	102	99	89
36	46	52	49	47	72	Malaysia	60	57	57	85	87	90
29	39	50	40	47	72	Jordan	70	65	60	98	89	91
.	.	.	44	48	72	Bahrain	.	.	.	92	84	92
.	.	.	50	53	71	Kuwait	.	.	.	82	92	93
9	42	42	45	46	70	Indonesia	101	60	73	91	106	94
.	29	48	38	47	70	Saudi Arabia	.	82	63	103	102	95
.	18	19	32	48	70	Bangladesh[a]	.	101	94	113	107	96
.	.	.	44	48	70	Belize	.	.	.	95	100	97
19	27	35	34	45	70	India	86	85	81	110	110	98
.	.	.	29	47	70	Oman	.	.	.	114	108	99
.	40	47	35	45	70	Korea, North	.	63	66	109	109	100
.	.	.	36	53	70	Qatar	.	.	.	106	115	101
.	.	.	44	42	69	Botswana	.	.	.	93	86	102
.	.	.	33	43	69	Fiji	.	.	.	111	101	103

(continued)

Table 6.3 (continued)

WISP70 (N = 107)	WISP80 (N = 124)	WISP90 (N = 124)	WISP00 (N = 162)	WISP10 (N = 162)	WISP18 (N = 162)	COUNTRY (N = 162)	WSPRNK70 (N = 107)	WSPRNK80 (N = 124)	WSPRNK90 (N = 124)	WSPRNK00 (N = 162)	WSPRNK10 (N = 162)	WSPRNK18 (N = 162)
42	41	51	49	47	69	Philippines	55	61	58	83	96	104
40	35	50	44	48	68	Honduras	56	75	61	94	83	105
35	37	47	48	49	68	Egypt	62	68	65	87	93	106
.	.	.	54	50	67	Turkmenistan	.	.	.	71	95	107
.	.	.	36	40	67	Namibia	.	.	.	107	105	108
23	12	12	28	40	67	Cambodia [a]	81	108	108	116	113	109
.	.	.	50	44	67	Tajikistan	.	.	.	81	103	110
.	.	.	22	39	65	Comoros [a]	.	.	.	124	132	111
13	17	17	22	43	65	Nepal [a]	96	104	97	123	134	112
30	30	36	33	42	65	Guatemala	68	80	77	112	112	113
.	.	.	13	40	64	Bhutan [a]	.	.	.	136	122	114
36	27	36	35	41	64	Myanmar [a]	59	84	78	108	119	115
.	36	36	36	40	64	Lesotho [a]	.	71	79	105	98	116
32	40	39	39	45	63	Syria	64	64	74	101	104	117
22	18	16	26	43	63	Ghana	83	99	98	118	116	118
32	35	35	28	28	62	Iraq	66	76	80	115	143	119
.	.	.	28	41	61	Gabon	.	.	.	117	114	120
27	26	24	12	35	61	Kenya	74	86	90	141	121	121
.	20	15	21	42	61	Lao PDR [a]	.	96	101	126	118	122
20	18	24	23	39	61	Pakistan	85	103	88	120	125	123
28	25	28	23	33	60	Haiti [a]	72	89	83	121	127	124
17	18	21	19	44	59	Rwanda [a]	89	102	93	130	123	125
30	31	23	19	41	59	Madagascar [a]	69	79	91	128	120	126
.	.	.	12	33	59	Djibouti [a]	.	.	.	142	142	127
.	22	27	22	36	58	Congo, Republic	.	91	86	122	136	128

						Country						
27	18	24	19	39	58	Senegal[a]	75	98	89	131	129	129
5	8	18	3	36	58	Burundi[a]	104	117	95	149	147	130
23	10	13	12	38	58	Mauritania[a]	80	113	106	140	131	131
			37	40	58	Swaziland				104	111	132
	29	28	14	39	57	Papua New Guinea		83	85	134	133	133
11	4	13	9	43	57	Malawi[a]	98	120	104	144	117	134
			5	27	56	Guinea-Bissau[a]				147	156	135
24	20	12	-6	24	56	Liberia[a]	78	97	109	157	161	136
14	17	8	19	39	56	Benin[a]	92	105	112	129	135	137
			13	34	56	Gambia, The[a]				139	137	138
14	5	-1	-4	32	56	Guinea[a]	94	118	120	155	149	139
	2	-4	4	33	55	Mozambique[a]		122	123	148	145	140
9	15	17	14	34	55	Togo[a]	100	106	96	135	146	141
			-15	29	55	Eritrea[a]				161	159	142
3	11	8	3	40	54	Burkina Faso[a]	107	111	113	150	126	143
15	21	14	-2	26	54	Congo, Demo Repub[a]	91	94	103	153	154	144
23	22	21	15	36	54	Cameroon	82	92	92	132	141	145
12	20	15	20	42	54	Tanzania, Republic	97	95	102	127	128	146
27	25	28	22	39	54	Zambia[a]	76	88	84	125	130	147
13	8	4	13	39	52	Mali[a]	95	115	115	137	139	148
	5	-3	-10	26	52	Angola[a]		119	122	158	157	149
24	24	16	12	35	52	Cote D'Ivoire	79	90	99	143	151	150
32	29	37	24	37	51	Zimbabwe	65	81	76	119	124	151
4	-10	-10	-12	38	51	Ethiopia[a]	105	124	124	160	140	152

(continued)

Table 6.3 (continued)

WISP70 (N = 107)	WISP80 (N = 124)	WISP90 (N = 124)	WISP00 (N = 162)	WISP10 (N = 162)	WISP18 (N = 162)	COUNTRY (N = 162)	WSPRNK70 (N = 107)	WSPRNK80 (N = 124)	WSPRNK90 (N = 124)	WSPRNK00 (N = 162)	WSPRNK10 (N = 162)	WSPRNK18 (N = 162)
.	4	3	−19	17	51	Afghanistan[a]	.	121	116	162	162	153
6	8	3	14	35	50	Niger[a]	103	116	117	133	148	154
18	18	13	13	35	49	Sudan[a]	88	100	105	138	150	155
14	14	12	7	37	49	Uganda[a]	93	107	107	146	144	156
6	26	11	−4	37	48	Nigeria	102	87	110	156	152	157
19	10	1	1	17	48	Somalia[a]	87	112	119	152	158	158
.	.	.	8	35	48	Yemen[a]	.	.	.	145	138	159
25	12	2	−10	25	48	Sierra Leone[a]	77	110	118	159	155	160
3	−4	−2	−4	26	47	Chad[a]	106	123	121	154	160	161
10	12	9	2	32	41	Central African Rep[a]	99	109	111	151	153	162

[a]Countries officialy identified by the United Nations as "least developed country" (United Nations Conference on Trade and Development, 2018)

The current list of the highest (and lowest) net social performers, however, is closely associated with the lessons learned from World War II, which significantly influenced the shift toward peace and enhanced the provision of social welfare for people situated everywhere within their societies. The major lesson learned, of course, is that steadily progressive social and economic development is a precondition for the attainment of peace; war, in turn, is the product of social, political, and economic chaos in combination with limited opportunities for access to well-paying jobs and social mobility (for at least their children and communities at large).

A careful review of the nations identified in Table 6.1 confirms that 21 of the 25 countries listed are European nations, many of which are member states of the European Union or of the European Commission or both. All 25 of these countries are members of the Paris-based Organization for Economic Cooperation and Development (Organization for Economic Cooperation and Development, 2018). The remaining four are located either in Asia (Japan), North America (Canada), or Oceania (Australia, New Zealand). The United States, as has been the case for more than two decades, retained its rank order position relative to all 162 countries studied at between 35 and 40. These countries function as role models for other nations that seek to attain and achieve progressively higher levels of social development and well-being for their already highly advantaged populations (Estes, 2019).

Twenty of the world's leading 25 SL identified in Table 6.1 are major sponsors of both uni- and multilateral programs of international foreign assistance and, in most cases, operate their own "in the field" programs of international development assistance like the American Peace Corps. The SL, in turn, are sponsors of major international exchange initiatives between scholars and undergraduate and graduate students with the ability to compete successfully in rigorous programs of international study. Innovative and highly productive programs of international research and cooperation are also hallmarks of this remarkable list of nations, which includes countries that award the most sought after and honorific awards including those given by the Swedish Academy of Science (https://www.nobelprize.org/) and, in the case of peace and the abolition of nuclear weapons, by the Norwegian Academy of Science (https://www.nobelprize.org/nobel_prizes/peace/)

Many of the world's SL tend to have comparatively small populations and, with exceptions, are predominately white and Protestant, although all of these demographic patterns are changing rapidly (Central Intelligence Agency, 2018). Further, SL distinguish themselves on the basis of their sustained high levels of social, political, and economic development *over time*. In comparison with other countries, SL enjoy consistently lower population growth rates, longer average life expectation, low rates of infant and child deaths, high levels of child and adult literacy, and remarkable levels of technological innovation including robust patent and copyright programs (United Nations Development Programme, 2017).

The majority of SL also have strong, dynamic economies. Employment rates are high in some of the European SL even in the presence of large-scale, often unwanted immigration. In general, inflation patterns within these nations tend to be comparatively low even as the rate of economic expansion is comparatively high. As a result, SL per capita income levels are high, and nearly all SL have access to more favorable exchange rates for their domestic currencies (World Bank, 2018). In addition, SL per capita debt levels, though high for some countries, are substantially lower than those which exist for the majority of developing countries (Organization for Economic Cooperation and Development, 2018).

World Socially Least Developing Countries

The world's 25 SLDC are identified in Table 6.2; all but two are deeply impoverished African nations (United Nations Development Programme, 2016). Only two of the world's SLDC are not located in Africa—both of which are Asian nations (Afghanistan and Yemen). Unfortunately, many of this same group of SLDCs are predominately Islamic in their cultural traditions and religious beliefs (Tiliouine & Estes, 2016).

Of the 162 countries included in this analysis, the world's countries that are least able to provide for at least the basic needs and well-being of their populations are the Central African Republic* (WISP18 = 41, rank = 162), Chad* (WISP18 = 47, rank = 161), Sierra Leone* (WISP18 = 48, rank = 160), Yemen* (WISP18 = 48, rank = 159), and Somalia* (WISP18 = 48, rank = 158).[2] Other similarly situated SLDC are Nigeria* (WISP18 = 48, rank = 157), Uganda* (WISP18 = 49, rank = 156), Sudan* (WISP18 = 49, rank = 155), Niger* (WISP18 = 50, rank = 154), and Afghanistan* (WISP18 = 51, rank = 153). All ten of these countries are desperately poor and experience high levels of internal or external migration of persons who are seeking improved economic opportunities and access to higher levels of health care, education, technology, and income security programs that are financed in part by their own labor. Many have been forced to travel to nearby or distant countries in order to have these high priorities met, often at the cost of losing solidarity with their families and communities of origin (United Nations High Commissioner for Refugees, 2017).

The composition of the nations that make up the group of SLDC, as reflected in the 20 years of rank order data summarized in Table 6.2, has remained stable despite the sometimes-dramatic increases in levels of social progress and well-being summarized for Africa in the author's earlier studies (Estes & Sirgy, 2017). The reason for these failures in social progress relative to the majority of the African region's 50 countries is that the national social performances of these countries, relative to all 162 countries included in the study, remained more or less the same from one period in the series to another.

---

[2] *Countries officially designated by the United Nations as "least developed countries," many of which are either land- or ocean-locked nations with a very limited array of products for sale on international markets (United Nations Commission on Trade and Development, 2018). Rounding of decimals to whole numbers accounts for some countries being assigned a whole number score on the WISP18.

The majority of the world's SLDC are characterized by lower levels of life expectancy relative to the gains achieved by other African nations and still high, but appreciably lowered, rates of infant, child, and maternal mortality. Technological innovation, even within their important agricultural sectors, remains low (especially in the storage and shipping of valued products), which significantly interferes with their ability to bring their goods for sale to international markets (Selian & McKnight, 2017). Though many children receive primary school credentials, substantially fewer of these countries facilitate moving children toward advanced secondary and, fewer still, toward postsecondary education, given the comparatively low level of technological economic production that characterizes many of these nations (Estes & Sirgy, 2018).

The world's SLDC are the primary recipients of the generous amounts of international development assistance provided by the United Nations and its specialized agencies (e.g., the United Nations Development Programme, the World Health Organization), other intergovernmental bodies such as the Organization for Economic Cooperation and Development, as well as through the flow of bi- and multinational development assistance bodies and the generous amount of financial aid provided by philanthropists and the charitable foundations they have created. Much of this aid is provided as part of the public-private partnership reflected in the United Nations' Sustainable Development Goals campaign. Despite some limited but important gains by a few SLDC since 1970, the pace of social progress remains painfully sluggish. Their situation continues to be much the same as that described by the Brandt Commission in 1980 (Quilligan, 2002):

> Many hundreds of millions of people in the poorer countries are preoccupied solely with survival and elementary needs. For them work is frequently not available or, when it is, pay is very low and conditions often barely tolerable. Homes are constructed of impermanent materials and have neither piped water nor sanitation. Electricity is a luxury. Health services are thinly spread and in rural areas only rarely within walking distance. Primary schools, where they exist, may be free and not too far away, but children are needed for work and cannot be easily spared for schooling. Permanent insecurity is the condition of the poor. There are no public systems of social security in the event of unemployment, sickness or death of a wage-earner in the family. Flood, drought or disease affecting people or livestock can destroy livelihoods without hope of compensation.
>
> The poorest of the poor...will remain outside the reach of normal trade and communication. The combination of malnutrition, illiteracy, disease, high birth rates, underemployment and low income closes off the avenues of escape... (p. 49).

Approximately 20% of the world's population—about 1000 million people in 2018—currently reside in SLDC. Their numbers are expected to continue to increase until at least the year 2030, by which time an even larger percentage of the world's population will reside in these deeply impoverished nations (World Bank, 2018). To resolve the challenges imposed by this reality will require a substantial combination of public and private resources. Nations with DME and member states of the Commonwealth of Independent States will need to redirect their foreign assistance, both money and human resources, to help move these countries toward a fuller sense of need satisfaction and well-being. All of these investments are warranted in the interest of reducing conflict and promoting peace and positive development within and between these nations. Without these more substantial well-being investments by Western countries and those of the Commonwealth of Independent States, the SLDC can be expected to continue their slide downward in socioeconomic-political development and high levels of internal and external dysfunction associated with their low levels of development and sense of collective well-being.

Dramatic Social Gains and Losses

Figures 6.1 and 6.2 show WISP scores and WISP rank positions for 20 countries that have experienced the most rapid social changes (Fig. 6.1) and social losses since 2000 (Fig. 6.2). Rank scores on the WISP are presented separately for the periods 2000 and 2018 and for the 20-year period 2000–2018 and have been converted into rank order positions based on the WISP scores.

Positive Social Change

A history of European colonization for many of these nations also has had an impact on the well-being scores for each country inasmuch as the WISP directly reflects a number of the forces associated with well-being. The presence of corrupt governments (Transparency International, 2018), the scarcity of new technologies (Selian & McKnight, 2017), and the absence of critically needed quality health care, education, and income security programs (International Social Security Association, 2018) are direct components of the WISP itself.

Even with all of the preceding qualifications to the impressive rates of social growth occurring in the study's 162 countries, the data reflected in Fig. 6.1 reinforce the patterns previously reported. Net social gains for the following 5 countries are especially impressive given their population size (either very small or very large), political and cultural complexity, and income security programs associated with the WISP, which measures the age and comprehensiveness of such programs: *Brazil* (net social gain = 39 ranks between 2000 and 2018), *Cape Verde* (net social gain = 38 ranks between 2000 and 2019), *Lebanon* (net social gain = 35 ranks between 2000 and 2018), *Lithuania* (net social gain = 33 ranks between 2000 and 2018), and *Algeria* (net social gain = 33 ranks between 2000 and 2018).

The five countries just listed are distributed across nearly all of the world's major continents. The fuller list identified in Table 6.3 reflects the same pattern. These findings add substantially to the impressive nature of the dramatic social gains for socially developing countries presented throughout this book. Further, all 20 of these countries are on the verge of moving into a more advanced socioeconomic cluster of countries given the broad-based nature of the social advances that have already taken place.

Negative Social Change

The 20 countries with the most significant net social losses on the WISP between 2000 and 2018 are identified in Fig. 6.2. Table 6.2 also identifies the 25 lowest performing countries of the 162 countries included in this study. These countries, referred to as SLDCs throughout this chapter, range from large countries to small nations, some of which are land- or ocean-locked countries (United Nations, 2014, 2017), but all are characterized by weak health, education, income security, technology development, environmental, and community development systems (United Nations Development Programme, 2017; World Bank, 2018). Many of these countries also are struggling with the serious problems associated with diversity-related social conflict, and a few are engaged in intraregional wars (Stockholm International Peace Research Institute, 2018).

The majority of these countries have been included in the WISP database since at least 2000, most since as early as 1970. Numerous reports on the unique well-being challenges confronting these nations have been issued by this author (Estes, 2012b, 2014, 2015a) and have been the subject of important national reports prepared by major international development research units (United Nations, 2014; World Bank, 2018) as well as by individual scholars (Helliwell, Layard, & Sachs, 2017).

Nineteen of the 20 countries (Luxembourg has been excluded) have been major recipients of international development assistance (Organization for Economic Cooperation and Development, 2018), including preferential development assistance from the United Nations, the World Bank, and other international intergovernmental bodies such as the Organization for Economic Cooperation and Development and the European Commission. The levels of aid provided to these countries have been substantial and likely have slowed, perhaps halted, their gradual decline over time. In any case, the following 10 countries lost substantial social ground, as represented in changes in their WISP rank positions, over the past 20 years: *Turkmenistan* (net social loss = −36 ranks between 2000 and 2018), *Taiwan* (net social loss = −32 ranks between 2000 and 2018), *Zimbabwe* (net social loss = −32 ranks between 2000 and 2018), *Tajikistan* (net social loss = −29 ranks between 2000 and 2018), *Swaziland* (net social loss = −28 ranks between 2000 and 2018), *Zambia** (net social loss = −22 ranks between 2000 and 2018), *Luxembourg* (net social loss = −21 ranks between 2000 and 2018), *Kazakhstan* (net social loss = −21 ranks between 2000 and 2018), *Philippines* (net social loss = −21 ranks between 2000 and 2018), and *Niger* (net social loss = −21 ranks between 2000 and 2018).

The Next Chapter

Chapter 7 provides a brief overview of the advances in well-being that have been achieved since 1970 in providing more adequately for the basic social and material needs of some of the populations in all societies that are at high risk of social failure, i.e., children and youth, women, and the aged. In all, these three population subgroups make up nearly 80% of the population of every society. Both narrative and objective data are presented in support of the thesis of major advances occurring worldwide since at least 1970 (Estes & Sirgy, 2018).

References

Central Intelligence Agency (CIA). (2018). *World factbook, 2018*. Washington, DC: U.S. Department of State.

El-Aswad, E. (2019). *Quality of life and policy issues among the Middle East and North African countries*. Cham, Switzerland: Springer International. in press.

Estes, R. J. (1976). *The social progress of nations*. New York: Praeger.

Estes, R. J. (1988). *Trends in world social development: The social progress of nations, 1970– 1987*. New York: Praeger.

Estes, R. J. (1998a). Social development trends in the successor states to the former Soviet Union: The search for a new paradigm. In K. R. Hope (Ed.), *Challenges of transformation and transition from centrally planned to market economies* (UNCRD Research Report Series No. 26) (pp. 13–30). Nagoya, Japan: United Nations Centre for Regional Development.

Estes, R. J. (1998b). Trends in world social development, 1970–95: Development prospects for a new century. *Journal of Developing Societies, 14*(1), 11–39.

Estes, R. J. (2007). Development challenges and opportunities confronting economies in transition. *Social Indicators Research, 83*(3), 375–411.

Estes, R. J. (2010). The world social situation: Development challenges at the outset of a new century. *Social Indicators Research, 98*, 363–402.

Estes, R. J. (2012a). Economies in transition: Continuing challenges to quality of life. In K. Land, A. C. Michalos, & M. J. Sirgy (Eds.), *Handbook of quality of life research* (pp. 433–457). Dordrecht, The Netherlands: Springer International Publishers.

Estes, R. J. (2012b). Failed and failing states: Is quality of life possible? In K. Land, A. C. Michalos, & M. J. Sirgy (Eds.), *Handbook of quality of life research* (pp. 555–580). Dordrecht, The Netherlands: Springer International Publishers.

Estes, R. J. (2014). Disadvantaged populations. In A. C. Michalos (Ed.), *Encyclopedia of quality of life and well-being research* (pp. 1654–1658). Dordrecht, The Netherlands: Springer International Publishers.

Estes, R. J. (2015a). Development trends among the world's socially least developed countries: Reasons for cautious optimism. In B. Spooner (Ed.), *Globalization in progress: Understanding and working with world urbanization*. Philadelphia: University of Pennsylvania Museum Press.

Estes, R. J. (2015b). Trends in world social development: The search for global well-being. In W. Glatzer, L. Camfield, V. Møller, & M. Rojas (Eds.), *Global handbook of quality of life: Exploration of well-being of nations and continents*. Dordrecht, The Netherlands: Springer International Publishers.

Estes, R. J. (2018). Disparities and wealth. In G. Brule & C. Suter (Eds.), *Wealth and Subjective well-being*. Dordrecht, The Netherlands: Springer. in preparation.

Estes, R. J. (2019). *The Social Progress of Nations Revisited: 1970–2018*. Cham, Switzerland: Springer International Social Indicators Research Book series. in preparation

Estes, R. J., & Sirgy, M. J. (2017). *The pursuit of human well-being: The untold global history*. Cham: Switzerland: Springer.

Estes, R. J., & Sirgy, M. J. (2018). *Advances in human well-being: Towards a better world*. London/New York: Rowman & Littlefield Ltd.

Helliwell, J., Layard, R., & Sachs, J. (2017). *World happiness report, 2017*. New York: Sustainable Development Solutions Network.

International Social Security Association. (2018). *Social security programs throughout the world*. [Publication Web site.] Geneva, Switzerland: International Social Security Association. Retrieved August 29, 2018 from https://www.ssa.gov/policy/docs/progdesc/ssptw/

Organization for Economic Cooperation and Development. (2018). *OECD. Stat*. [Database]. Retrieved August 29, 2018 from https://stats.oecd.org/

Quilligan, J. B. (2002). *The Brandt equation: 21st century blueprint for the new global economy*. Philadelphia: Center for Global Negotiations. Retrieved August 29, 2018 from http://www.brandt21forum.info/Report_TableofContents.htm

Selian, A. N., & McKnight, L. (2017). The role of technology in the history of well-being: Transformative market phenomena over time. In R. J. Estes & M. J. Sirgy (Eds.), *The pursuit of human well-being: The untold global history* (pp. 639–687). Cham, Switzerland: Springer International.

Sirgy, M. J., Estes, R. J., & Rahtz, D. R. (2018). Combatting jihadist terrorism: A quality-of-life perspective. *Journal of Applied Research in Quality of Life*. (on; line). https://doi.org/10.1007/s11482-017-9574-z

Stockholm International Peace Research Institute (SIPRI). (2018). *SIPRI yearbook 2018: Armaments, disarmament and international security*. Stockholm: Stockholm International Peace Research Institute.

Tiliouine, H., & Estes, R. J. (2016). *The state of social progress of Islamic societies: Social, political, economic, and ideological challenges*. Dordrecht, The Netherlands: Springer.

Transparency International. (2018). *Corruptions perception index*. [Organization Web site.] Berlin: Transparency International. Retrieved August 24, 2018 from https://www.transparency.org/research/cpi/overview

United Nations. (2014). *"Sea-locked countries" face up to climate change*. UN News, September 2. Retrieved from https://news.un.org/en/audio/2014/09/591762/

United Nations. (2017). *Enhancing the participation of the landlocked states in the implementation of Sustainable Development Goal (SDG) 14*. [Meeting]. Retrieved August 29, 2018 from http://unohrlls.org/event/enhancing-participation-landlocked-states-implementation-sustainable-development-goal-sdg-14/

United Nations Commission on Trade and Development (UNCTAD). (2018). *List of least developed countries*. Geneva, Switzerland: United Nations Commission on Trade and Development. Retrieved August 29, 2018 from http://unctad.org/en/pages/ALDC/Least%20Developed%20Countries/UN-list-of-Least-Developed-Countries.aspx

United Nations Development Programme. (2016). *Ending poverty: Millennium development goals and beyond 2015*. New York: United Nations Development Programme. Retrieved August 29, 2018 from http://www.un.org/millenniumgoals/

United Nations Development Programme. (2017). *Human development reports, 2017*. New York: United Nations Development Programme. Retrieved August 29, 2018 from http://hdr.undp.org/en/year/2017

United Nations High Commissioner for Refugees. (2017). *Refugee and migrant report* (p. 2017). Geneva, Switzerland: United Nations High Commissioner for Refugees.

World Bank. (2018). *World development report 2018: Learning to realize education's promise*. Washington, DC: World Bank. Retrieved August 29, 2018 from http://www.worldbank.org/en/publication/wdr2018

Part VI

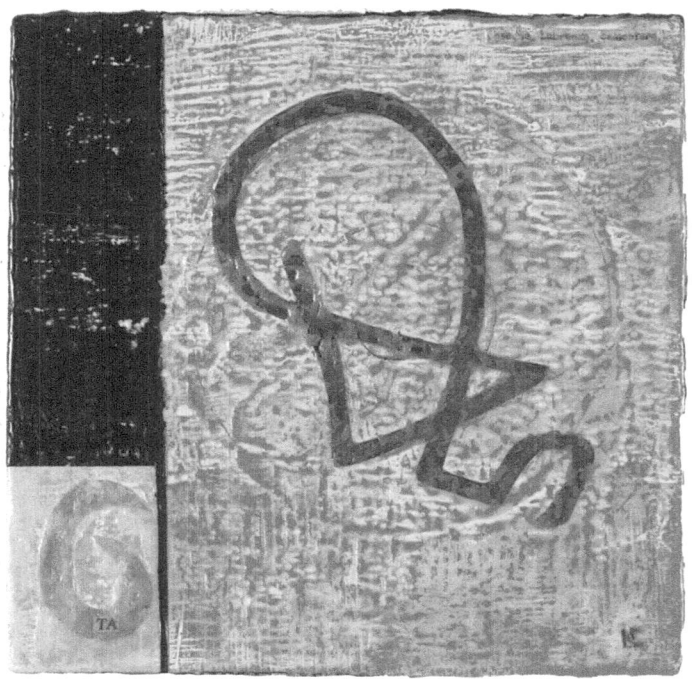

Image 6: © Lylia Ferero Carr: Muysca, Ta

Chapter 7
Advancing Well-Being of "At Risk" Populations

The central goal of well-being research, policy, and practice is to improve the conditions under which people live, especially those population groups that are "at risk" of failing to achieve a reasonable level of quality of life and well-being. The population groups at high risk of negative levels of well-being historically have been children and youth, the elderly, women, persons with serious emotional or physical limitations (often both), the extremely poor, and those living on the margins of society because of race, ethnicity, religious beliefs, and other "socially crushing" factors. Fortunately, in recent decades, both nations and global organizations have promulgated a rich series of policies and regulations, resolutions, declarations, and covenants that have been focused on the special well-being needs of each of these marginalized population groups. This situation has been the case for each of the population groups identified below as well as for others whose well-being societies share major responsibilities.

Children and Youth

The all-important United Nations *Convention on the Rights of the Child* (United Nations Human Rights Office of the High Commissioner, 1989) granted children the same rights and protections given to all other members of society beginning with the right to life itself. The document is very comprehensive and carefully weaves together the principles of child rights with those already formulated in the originating *Universal Declaration of Human Rights* (1948) (https://www.ohchr.org/EN/UDHR/Documents/UDHR_Translations/eng.pdf) and the whole series of universal rights documents that have been proclaimed by the United Nations for a wide array of minority populations.

© Springer Nature Switzerland AG 2019   113
R. J. Estes, *The Social Progress of Nations Revisited, 1970–2020*, Social
Indicators Research Series 78, https://doi.org/10.1007/978-3-030-15907-8_7

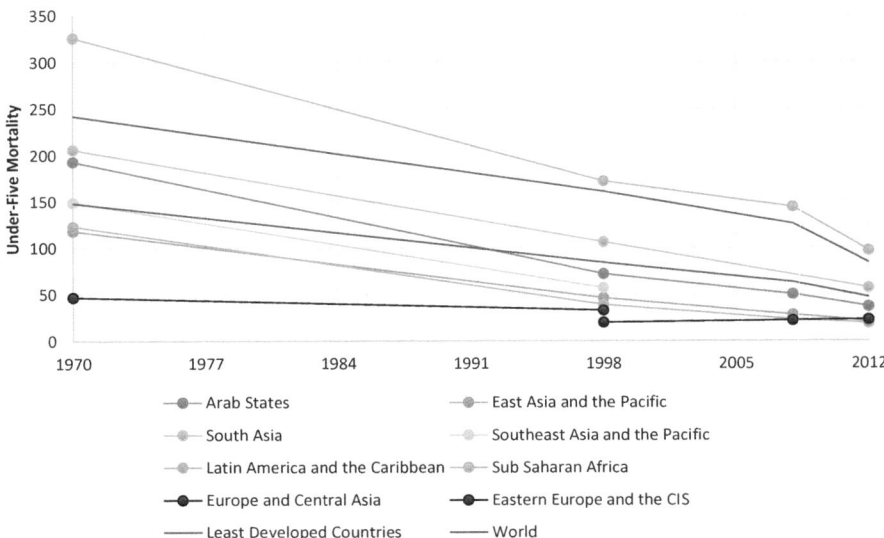

Fig. 7.1 Child mortality rates by major world region. *CIS* Commonwealth of Independent States. (Data from World Bank, 2017; figure © *Advances in Well-Being: Towards a Better World*, by Richard J. Estes and M. Joseph Sirgy, published by Rowman & Littlefield International, 2018; reprinted with permission)

Children and Health

Figure 2.1 (in Chap. 2), summarizes the major advances that have been made since 1950 in reducing rates of infant mortality for each of the world's major development zones and for the world (Estes & Sirgy, 2017, 2018). Figure 7.1 reports worldwide successes in reducing child mortality rates, including children aged one to five years (Estes & Sirgy, 2017). The data presented in both figures are impressive and reflect the depth of the positive outcomes that have been achieved through close working partnerships between governments, corporations, other business leaders and, certainly, international and national nongovernmental organizations in pooling their efforts on behalf of children (Estes & Zhou, 2014; United Nations Development Programme, 2018a, 2018b). The partnerships have proven to be highly effective in generating the multilayered fiscal and other resources needed to improve the lives of children.

Key Facts

- Nearly 9 million children under the age of five die every year, according to 2007 figures.
- Around 70% of these early child deaths are due to conditions that could be prevented or treated with access to simple, affordable interventions.
- Leading causes of death in children under five years of age are pneumonia, diarrhea and health problems during the first month of life.

- Over one third of all child deaths are linked to malnutrition.
- Children in developing countries are ten times more likely to die before the age of five than children in developed countries.

Key Facts: Uneven and Insufficient Progress

- More than one billion children are severely deprived of at least one of the essential goods and services they require to survive, grow, and develop—these include nutrition, water, sanitation facilities, access to basic health-care services, adequate shelter, education, and information. As a result almost 9.2 million children under five die every year. A further 3.3 million babies are stillborn.
- Most of the 25,000 children under five that die each day are concentrated in the world's poorest countries in sub-Saharan Africa and South Asia. There, the child mortality rate is 29 times greater than that in industrialized countries: 175 deaths per 1000 children compared with 6 per 1000 in industrialized countries.

Why Are Death Tolls Still High?

- Poor families are often unable to obtain even the most basic health care for their children. Poor or delayed care-seeking contributes to up to 70% of all under-five child deaths.
- Of the 12 countries where more than 20% of children die before their fifth birthday, nine have recently suffered a major armed conflict.
- Countries with weak and fragile health systems have not been able to provide effective child survival strategies that are crucial to reduce under-five child deaths, especially neonatal deaths. Basic health services have been lacking as well as nutrition, water supplies, and sanitation facilities.
- Almost half a million deaths each year due to malaria in children under five in sub-Saharan Africa could have been prevented with the use of insecticide-treated bed nets, shown to reduce under-five mortality rates by up to 20%

What Can Be Done?

- Scaling up effective health services: more than 60% of all under-five child deaths can be avoided with proven, low-cost preventive care and treatment. Preventive care includes continuous breast-feeding, vaccination, adequate nutrition, and, in Africa, the use of insecticide-treated bed nets. The major causes of under-five deaths need to be treated rapidly: for example, with salt solutions for diarrhea or simple antibiotics for pneumonia and other infections. To reach the majority of children who today do not have access to this care, we need more and better trained and equipped health workers. Families and communities need to know how best to bring up their children healthily and deal with sickness when it occurs.
- Political awareness, commitment, and leadership are needed to ensure that child health receives the attention and resources needed to accelerate progress towards Millennium Development Goal #4. Better information on the number and causes of under-five child deaths will help leaders to decide on the best course of action.

Causes of Under-Five Child Deaths

Six conditions account for about 70% of all child deaths: acute lower respiratory infections, mostly pneumonia (19%), diarrhea (18%), malaria (8%), measles, (4%), HIV/AIDS (3%), and neonatal conditions, mainly preterm birth, birth asphyxia, and infections (37%). The relative contribution of HIV/AIDS to the total mortality of children under five, especially in sub-Saharan Africa, has also been increasing steadily. Malnutrition is a factor in more than half of the children who die after the first month of life. (See http://www.who.int/pmnch/media/press_materials/fs/fs_mdg4_childmortality/en/ for more information.)

Situation

A total of 5.4 million children under age five died in 2017.

The risk of a child dying before completing five years of age is still highest in the World Health Organization (WHO) African Region (74 per 1000 live births), around 8 times higher than that in the WHO European Region (9 per 1000 live births). Many countries still have very high under-five mortality rates—particularly those in WHO African Region, home to five of the six countries with an under-five mortality rate above 100 deaths per 1000 live births. In addition, inequities in child mortality between high-income and low-income countries remain large. In 2017, the under-five mortality rate in low-income countries was 69 deaths per 1000 live births—around 14 times the average rate in high-income countries (5 deaths per 1000 live births). Reducing these inequities across countries and saving more children's lives by ending preventable child deaths are important priorities.

Children and Education

The impressive social gains achieved for infants and children in the health sector are mirrored in the educational sector; together, they have added to the substantial improvements in the quality of life of people living in both rural and urban areas everywhere in the world. Figure 2.1 (see Chap. 2), for example, shows the total number of years of formal education completed by all people living in each of the world's major geopolitical regions and in the world as a whole. The data include school completion rates for primary, secondary, and postsecondary education. The data also include people who have successfully completed formal programs of vocational training (Estes & Sirgy, 2018). The regional and world gains reported in this figure are exceptional and reflect a renewed global strategy to advance education for all people everywhere in the world.

People living today, including children and youth, are better educated and more highly trained that any populations of the past. Today, the human capital resources of our planet are deeper and richer than at any other time in the past, and they continue to be enriched each year. These patterns, unlike in the past, apply equally to boys and girls and men and women. Indeed, the students of most universities located in economically advanced countries today are women rather than men; a portion of the latter choose to enter the military or the workforce rather than to pursue higher education. Education will continue to be a driving force in advancing universal well-being, especially in the sciences and technological innovation. The most dramatic changes are expected to take place in the developing countries of Africa, Asia, and Latin America, where more than 59.7%, 16.0%, and 8.6%, respectively, of the world's total population in 2018 are located. These regions will shift quickly from being consumers of world resources to being producers of world resources, which is nearly the case, and, by 2050, almost certainly will be the developers of leading technologies that contribute to the well-being of people everywhere in the world (Selian & McKnight, 2017).

Population Growth, Children, and Social Vulnerability

A final note on the status of child and youth especially regarding their health and educational vulnerabilities and the rapid rates of population growth that continue to characterize many developing countries. This situation rises to critical proportions in areas where the percentage of the total population becomes child-dominated and the share of people in the total population to care for them declines. The situation is especially acute among the countries of the Middle East and West Asia, where children and youth younger than 15 years of age comprise more than 40% of the total population. The result is that many children, especially during their teenage years, must take responsibility for their own rearing, some of which becomes antisocial, especially in situations in which large numbers of these children live in poverty or under highly unfavorable social conditions.

Many countries in Latin America also struggle with the combined challenges associated with rapid population growth and, following the successes in the health and education sectors reported previously, are characterized by high percentages of concentrations of infants, children, and youth. This trend is illustrated in the population trends reported for Mexico for 2016 earlier in the book. Of special note in this figure is the comparatively small percentages of working age adults available to provide for these large numbers of children, although in Latin America at least, communities share actively in caring for families with large numbers of children. As among most African nations, Latin Americans also place families at the center of community life and regard the care of all children as a shared responsibility. These values predominate in Latin America's many rural communities but also are shared among its increasingly more concentrated urban populations.

The Aged and the Elderly

Since ancient times, one of the major aspirations of people everywhere has been to live a long, healthy, and enjoyable life. The Book of Genesis in the Hebraic texts speaks to a promise of 70 years of life expectancy on average. Genesis also lists the ages of many of its early prophetic leaders at the time of their deaths, and many exceeded 100 years. The same aspiration is found in the ancient texts of the East, which include the writings of Confucius, Buddha, and other great teachers of South and Southeast Asia. All these societies value aging and the aged and have in place long-standing traditions and norms that promote their inclusion in all aspects of collective life.

Successful aging also depends on good health, a reasonable level of financial security, and the presence of functional family and kinship relationships in combination with strong communities that place a value on the aged and on the rich knowledge that older persons contribute to collective life. However, aging is most difficult for the solitary elderly, especially those who have no biological children of their own and who have few or no ties to extended kinship or community networks. Older persons living in poverty and the seriously ill elderly, even though they have gained longevity, experience low levels of well-being and quality of life. This issue is especially pronounced among impoverished persons living in remote rural communities and those living in societies with weak systems of income security (International Social Security Association, 2018). Significant social gains are being made both in extending the lives of people and in ensuring more successful aging among the elderly (Organization for Economic Cooperation and Development, 2018).

Social advances in aging are the result of the growing numbers of aging persons in all societies, the extraordinarily long lives that many enjoy, and the increasing sophistication and inclusiveness of income security systems in nearly all countries (International Social Security Association, 2018). The outcome of these advances in population growth and social provision for both men and women is illustrated in Fig. 2.2, which reports population size and aging data for the world's 10 most populous countries in 2016. In all, the ten countries included in the figure total approximately 4.21 thousand million people or approximately 57% of the world's total population. Comparable patterns exist in other large countries of the world, but virtually everywhere years of average life expectancy and aging have increased substantially just since 1970.

Women

Though often identified as a "minority," in fact, girls and women make up more than half of the world's total population. They are not only the mothers who give birth to all of us but also are the major carriers of cultures. Women also are justifiably credited with setting the emotional tone within families and, not infrequently, are the arbiters of conflicts between family members of subgroups within their villages and local communities. However, women also are the major victims of domestic violence and, unlike their sons and husbands, have had comparatively limited opportunities to advance their personal independence, their economic and educational status, and their ability to vote and to represent the needs of their communities in local, regional, and national political bodies (Eckermann, 2014).

The situation of women has been changing rapidly everywhere in the world with the result that their health, education, and more comprehensive social status have improved significantly since the close of the *4th Global Conference on Women* held in Beijing in 1995 (http://www.un.org/womenwatch/daw/beijing/). The speed of improvements in the health of women since 1995 has been almost breathtaking (UN Women, 2018). Because of their close relationship, the health of children, as discussed previously, also has advanced dramatically. Until 1970, the image on a grave stone in Dresden, Germany (Fig. 7.2) was an all too common one throughout both developing and more economically advanced countries of the period. The image, as the title indicates, depicts a dying mother after having just delivered her child.

Figure 7.3 reports in detail rates of maternal mortality for countries grouped by major aggregations for the almost 30-year period between 1990 and 2018. Though

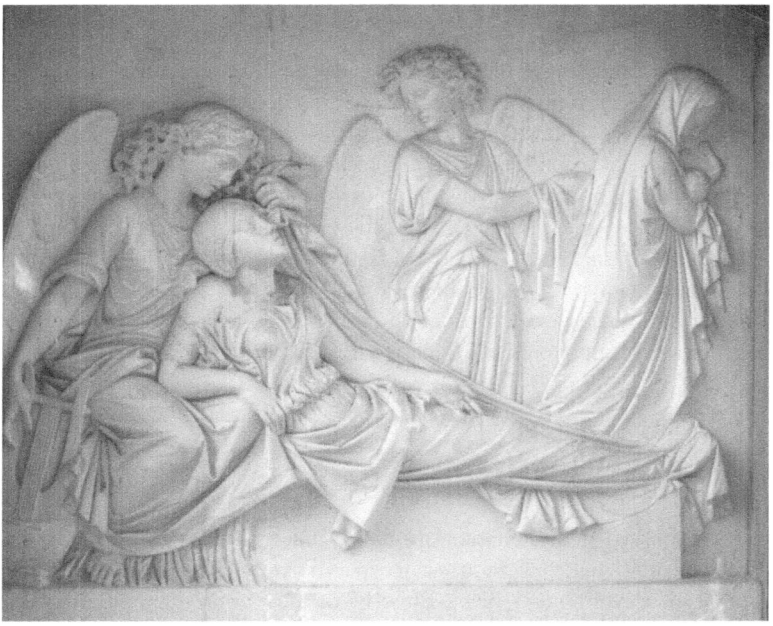

Fig. 7.2 A mother dies and is taken by angels as her new-born child is taken away. A grave from 1863 in Striesener Friedhof in Dresden. (Photo by Stephen C. Dickson; at https://en.wikipedia.org/wiki/Maternal_death#/media/File:A_mother_dies_and_is_taken_by_angels_as_her_new-born_child_is_taken_away,_A_grave_from_1863_in_Striesener_Friedhof_in_Dresden.jpg; Creative Commons Attribution-Share Alike 4.0 International license)

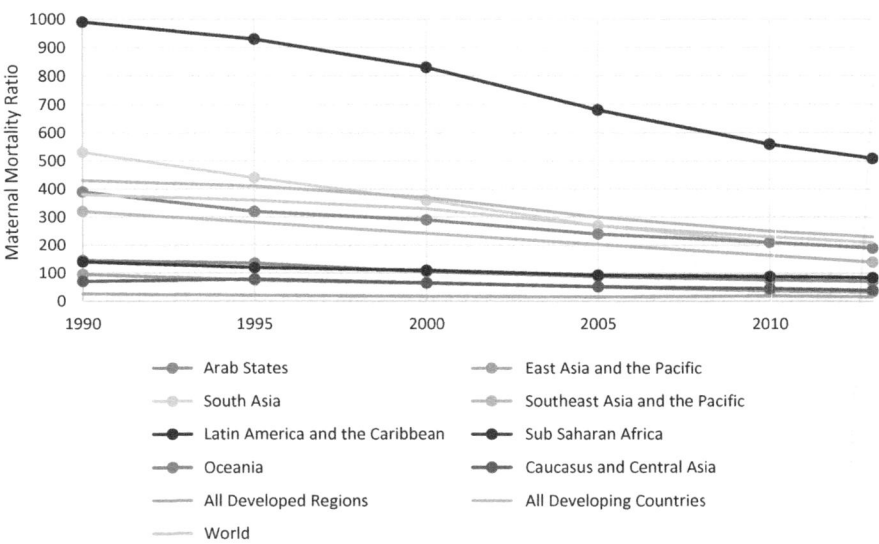

Fig. 7.3 Changes in maternal mortality, 1990–1920. (Figure © *Advances in Well-Being: Towards a Better World*, by Richard J. Estes and M. Joseph Sirgy, published by Rowman & Littlefield International, 2018; reprinted with permission)

seemingly not as dramatic as the improvements reported previously for infants and children, in fact, maternal mortality rates are also declining at a rapid pace. These advances have been achieved through carefully organized partnerships between state and nonstate actors and, as expected, have involved substantially higher levels of fiscal and human resource investments in the well-being of women (Save the Children, 2017). These heightened levels of developmental investments have proven to be especially critical, given the key roles that women play in families, communities, and, at least, local markets. Women, now as in the past, are central to the smooth functioning of all these institutions and that of the religious, cultural, and community development components of collective life (Eckermann, 2014).

This Chapter and the Next

The issues discussed in this chapter are highly interdisciplinary and cross-cutting. Such is the result when one focuses on specific population groups inasmuch as every sector of development bears directly on the well-being of all population groups (United Nations Development Programme, 2018a). This chapter just touches the surface of the drivers of well-being that influence the quality of life of those population groups identified in this chapter and other population groups as well (United Nations Development Programme, 2018b).

Chapter 8 examines the critical role of women in promoting the quality of life and well-being of their families, their economic contributions to the family, and their involvement in the social, political, economic, technological, and intellectual lives of their families, society, and the world as a whole. Chapter 9 focuses on variety of topics related to global poverty and its alleviation, with a special focus on the major sectors and actors that are seeking to incorporate the extreme poor into the mainstream of society.

References

Eckermann, L. (Ed.). (2014). *Gender, lifespan and quality of life: An international perspective.* Dordrecht, The Netherlands: Springer.

Estes, R. J., & Sirgy, M. J. (Eds.). (2017). *The pursuit of human Well-being: The untold global history.* Cham, Switzerland: Springer International.

Estes, R. J., & Sirgy, M. J. (2018). *Advances in Well-being: Toward a better world for all.* London: Rowman and Littlefield.

Estes, R. J., & Zhou, M. H. (2014). A conceptual approach to the creation of public–private partnerships in social welfare. *International Journal of Social Welfare, 24*(4), 348–363.

International Social Security Association. (2018). *Social security programs throughout the world, 2018.* Geneva, Switzerland: International Social Security Association. Retrieved August 30, 2018 from https://www.ssa.gov/policy/docs/progdesc/ssptw/

Organization for Economic Cooperation and Development. (2018). *Receipts and distributions of the development assistance committee, 2018.* Paris: Organization for Economic Cooperation and Development, Development Assistance Committee.

Save the Children. (2017). *2017 Annual report: Results for children.* Retrieved August 12, 2018 from https://www.savethechildren.org/us/about-us/resource-library/annual-report

Selian, A., & McKnight, L. (2017). The role of technology in the history of Well-being: Transformative market phenomenon over time. In R. J. Estes & M. J. Sirgy (Eds.), *The pursuit of human Well-being: The untold global history* (pp. 639–690). Cham, Switzerland: Springer.

United Nations Development Programme. (2018a). *Human development reports, 2018.* [Collection of documents]. New York: United Nations Development Programme. Retrieved August 30, 2018 from http://hdr.undp.org/en/year/2018

United Nations Development Programme. (2018b). *Sustainable development goals, 2018.* New York: United Nations Development Programme. Retrieved August 30, 2018 from http://www.undp.org/content/undp/en/home/sustainable-development-goals.html

United Nations Human Rights Office of the High Commissioner (1989). *Convention on the rights of the child.* Retrieved August 29, 2018 from https://www.ohchr.org/en/professionalinterest/pages/crc.aspx

UN Women. (2018). Turning promises into action: Gender equality in the 2030 sustainable development goals.. Retrieved August 11, 2018 from http://www.unwomen.org/en/digital-library/publications/2018/2/gender-equality-in-the-2030-agenda-for-sustainable-development-2018.

Chapter 8
Women and Development: From Homemakers to Nation Builders

A widely cited Chinese saying of Mao Zedong states that "women hold up half the sky." Readers who are married, have children, parents, or in-laws likely would argue that the gender-defined responsibilities carried by women are greater than those of men, especially when they have to care for the short- or long-term needs of infirm spouses, children, or aged parents. More accurate from the perspective of these persons is the commonly heard proverb, "a woman's work is never done."

The second statement captures more fully the multiple roles that women carry as wage earners, business owners, emotional tone setters for families, providers of child care and, more generally, as "home makers" even when they hire women to help them carry out these functions. Women working outside of the home, of course, have even greater demands placed on them, and their occupational and gender-defined responsibilities far exceed those assigned to men (Eisenchlas, 2013; UN Women, 2018a). Eckermann (2014) and her colleagues have provided ample evidence that women work far longer hours than do men and, typically, the nature of the work is extremely demanding physically and emotionally. And, they must repeat the schedule all over again day after day, especially in societies in which equality between men and women and women working outside of the home is frowned upon, even within economically advanced societies (Verloo, 2018).

Despite the importance assigned to women's development in most regions of the world, today, the contribution of women to national and international development, as well as to their own development, remains relatively absent from many national 5-year and other planning documents (Estes, 2010, 2019; United Nations Development Programme, 2018). Even when discussed, the role of women often is relegated to just a few paragraphs, a special subsection or, in the most egregious situations, to footnotes that discuss the role of families and communities in development. The socioeconomic advancement of men remains central in most development plans, this despite recognition that the most significant gains in human

© Springer Nature Switzerland AG 2019
R. J. Estes, *The Social Progress of Nations Revisited, 1970–2020*, Social Indicators Research Series 78, https://doi.org/10.1007/978-3-030-15907-8_8

development over the past century have resulted from educational, health, and related opportunities made available to women (Nearing & Nearing, 1912). The situation is especially egregious in the nations of the Middle East and North Africa (MENA region), where strict controls are placed on the independence of women, including their ability to receive inheritances directly, to open bank accounts in their own name, to initiate divorce, and even in the matter of the clothing they must wear in public. The social progress of women in the MENA region has been among the slowest worldwide and likely will continue to remain so until men truly recognize the special talents and resources that women bring to the planning process (Tiliouine & Estes, 2016; United Nations Development Programme, 2005).

This chapter explores the critical role that women play in promoting the quality of life and well-being of families, their roles as economic partners with their spouses when present or as solitary income earners when not, and the myriad contributions that they make to the social, political, economic, technological and, yes, intellectual lives of their families, societies, and to the world as a whole. The chapter addresses the following issues relating to the changing status of the women in the world:

- The status of women at the turn of the twentieth century relative to their status in world;
- The major factors that have accounted for the progress of women worldwide and from subregions;
- Factors that inhibit the progress of women in achieving social and economic parity with men;
- Action steps that need to be taken in stabilizing the social gains made by women and in propelling their further development into the future (World Health Organization et al., 2015).

The Status of Women at the Turn of the Twentieth Century

The social status of women and girls at the outset of the nineteenth and early twentieth centuries was much more limited than that which existed for men and boys. Apart from women who occupied roles as queens or as senior members of royal families, the majority of women (a) occupied roles and performed functions that were far less valued than those performed by men and boys; (b) could not visualize themselves as active members of the voting classes; (c) rarely owned property outright, or at least in their own names, even when they brought that property or wealth with them into marriages (Martin, 2007); (d) were often coerced into initially loveless marriages of convenience that suited the preferences of their parents or

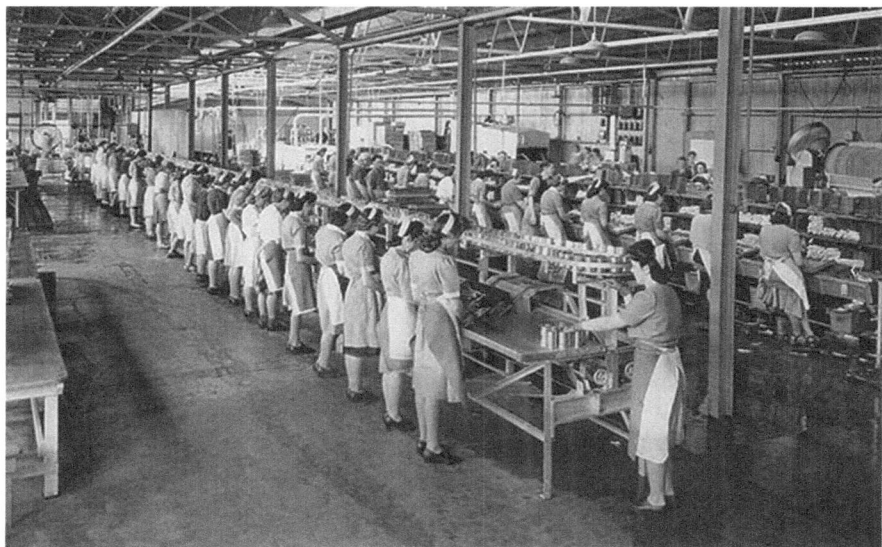

Fig. 8.1 Women working in an asparagus cannery, Bathurst (New South Wales, Australia). (https://commons.wikimedia.org/wiki/File:Women_working_in_a_cannery.jpg;   this   file   is licensed under the Creative Commons Attribution 2.0 Generic license)

guardians; (e) received little or no education; (f) received little or limited health care even when pregnant; (g) unless in the lower classes, could not perform services for which they could be paid unless such services were tied to being indentured or even a slave (Jones-Rogers, 2019) or to the performance of household services for the financially advantaged classes. Because of these conditions women died far earlier than is the situation today, lost many of their children through infant and child deaths and gave birth under the most risk-prone conditions, often without the assistance of midwives, nurses, or doctors. Women with complex pregnancies frequently lost not only their newborn infants but their lives as well. A walk through most cemeteries of the period will readily confirm the frequent early deaths of women from childbirth, hard labor, and related disadvantaged social conditions (Loudon, 1993). Such was the status of women until the *Great War* (1914–1918) and the beginning of their entry into the paid labor force to compensate for the shortage of available men to work in the massive factories constructed as part of the *Industrial Revolution* (1790–1870) (Fig. 8.1). After these global events, the status of women and that of the men and boys in their lives would never be the same (Essays UK, 2013).

Social Progress and Change in the Status of Women: The War Years and Beyond

The social and economic progress of women increased dramatically during the periods of the *Great War* (1914–1918) and, then again, during the years of the *Second World War* (1939–1945) and the decades of dramatic social and technological changes that followed these wars. The changes that occurred during and following the war years took place on the heels of the *Industrial Revolution* (1790–1870), which resulted in the emergence of large paid work force, competitive employment opportunities, widescale migration from rural to urban communities, new approaches to living situations, and the foundations of the beginnings of an income security system in Germany and England (Wilensky & Lebeaux, 1965). The United Nations also emerged during this period (1945) and, early on, created a large network of specialized departments and agencies focused on the needs of vulnerable and economically dependent population groups including those of women and girls. Indeed, promotion of health, education, economic, and general well-being of women and girls was and continues to be a central objective of virtually all the United Nations specialized agencies. And, these agencies have been largely successful in achieving their gender-based goals and objectives.

Of importance, too, is the fact that tens of millions of women entered the paid workforce during the war years…never to fully return to the home after achieving a high level of social and economic self-sufficiency for themselves. Even so, the time demands placed on women did not change because of their economic contribution of well-being of families since women still were, and largely continue to be, expected to perform, or at least arrange for, the bulk of child care, home making, and other tasks that they traditionally have carried out for millennia.

The pluses and minuses of the social changes that impacted the economic and social autonomy of women following the war years for the period 1946–1960 in the United Kingdom are summarized in Box 8.1. Though these processes changed even more dramatically, and for the positive, during subsequent decades, the historical patterns reported in Fig. 8.1 demonstrate the nature of the struggles that women experienced as they entered the paid workforce. And these struggles were rooted in long-standing socio-cultural values that were not easily changed. But, suffragette and other women's national and international movements (Harper, 1922: Volume 6), helped women achieve advanced social status at levels never previously thought possible.

Box 8.1 Early Social Gains and Losses for Women Immediately After WWII, 1946–1960 (Striking Women, 2017)

- The *welfare state* created many job opportunities in what was seen as "women's work."

  - Jobs were available in the newly created National Health Service for nurses, midwives, cleaners, and clerical staff.
  - Banking, textile, and light industries such as electronics also expanded during this period and provided women with opportunities in clerical, secretarial, and assembly work.
  - Jobs were still strictly segregated by gender and routine repetitive work was categorized as women's work for women's (lower) wages.

- The proportion of women in the labor force as a percentage of women of working age (15–64) increased from 45.9% in 1955 to 51% in 1965.

  - Despite this increase in the rate of women's employment, women were still considered to be "secondary workers."
  - Women's wages were not considered central to families' income, instead it was thought that women's wages were for "extras" such as holidays or new consumer durables.
  - Mothers of young children were once again discouraged from working and most of the state funded nurseries set up during WWII were closed by the post-war Labour government.
  - Welfare payments for families assumed that a man's income supported his wife and children who were his dependents (the "family wage"). The benefit rates for married women were set at a lower level than those for married men.

- In the early 1950s, many employers still operated a "Marriage bar," whereby married women were barred from certain occupations like teaching and clerical jobs (but not lower paid jobs) and those working were sacked upon marriage.
- But throughout the 1950s and 1960s it became more common for married women to work for wages - at least part-time. By the 1960s, 38% of married women worked but women were routinely sacked when they got pregnant and continued to be paid less than men even if they did the same jobs.

The development challenges confronting women in the post-war United Kingdom were not very different from those that confronted women in other economically advanced countries. Everywhere women faced a complex set of social and cultural obstacles in moving toward self-sufficient roles within their respective societies. Deep-seated social patterns rooted in the societal norms, values, traditions, and history prevented substantial numbers of women from achieving the new, more independent status they desired (Eisenchlas, 2013). Only in the four Nordic countries of Scandinavia, which already had a tradition of strong and powerful women, were women able to achieve parity with their partners with a high degree of mutual satisfaction (Bazilchuk, 2018).

In developing Africa, Asia, and Latin America the pace of women's social progress in the decades that immediately followed the war years continued to move slowly and, in most cases, remained within a traditional context (UN Women, 2000). But as time passed the progress of women living in developing societies also moved forward at a steady and positive pace (United Nations Development Programme, 2018). The difficulties associated with social progress in these countries were complex. Changes in traditional roles required permission not only from spouses but also from mothers-in-law and, not unusually, from local priests or other clerics who maintained strong control over the personal lives of families.

These changes also had to be supported by members of the larger civilian community, including other female family members, members of their extended kinship system and, often, their mothers-in-law, who were considered to be the chief architects of social life *within* families even as men maintained responsibility for relationships *outside* the social lives of families and their interactions with other families and with other women in the community (Eisenchlas, 2013; Wilensky & Lebeaux, 1965).

With considerable difficulty and with some qualifications, women eventually achieved their independence and, with it, the right to be recognized as their own person, the right to produce their own wealth, the right to accumulate savings and property, the right to make decisions concerning marital choices, the right to divorce, and the right to continue to be identified as, whether single, married, or divorced, an autonomous person (Eckermann, 2014).

Women and Family During and After the War Years

The decades that followed the war years had a transformational impact on the structure of families, especially on the relationship between women and their spouses. The changes were less impactful on children who had not known any other type of family structure but children did both benefit from and struggle with the changing roles of their mothers.

Another of the dramatic changes that impacted families was the increasing ability of women exercise control over their own reproductive cycles. The introduction of condoms and the Food and Drug Administration's approval in 1960 of the birth control pill, provided women with a new level of sexual freedom. Women no longer needed to fear sex with their partners but could control the outcomes of these unions with the assistance of a small pill taken daily. For the first time, women could decide when and if they would have children and those who were already parents could limit the size of their families to fit with their economic ability to care for their children. The concerted efforts of women for more than a century to develop an effective and safe mechanism for controlling their fertility, without depending on the decisions made by their sexual partners, freed women to try to become full and equal partners in the workforce as well as co-equal heads of their families.

This freedom of choice continues for women worldwide as increasing numbers of at least married women have access to medically prescribed and monitored drugs that offer new aspirations and opportunities.

From the War Years to the Beijing World Conference on Women, 1995

The United Nations *Fourth World Conference on Women* was held in Beijing, China in September 1995 (http://www.un.org/womenwatch/daw/beijing/platform/). The conference was one of the most important in bringing women together from around the world to formulate and strategize a realistic plan for global action with the goal of advancing the status of women (and girls) worldwide. The central theme of the 163-nation conference was *Action for Equality, Development and Peace*. The plan of action that resulted from the conference carefully linked all three outcomes with one another and with other sectors critical to comprehensive socio-economic development. In addition to all member state governments of the United Nations, the meeting, and the resulting Plan of Action, included representatives of hundreds of major international development assistance organizations as well as less formal organizations that represented the needs of women and girls more directly. Also included in the conference were representatives of major international development assistance organizations, philanthropic organizations, and private philanthropists. The meeting was a major hallmark in planning for the advancement of women worldwide and brought together women from societies, cultures, religious beliefs, and informal organizations that otherwise would never have met let alone created a working network of international exchange and development (United Nations, 1995; UN Women, 2000).

Some of the major social gains experienced by women after 1960 were even more dramatic than those take took place between 1946 and 1960 (Box 8.2). The post-1960s gains were built on the solid achievements realized during early decades...*but with a difference*. By 1960 and, with it, the reproductive freedom of women, women entered the workforce as full-time, career-oriented workers. Women's traditional roles as teachers, social workers, nurses, and other care-giving professionals expanded dramatically as did the lower average salaries associated with these occupations. At the same time, however, universities across the world opened their doors to women at all levels of education and in all disciplines, including medicine, veterinary medicine, law, engineering, dentistry, and related professional disciplines that traditionally have been male dominated. Most of these disciplines now are heavily populated by women, a trend that is expected to continue well into the future (United Nations Educational, Scientific, and Cultural Organization, 2018).

Box 8.2 Major Social Gains for Women for the United States, 1960–2015 (Vagianos, 2016)

- 1960: Women were finally able to purchase the birth control pill.
- 1968: Women gained the right to have equal access to job listings.
- 1970: Women gained the right to be paid the same as men for the same work.
- 1973: Women could legally get abortions.
- 1974: Women gained the right to get a credit card in their own name
- 1978: Women gained the right to work without discrimination due to pregnancy.
- 1985: Women could divorce their husbands because of "irreconcilable differences."
- 1986: Women could finally seek damages for sexual harassment in the workplace.
- 1993: Marital rape became a criminal offense in all 50 states.
- 1998: Women could access the morning-after pill.
- 2009: Women could file a complaint about pay discrimination.
- 2013: Women in the military could fight on the front lines.
- 2015: Women could finally marry other women.

The legal reforms that made possible the major breakthroughs achieved by women from 1960 to the present are summarized in Fig. 8.5. The policy reforms reported in Box 8.5 are for the United States but, in fact, reflect equivalent changes that have occurred in most economically advanced countries as well as in the upper tier of developing countries. They also reflect changes that are beginning to gain momentum in most other world nations with the result that by 2050 the more favorable social situation of women will differ dramatically from those that exist for most of the world's nations today. And, these transformational social advances that are occurring for women are benefitting men and boys as well, especially in the socio-political-economic sectors, which affect all aspects of collective life.

At the same time, the overall health, social, political, and economic status of women began to improve at a dramatic pace beginning as early as 1970. The figures that follow are illustrative of these and other shifts forward with respect to women, in some cases, with comparable changes that were taking place for men along the same dimensions—life expectancy and health, educational opportunities, employment and income levels and, most importantly, the contributions made by women to the intellectual life of their societies and that of the world through science and technology. Many other indicators of advances in gender equality also could have been used to illustrate this discussion, but those presented here are critical to identifying the major drivers of increased progress in advancing equity and equality between men and women.

The Millennium Development Goals Following the Beijing Conference on Women (2005–2015)

The action agenda of the *Beijing Conference on Women*, at least in part, was converted into Goal 3 of the United Nations seven *Millennium Development Goals*: "to **promote gender equality and empower women.**" The objectives of this goal are listed in Box 8.3. These objectives are part of the operational targets described in greater detail in Box 8.4.

Box 8.3 MDG 3. Eliminate gender disparity in primary and secondary education, preferably by 2005, and in all levels of education by no later than 2015 (World Health Organization, 2018a)

- Girls' education is critically linked to self-determination, improved health, social, and economic status as well as positive health outcomes for the mother and the child. Yet, girls still account for 55% of the out-of-school population.
- Maternal deaths and pregnancy-related conditions cannot be eliminated without the empowerment of women. Maternal mortality is the number one cause of death for adolescents 15–19 years old, and in many countries, sexual and reproductive health services tend to focus exclusively on married women and ignore the needs of adolescents and unmarried women.
- Empowerment of women, including ensuring access to health information and control of resources such as money, is important for achieving gender equality and health equity. However, the ratio of female-to-male earned income is well below parity in all countries for which data are available.
- Up to one in three women worldwide will experience violence at some point in her life, which can lead to unwanted pregnancy and abortion, among other things.

Box 8.4 MDG Goal 3, Target 3A: Promote Gender Equality and Empower Women (United Nations, 2015)
Target 3.A: Eliminate gender disparity in primary and secondary education, preferably by 2005, and in all levels of education no later than 2015

- The developing countries have achieved the target to eliminate gender disparity in primary, secondary and tertiary education.
- Globally, about three quarters of working-age men participate in the labour force, compared to half of working-age women.
- Women make up 41 per cent of paid workers outside of agriculture, an increase from 35 per cent in 1990.
- The average proportion of women in parliament has nearly doubled over the past 20 years.
- Women continue to experience significant gaps in terms of poverty, labour market and wages, as well as participation in private and public decision-making.

Selected Gains of Millennium Development Goal 3A

The data reported in Fig. 8.5 identify some of the gains that were achieved in the political and representational status of women for the period of at least 2005 to 2015, albeit many of the changes identified cover longer time periods.

Data reported in the next section provide considerable detail regarding the comparative social gains and social losses experienced by women from 1960 or 1970 to the present. The data reported in all the figures reflect the tremendous social progress experienced by women over a 40–50 year time…a period sufficiently long to assess the stability of these changes over the long expanse of recent human history.

Major Social Changes in Advancing the Progress of Women Since 1960 and Later

Women, despite the high death rates associated with pregnancy and delivery, always have had the demographic advantage over men. They still do in that, on average, women live 5–8 years longer than men, many even longer (United Nations Population Division, 2017). The reasons for women's advantaged life expectancy are not fully understood but most likely result from a combination of genetics, a tendency to seek health care for new or emergent problems sooner and more often than do men, the generally safer nature of their work and work environment even in the presence of long hours, and the availability of midwives and other medically

Box 8.5 Millennium Development Goal −15 Achievements on Gender Equality (Ford, 2015)

- The number of female MPs globally has doubled over the past 20 years, according to the Inter-Parliamentary Union.
- By 2012, significantly more girls were enrolled in, or had attended, primary school, globally.
- Southern Asia has made strong gains in getting more girls into primary school. In 1990, 74 girls for every 100 boys were enrolled in school. By 2012, equal numbers of girls and boys were enrolled.
- Benin, Burkina Faso, Senegal and Sierra Leone are among the countries in sub-Saharan Africa that have made the greatest improvements in enrolling more girls into school. Over this period, between 30 and 40 additional girls were enrolled in school for every 100 boys.
- Rwanda has the most female lawmakers in the world. Women now make up 64% of MPs in the lower house.
- More girls than boys are enrolled in secondary schools across Latin America and the Caribbean.
- The number of women employed in paid work in non-agricultural jobs increased, with the global share rising from 35% to 40% between 1990 and 2012.
- In 2012, Nicaragua recorded the most women holding ministerial positions in the world – 57% – ahead of Sweden, Finland, France, and Norway.
- In February, Malawi passed a bill that increased the age of marriage from 15 to 18. Early marriage is a prime reason why girls do not attend secondary school.
- Bolivia has revoked laws that did not allow women to work at night.
- According to the International Labour Organisation, the number of UN member states that have ratified the equal remuneration convention has risen from 126 in 1995 to 171 today.
- The number of countries that have ratified the discrimination (employment and occupation) convention has risen from 122 to 172, according to the International Labour Organization.

trained personnel to assist them with routine childbirths (ICM, 2018). The higher levels of spirituality reported for women likely also contribute to a higher life quality as does their increased willingness to participate in support and social groups of other women for advancing their social and recreational health (World Health Organization, 2017).

By contrast, men often engage in dangerous work (including warfare, mining and other extraction industries), generally seek medical assistance in only the most serious situations and then often become non-compliant patients (who are reluctant to give up smoking or other substances that place them as risk of illness), tend to be more isolative, and engage in sports and other activities that are more competitive

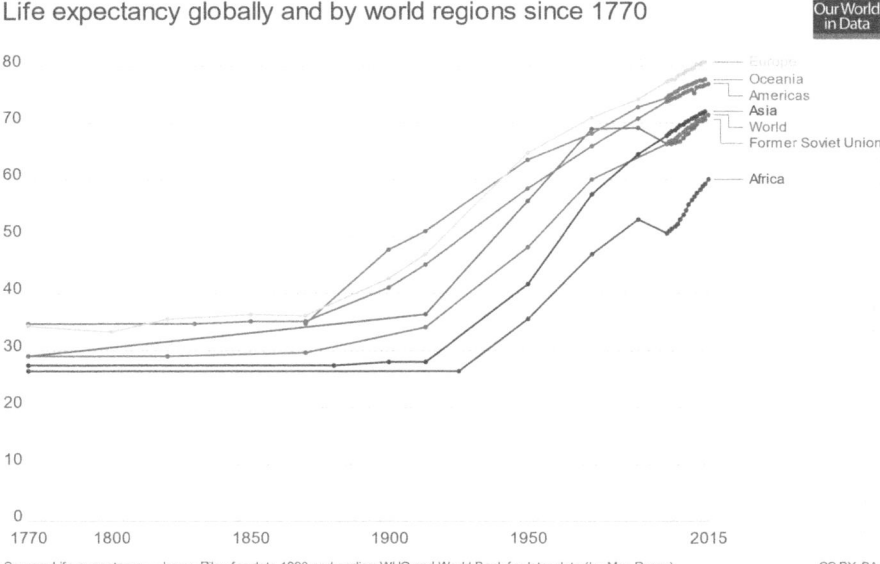

Fig. 8.2 Life expectancy globally and by world regions since 1770. (Source: Life expectancy – James Riley for data for 1990 and earlier; World Health Organization and World Bank for later data [by Max Roser] https://ourworldindata.org/life-expectancy)

and transactional in nature (Bertakis, et al., 2000). In short, men engage in many more unhealthy activities than do women and, apart from exposure to infectious and contagious diseases or affliction with an incurable illness, frequently succumb to death earlier than women (World Health Organization, 2017). Such has been the case throughout all recorded human history and continues into the present.

Figure 8.2 summarizes years of average life expectancy for men and women from 1770 to the present. The figure reflects the dramatic changes that have taken place for men and women during the period just prior to the American independence from Britain. The figure also reflects all of world's major regions that, together, reflect a steady, progressive movement forward in life extension for men and women, but with higher gains in years of life expectancy for women than for men. The data reported in the figure come from the World Health Organization and the World Bank and were assembled by Max Roser of the *Our World in Data* think tank for the period 1770–2015 (Roser and Ortiz-Espina, 2018). The data are disaggregated by major world region (N = 7).

Several patterns regarding the advancement of the average years of life expectancy by major world region are reflected in the figure: (1) very appreciable gains have been realized in years of average life expectancy for men and women alike from 1770 to the present; (2) these gains in years of average life expectancy have been the most significant among the world's already economically advanced societies, especially those of Europe, Oceania, and the Americas; (3) substantial gains also have been made in years of average life expectancy among the developing nations of Africa, Asia, and Latin America; and (4) Africa continues to be the continent that lags behind the others in gains in years of average life expectancy but the rate of gain along this dimension is quite rapid and, in time, will be comparable to that achieved by the nations of Latin America (Estes, 2019).

The net progress in years of average life expectancy is the result of gains in nutrition, earlier medical intervention, especially prenatal care, improved level of education and literacy, and improved sanitation including the introduction of indoor plumbing (World Health Organization, 2018a, 2018b). These significant social advances added appreciably to gains on the part of women and girls in average years of life expectancy as well as setting the framework for successful implementation of the United Nations' *Millennium Development Campaign* and the global efforts of major international development assistance organizations, including those of private philanthropists and charitable foundations. These gains in social progress are well documented and demonstrate the close interrelationship that exists between health, other sectors of development, quality of life, and a heightened sense of well-being (Cohen, 2011).

Figure 8.3 reports average years of life expectancy for men and women for 25 of the world's nations with the longest overall life expectancy. Not all these nations are among the world's most economically advanced nor are they the largest or smallest nations. What they do share with one another, however, is average years of life expectancy of at least 80 with the longest in all cases being that of women in these societies. In most cases, approximately seven to eight years separate men and women in terms of overall years of life expectancy. The same pattern predominates throughout much of the world.

Under-Five, Infant, and Neonatal Mortality

Figure 7.1 of Chap. 7 summarizes changes in the combined rates of infant and child mortality for the period 1970–2012 for nearly all the world's regions and subregions (United Nations Inter-Agency Group for Child Mortality Estimation, 2018). Only data for the small island nations of the Pacific and parts of Oceania have been excluded because of problems of data availability and timeliness. The positive trends vis-à-vis reductions in death rates for infants and children five years of age and under for the 95% of the world's population covered by Fig. 7.1 are quite dramatic and positive. These advances in early child survival rates impact directly on the quality of lives of women and their families and have contributed appreciably to worldwide reductions in the sizes of families, given that more offspring survive well into adulthood. Therefore, large families are no longer needed to provide a sense of social insurance for parents as they age or become seriously ill (Mettrop, 1974).

The levels of social progress associated with contemporary child survival rates reverse patterns that have existed for centuries, indeed, millennia, during which scores of just born children died from a lack of medications and medical care that now are readily available nearly everywhere in the economically developed and

Life expectancy at birth (years), UN World Population Prospects 2015

Rank	State/Territory	Overall	Male	Female
1	Japan	83.74	80.91	86.58
2	Italy	83.31	80.00	86.49
3	Switzerland	82.84	80.27	85.23
4	Singapore	82.66	80.43	84.74
5	Israel	82.64	79.59	85.61
6	Iceland	82.30	80.73	83.84
7	Spain	82.28	79.42	85.05
8	Australia	83.42	80.33	86.56
9	Hong Kong	82.07	80.18	83.82
10	Sweden	81.93	80.10	83.71
11	France (metropole.)	81.85	78.76	84.87
12	Canada	81.78	79.69	83.78
13	New Zealand	81.56	79.71	83.35
14	South Korea	81.43	77.95	84.63
15	Luxembourg	81.34	78.94	83.65
16	Norway	81.32	79.22	83.38
17	Netherlands	81.31	79.36	83.14
18	Chile	81.21	78.09	84.12
19	Martinique (France)	81.18	77.79	84.36
20	Austria	81.09	78.47	83.59
21	Germany	80.66	78.18	83.06
22	Greece	80.60	77.64	83.60
23	Ireland	80.57	78.40	82.74
24	Guadeloupe (France)	80.56	76.83	83.98
25	Portugal	80.55	77.43	83.50

Fig. 8.3 Advances in years of average life expectancy for the top 25 countries by gender, 2015. (Source: *World Population Prospects: 2015*. Revision. New York: UN Population Division. Retrieved November 12, 2018 from https://esa.un.org/unpd/wpp/Publications/Files/WPP2015_Volume-I_Comprehensive-Tables.pdf)

developing worlds. The contributions of better trained and more skilled midwives in rural communities have played a big role in achieving the higher child survival rates as has the availability of more visiting nurses, nurse practitioners, specially trained obstetricians, and neonatal intensive care units in most large urban general hospitals and virtually all university affiliated hospitals. Many countries also are fortunate in having a sizeable network of children's hospitals where near miraculous lifesaving procedures are performed on infants and small children than cannot be adequately carried out in a general hospital, even in the highly specialized neonatal intensive care units.

Figure 7.2 of Chap. 7 is a photograph of a tombstone in Dresden, Germany reflecting the death of an infant immediately following birth as well as the emotional distress experienced by the mother as her now dead child is whisked hurriedly away by midwives. Fortunately, the occurrence of events such as this one is on sharp decline with the result that cemetery headstones of this type, however beautiful, have become increase rare nearly everywhere. Continuing advances in pre- and postnatal care, the availability of healthier food, improved housing and sanitation practices, and rapid medical emergency services will ensure the increased survival of infants and children born and raised in distant rural communities.

These gains, which are substantial, were not easily achieved and required enormous programmatic efforts and financial investments on the part of governments and private entities (Save the Children, 2018; UN Women, 2018a). And still more progress in reducing infant and child deaths is occurring even as this book is being written. With the introduction of the United Nations 17 Sustainable Development Goals in 2015, which will span a period of approximately 15 years, we can expect that, by 2050, the worldwide death rate of infants and young children should fall below 75/1000 live born to as few as 65/1000 live born, perhaps lower, within an increasing number of the world's most rapidly socially developing nations (UN, 2018; WHO, 2017). Parity between all blocks of nations likely will not be achieved during the remainder of this still young century but, almost certainly, will be realized as we begin a new period in which nations enjoy a much higher degree of equality with respect to the distribution of income, health care, education, technology and other conditions that have improved the situation so rapidly in the world's most economically advanced nations (Estes & Sirgy, 2018; Estes, 2019).

Maternal Mortality

By far, the most significant advance in the well-being of women is reflected in the significant, in some countries dramatic, decline in maternal mortality rates. The extent of these declines is reported in Fig. 8.4, which provides clear evidence of this progress for all the world's regions for three critical time periods: 1990, 2000, and 2015 (World Health Organization et al., 2015). In effect, maternal deaths have been cut in half in just 15 years with the most significant gains reported for the world's least

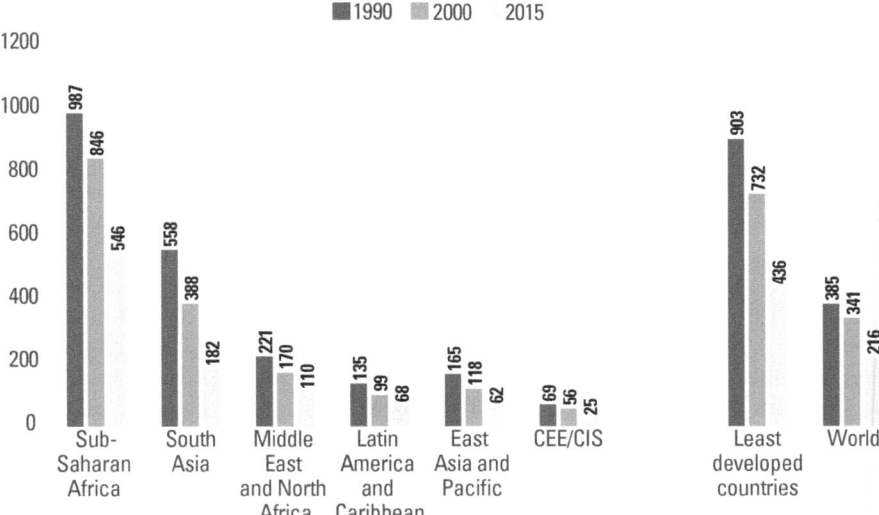

Fig. 8.4 Maternal mortality declined by almost half between 1990 and 2015 in the world's developing nations, per 100,000 (World Health Organization et al., 2015) (*CEE/CIS: Central and Eastern Europe and the Commonwealth of Independent States)

economically advantaged nations, from more than 900/100,000 live births in 1990 to about 425/100,000 live births in 2015. Appreciable gains in reducing maternal mortality rates also are taking place in the world's most economically advanced countries, with maternal death rates in 2015 averaging well under 10 per 100,000 live born (World Health Organization, 2018c).

The important gains in protecting the lives of women from the risks of premature death associated with childbirth have come from a combination of early and effective prenatal care, much more aggressive immunization outreach programs, the establishment of community health centers within reachable distance for most women in rural communities, in-home midwifery and medical care prior to and following the births of their children. Improved literacy has allowed women to educate themselves about their bodies and the symptoms associated with premature birth and post-delivery issues and about broad-based social developments (including access to safe drinking water, improved sanitation, improved roads, the introduction of communications technology, and the like).

Key Factors Associated with Maternal Mortality Rates Since 1990

Death is not a normal or usual outcome of pregnancy and delivery, even complex deliveries involving irregularly placed or multiple newborns. Rather, maternal deaths result from a broad range of factors, nearly all of which are preventable or at least minimized if not entirely preventable. The World Health Organization has recently published a fact sheet that provides useful information for midwives and other health care professionals to be cognizant of when providing preventive services to pregnant women and their babies. The fact sheet also alerts care providers to the major risks that threaten the lives of women when giving birth. Some of the most important facts and alerts pertainion to the protection of pregnant women when giving birth are summarized in Box 8.6.

Box 8.6 Selected Facts from the World Health Organization Associated with Maternal Mortality (World Health Organization, 2018c)
Key Facts

- Every day, approximately 830 women die from preventable causes related to pregnancy and childbirth;
- 99% of all maternal deaths occur in developing countries;
- Maternal mortality is higher in women living in rural areas and among poorer communities;
- Young adolescents face a higher risk of complications and death because of pregnancy than other women;
- Skilled care before, during and after childbirth can save the lives of women and newborn babies;
- Between 1990 and 2015, maternal mortality worldwide dropped by about 44%; and,
- Between 2016 and 2030, as part of the *Sustainable Development Goals*, the target is to reduce the global maternal mortality ratio to less than 70 per 100,000 live births

Why do women die?
Women die because of complications during and following pregnancy and childbirth. Most of these complications develop during pregnancy and most are preventable or treatable. Other complications may exist before pregnancy but are worsened during pregnancy, especially if not managed as part of the woman's care. The major complications that account for nearly 75% of all maternal deaths are *(4)*:

- severe bleeding (mostly bleeding after childbirth)
- infections (usually after childbirth)
- high blood pressure during pregnancy (pre-eclampsia and eclampsia)
- complications from delivery
- unsafe abortion.

The remainder are caused by or associated with diseases such as malaria, and AIDS during pregnancy.

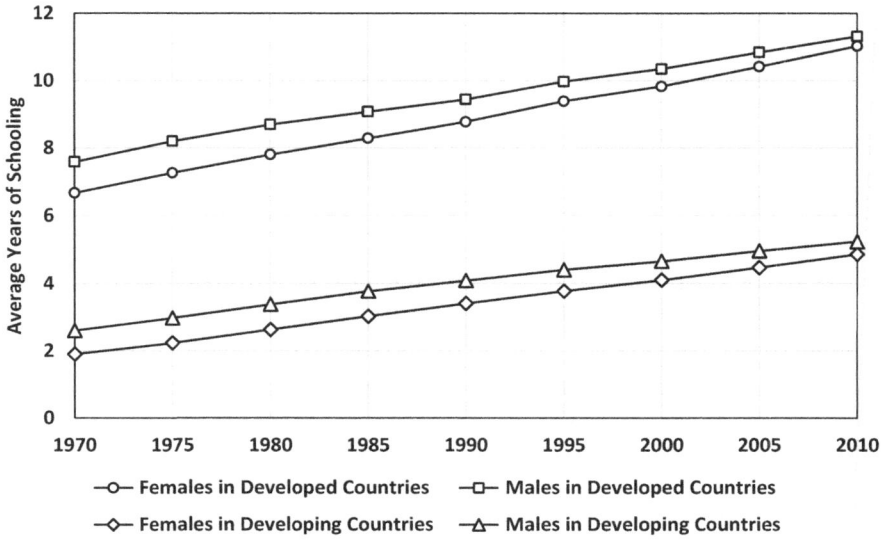

Fig. 8.5 Average years of total schooling, age 15+, males vs. females, developed vs. developing countries (Data from World Bank, 2017). Reprinted with permission from Estes, R. J. & Sirgy, M. J. (2018). *Advances in Well-Being: Toward a Better World for All*. London: Rowman & Littlefield

Female Literacy Rates

Not only are women and girls living longer but they also are more literate and better educated than at any time in human history. These accomplishments, too, represent major foundations on which greater progress for women and girls will be built. Not coincidentally, these gains for women also are taking place at a time when the informal and formal education of boys and men also is taking place. Thus, both genders are benefitting appreciably from actions that have been undertaken to promote the educational and overall social progress of women. This has been a "win-win" outcome for everyone, including the larger society, which benefits directly from a more literate and better educated population (and potentially workforce).

Figure 8.5 reports the total percentage of persons age 15+ years enrolled in formal programs of education for the years 1970–2010. The data are disaggregated by gender and level of overall socioeconomic development of nations and reflect several patterns that support the statements made above: (a) increasing numbers of boys, men, girls, and women are enrolled in full-time formal educational programs; (b) a tremendous disparity exists in the proportion of children and adults in developing countries enrolled in formal educational programs vis-à-vis those enrolled in such programs in more economically advanced nations, but the trajectories of the data summarized in the figure show that, in time, parity between the two groups of nations may eventually be reached but it will require many decades to achieve; (c)

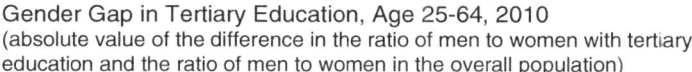

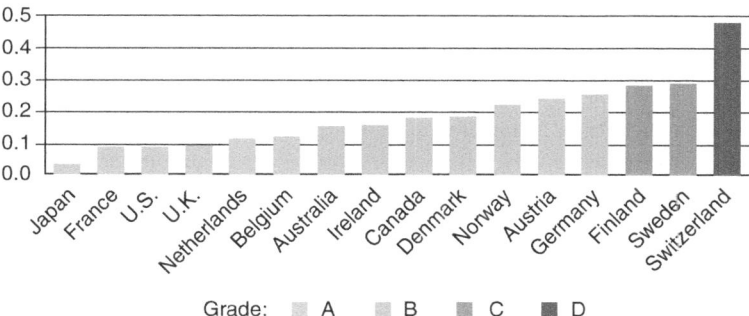

Fig. 8.6 Gender gap in tertiary education, age 25–64, 2010 (absolute value of the difference in the ratio of men to women with tertiary education and the ratio of men to women in the overall population). (Source: Conference Board of Canada (2013)

within developing societies boys and girls now are enrolled in formal educational programs but the rate growth in these programs is more rapid for girls and women than for boys and men; (d) by 2025, educational enrollment rates of girls and women in developing countries likely will exceed those of boys and men as more men enter the workforce and women enter secondary and post-secondary educational training.

Female Tertiary Education

Universities and other centers of post-secondary education are accepting increasing numbers of women in their student bodies. These programs are primarily academic and professional in nature and are opening opportunities for women to enter previously "male only" professions such as medicine, dentistry, law, and engineering, among others. Still other women are pursuing opportunities for more technical training in schools specifically set up to prepare people for practical professions such as nursing and dental assistants, teaching assistants, mechanics, computer technicians and the like. The opportunities for women have significantly raised the contributions of many to work force, ensured their own job and income security, and have filled labor market needs that otherwise would have remaining vacant. The varied nature of opportunities for officially recognized, usually accredited, post-secondary education has further increased the independence of women while enhancing their status at home and in the workplace (International Labour Organization, 2018; UN Women, 2018a, 2018b).

Figure 8.6 illustrates the social progress of women at the post-secondary educational level for 16 of the world's economically advanced countries. The figure was prepared by the *Conference Board of Canada* (2013) and focuses on the gap in higher education that existed between adult men and women for these 16 countries for the year 2010. The purpose of the figure was to rank order the educational performance of these countries using the educational attainment of women rather than that of men as the central focus. The following patterns are easily discernable from a review of the data summarized in the figure:

- Women's educational achievements at the post-secondary level are substantial and in many economically advanced countries are beginning to achieve parity with those of men, e.g., Japan, France, the United States, the United Kingdom, Netherlands, and Belgium;
- The six nations in the first tier, by promoting gender parity in higher education, have made higher levels of public and private investments in the sector and are reaping the benefits by ending centuries-old exclusionary practices designed to limit the educational choices of women;
- Increasing levels of gender parity in the remaining 10 countries identified in the figure are highly favorable though not at the same level as those of the first-tier group of nations;
- The admissions practices of institutions of higher learning in the second tier of ten nations still are inclusive of large numbers of women students, but these practices favor the admission of men over that of women;
- Thus, considerable effort remains to be taken to break the "glass ceiling" that continues to limit the advanced educational opportunities available to women from the initial point of entry into post-secondary schools to their eventual graduation. But progress is taking place and, for many, at a rapid if not quick enough pace.

Of significance regarding general post-secondary educational trends is the fact that the admission of large numbers of women to institutions of higher education has not been a "win-win" situation in most cases. Indeed, the number of available "seats" at many competitive colleges and universities tends to be fixed, with the result that men and women can occupy the same seat (Lopez & Gonzalez-Barrera, 2014). Thus, with the admission of large numbers of women into post-secondary programs, increasing numbers of men have to either join the labor force, enter military service, or undertake other types of work for which a post-secondary certificate or degree is not needed. In the United Kingdom, for example, researchers at *The Guardian*, citing research conducted by the Universities and Colleges Admissions Service, reported that,

> across the UK 27.3% of all young men are expected to go to university this year, compared with 37.1% of young women. That means 18-year-old women are 36% more likely to start degree courses this autumn than their male peers" (Editors, 2017).

Even with this new disparity in admissions outcomes in institutions of higher education, the percentage of college, university, and technical school men continues to far exceed the number of women with similar levels of education. Another century of concerted effort will likely be needed to achieve true educational parity even in the most economically advanced nations.

Women in Science and Technology

One of the major stumbling blocks in the progress of women has been their "admission" to the even more rigidly controlled fields of science and technology...even when much of the work for which male scientists claim credit depended on the long hours, hard work, and perspiration of women. Women always have carried critical responsibilities in science. They can legitimately be credited with major breakthroughs that have laid the foundation for even greater scientific advances. The 10 scientists identified in Box 8.7 have been among the most distinguished and contributive women in science during the early and mid-twentieth century to the present.

Box 8.7 Leading Women in Science and Technology (*Science*, 2018)
Marie Curie (1867–1934). Polish-born French physicist and chemist best known for her contributions to radioactivity.
   Jane Godall (1934–present). British primatologist and ethologist, widely considered to be the world's foremost expert on chimpanzees.
   Maria Mayer (1906–1972). German-born American physicist who received the Nobel Prize for suggesting the nuclear shell model of the atomic nucleus.
   Rachel Carson (1907–1964). American marine biologist and conservationist whose work revolutionzied the global environmental movement.
   Rosalind Franklin (1920–1958). British biophysicist best known for her work on the molecular structures of coal and graphite and X-ray diffraction.
   Barbara McClintock (1902–1992) American scientist and cytogeneticist who received the Nobel Prize in 1983 for the discovery of genetic transposition.
   Rita Levi-Montalcini (1909–2012). Italian neurologist who received the Nobel Prize in 1986 for the discovery of nerve growth factor.
   Gertrude Elion (1918–1999). American biochemist and pharmacologist who received the 1988 Nobel Prize in physiology or medicine.
   Elizabeth Blackwell (1821–1910). American physician who was the first woman to become a medical doctor in the United States.
   Christiane Nusslein-Volhard (1942–present). German biologist who received the Albert Lasker Award for Basic Medical Research in 1991.

One final measure that I shall use in discussing the social progress of women, in this case again in science, is the distribution by gender of those persons who make decisions concerning the publication of new areas of research, particularly in journals and other periodicals that reach large numbers of scientists and that, in turn, help to shape the direction that new areas of investigation may take. This issue is especially critical for academics who are working their way up the professorial career ladder as well as young and experienced scientists who seek to receive financial sponsorship from highly competitive sources. Traditionally, but also owing to their comparatively small numbers, women have been excluded from many of the most critical review and decision processes related to financial funding opportunities as well as from opportunities to serve as reviewers and decision makers concerning reports of research that already has been completed.

Despite appreciable progress in both dimensions of scholarly activity, women continue to be represented only in small numbers on the research and publication review panels of many of the most important journals in science and technology. Though the situation is improving steadily over the short term, still much ground needs to be gained if men and women are to achieve parity in making the most important decisions that impact the career paths of scientists, their funding and publications streams, and the opportunity for other scientists to become familiar with their work. These patterns are reflected in Fig. 8.7, which reports several trends related to members of selected scientific organizations that (a) performed a range of functions within the organizations; (b) were first authors of manuscripts submitted for review and eventual publication; and (c) the proportion of the members that are women who functioned in the capacity of reviewers of original research manuscripts submitted for publication (Botkin-Kowacki, 2017).

Several patterns pertaining to the changing status of women in science are readily discernable from the figure: (a) women comprise an increasing share of the total scientific community, albeit men still outnumber women in science by a factor of 2:1; (b) women are emerging with increased frequency as the first authors of scientific papers submitted for publication; and (c) as a percentage of reviewers of scientific papers submitted for publication, women continue to be underrepresented, given their contributions as first authors and as members of scientific societies. Judging by the latter trend, it likely will require several more decades for women to fill the seats vacated by male researchers on journal editorial boards as either first authors or as reviewers of original research manuscripts submitted for publication, the majority of which likely have been written by men.

The tremendous contributions made to humanity through science and technology by women continue to lay the foundation for younger men and women scholars, some of whom will be women whose contributions will equal or exceed those of the women who comprise the panel of remarkable women identified in Fig. 8.7.

Discussion and Conclusions

The twenty-first century is rapidly emerging as "the century of the women." The social achievements of women and girls during the century just ended and the beginnings of this century have been unparalleled in human history (UN Women, 2018b). Women today enjoy access to levels of health care previously unavailable either to those who preceded them or to even economically advantaged men and boys who lived during the same periods. For example, today a larger percentage of the world's women have completed primary and secondary education and a very high

Fig. 8.7 Gender distribution in various activities compared to the gender of reviewers. (Source: Botkin-Kowacki 2017)

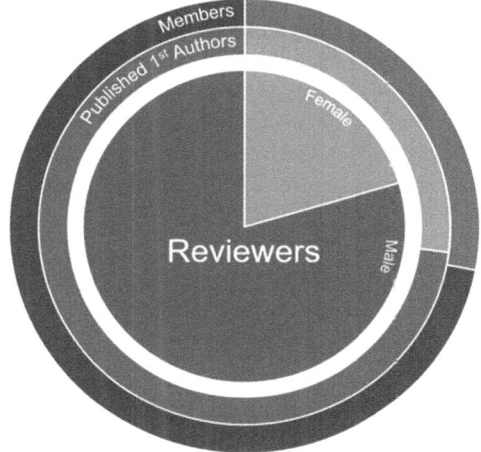

Fig. 8.7 Gender distribution in various activities compared to the gender of reviewers. (Source: Botkin-Kowacki 2017)

percentage of women are enrolled in post-secondary and university degree-granting institutions of higher education. Women also are rapidly emerging as leaders in corporate management, in research roles in applied science and technology, and in the major professions as doctors, veterinarians, lawyers, engineers, and the like. And, of course, they continue to be major contributors to the performing arts (Fidell & DeLamater, 1971).

Women, increasingly, are major scholars in universities and empirically based think tanks and have become major contributors to all fields of social, psychological, medical, and biological science and technology. Increasing numbers of journal articles and books are being authored by women, and, increasingly, the number of women on the editorial boards of prestigious journals and other periodicals also are increasing, Women working full time as mathematicians, "bench scientists," and engineers remain in comparatively short supply but their numbers are increasing rapidly in these and other previously male-dominated professions. Today, in many Western countries, the proportion of women enrolled in the professional schools of major universities approximates the share of men enrolled in the same programs, e.g., medicine, dentistry, law, communications, social work, and education.

In short, the social status of women and girls is changing, and all of these gains have worked to the benefit of women everywhere in the world. More women serve as popularly elected members of parliaments, as prime ministers and other heads of state, and have provided intellectual leadership in many areas of the theoretical and applied social and physical sciences. As a result, discrimination against women and girls *based on their gender* is rapidly declining and reflects a pattern that can be expected to continue well into the present century as women achieve increasing professional and economic parity with men. These advances will not be easily sustained but sustained they will be for many decades. No longer, for example, will women be denied opportunities routinely offered to men based on their gender alone. In the end, women truly will "hold up half the sky" and, in doing so, will bring new insights and dimensions into advancing not only their own well-being but that of men and boys as well. Women increasingly will be recognized as the full and equal partners in improvements in development, quality of life, and well-being that already are being achieved by female activities outside of the home. As these transformational changes are brought about, women and girls will have arrived at the point of personal and collective accomplishment sought after by suffragettes worldwide and summed up in a few words by the pioneering American feminist, Betty Friedan,

> It is ridiculous to tell girls to be quiet when they enter a new field, or an old one, so the men will not notice they are there. A girl should not expect special privileges, because of her sex, but neither should she "adjust" to prejudice and discrimination. The Feminine Mystique (1963)

Humanity is collectively and actively contributing to the inclusion of women in all aspects of community, national, and international development. The contributions of women to these processes are just too valuable to ignore, minimize, or leave out entirely. Women, as demonstrated by history, work toward more reconciliatory approaches to conflict resolution and peace than do men and, in doing so, make a unique contribution to recognizing that development depends fundamentally on peace and peaceful approaches for dealing with disagreements that occur with considerably frequency within and between large collectives of people. This unique contribution to peace promotion through development (and the reverse) is characteristic of most women in positions of major societal responsibility. However, women in positions of power can be confrontational in conflict situations in which the other parties fail to respond to more cooperative approaches to peace, development, quality of life, and well-being, e.g., Indira Gandhi fought off insurgent attacks initiated by Pakistani nationals; Golda Meier of Israel forcefully encouraged higher levels of intraregional cooperation in the Middle East; and Scandinavian women leaders forcefully promoted more secure social safety nets for highly vulnerable population groups. These processes and priorities are expected to continue well into the future (UN Women, 2018a, 2018b).

This author believes that widespread agreement exists that women, and even girls, will no longer remain silent about the prejudicial, discriminatory, and disadvantaged situation that has characterized their social status throughout much of recorded history. Nor should the expectation exist that they should. Humanity's future success depends on all people, of both genders, moving forward in making their best and fullest contribution to society. For girls and women to realize this objective poses no threat to boys and men but, instead, contributes to the realization of their objectives. We all, men and women alike, stand on the shoulders of the remarkable women who already have reshaped society and on whose shoulders we securely stand: Maria Sklodowska-Curie, physicist (1867–1934), Jane Addams, activist and philanthropist (1860–1935), Margaret Sanger, activist and philanthropist (1879–1966), Indira Gandhi, activist and politician (1917–1984), Golda Meir, politician (1897–1978), Margaret Thatcher, politician (1925–2013), Betty Friedan, activist and author (1921–2006), Aung San Suu Kyi, activist and politician (1945-present), among hundreds of others who are working as thought and political leaders everywhere in the world in the context of their own countries and those of neighboring states.

Women in critical leadership positions can be expected to continue to promote peace and development. The central focus of women in advancing the formulation and implementation of social policy traditional has been to advance the quality of life of all people, including the large numbers of the poor, aged, disabled, and jobless workers that exist in developed and developing societies alike. This priority is not genetically based but is anchored in recognition of the need for more progressive solutions to satisfy the needs of all people in society and not just the already advantaged minority people at the top of the social pyramids that exist in all societies. Women as mothers simply tend to be more nurturing than many men and more easily recognize the need for secure social safety nets that provide for the needs of all people in society, including those who live along its margins. Former Secretary-General of the United Nations, the Korean Ban Ki- Moon, emphasized the interrelationship that exists between the advancement of women and the resolution of other major social challenges that confront the world today. Said Ban Ki-Moon in an address before the United Nations General Assembly on September 21, 2011 (Moon, 2011),

> *Saving our planet, lifting people out of poverty, advancing economic growth… these are one and the same fight. We must connect the dots between climate change, water scarcity, energy shortages, global health, food security and women's empowerment. Solutions to one problem must be solutions for all.*

The social gains reported for women and girls in this chapter suggest that society is, at last, advancing some of the most critical actors needed to advance the well-being of people worldwide. Every expectation is that progress in this critical aspect of the social progress of nations will continue well into the future (National Organization for Women, 2018; UN Women, 2018b; World Health Organization, 2018a).

References

Bazilchuk, N. (2018, March 30). Family life makes Nordic men happy. *Science Nordic*. Retrieved November 12, 2018 from http://sciencenordic.com/family-life-makes-nordic-men-happy

Bertakis, K. D., Azari, R., Helms, L. J., Callahan, E. J., & Robbins, J. A. (2000). Gender differences in the utilization of health care services. *Journal of Family Practice, 49*(2) 147–152.

Botkin-Kowacki, E. (2017, January 25). Are women scientists overlooked by journals as peer reviewers? *The Christian Science Monitor*. Retrieved November 4, 2018 from https://www.csmonitor.com/Science/2017/0126/Are-women-scientists-overlooked-by-journals-as-peer-reviewers

Cohen, N. (2011, April 29). The top 40 most innovative international development organizations. *Nonprofit Quarterly*.

Conference Board of Canada. (2013). *Gender gap in tertiary education: International rankings*. Retrieved November 8, 2018 from https://www.conferenceboard.ca/hcp/Details/education/gender-gap-tertiary.aspx?AspxAutoDetectCookieSupport=1

Eckermann, L. (2014). *Gender, life span, and quality of life: An international perspective.* Dordrecht, The Netherlands: Springer Publishers.

Editors. (2017, August 27). University gender gap at record high as 30,000 more women accepted. *The Guardian.*

Eisenchlas, S. A. (2013). Gender roles and expectations: Any changes online? *SAGE Open,* October–December 2013: 1–11.

Essays, UK. (2013). *The effects on women during the industrial revolution history essay.* Retrieved from https://www.ukessays.com/essays/history/the-effects-on-women-during-the-industrial-revolution-history-essay.php?vref=1

Estes, R. J. (2010). The world social situation: Development challenges at the outset of a new century. *Social Indicators Research, 98*(3), 363–402.

Estes, R. J. (2019). The social progress of nations, 1970–2020. *Social Indicators Research* (under review).

Estes, R. J., & Sirgy, M. J. (2018). *Advances in well-being: Toward a better world for all.* London: Rowman & Littlefield.

Fidell, L. S., & DeLamater, J. D. (1971). *Women in the professions.* Beverly Hills, CA: Sage Publications.

Ford, L. (2015). Millennium development goal 3: 15 achievements on gender equality. *The Guardian,* March 26. Retrieved November 1, 2018 from https://www.theguardian.com/global-development/2015/mar/26/millennium-development-goal-3-15-achievements-on-gender-equality

Friedan, B. (1963). *The feminine mystique.* New York: W. W. Norton.

Harper, I. H. (1922). *The history of women suffrage.* 6 Volumes. Washington, DC: National American Women Suffrage Association.

International Confederation of Midwifery (ICM). (2018). *About our work.* Hague, The Netherlands. Retrieved November 26, 2018 from https://www.internationalmidwives.org/.

International Labour Organization (ILO). (2018). *Global commission on the future of work.* Geneva, Switzerland: ILO.

Jones-Rogers, S. E. (2019). *They were her property: White women as slave owners in the American South.* New Haven, CT: Yale University Press.

Lopez, M. H., & Gonzalez-Barrera, A. (2014, March 6). Women's college enrollment gains leave men behind. *Pew Research Center: Fact Tank.*

Loudon, I. (1993). *Death in childbirth: An international study of maternal care and maternal mortality 1800–1950.* London: Clarendon Press.

Martin, V. (2007). *Property.* New York: Vintage Books.

Mettrop, G. (1974). Child survival and family size. *World of Irish Nursing, 3,* 23–24.

Moon, B-K. (2011). *Address to the 66th general assembly: "We the Peoples."* Retrieved November 23, 2018 from https://www.un.org/sg/en/content/sg/speeches/2011-09-21/address-66th-general-assembly-we-peoples

National Organization for Women (NOW). (2018). *Help build a feminist future.* Retrieved November 1, 2018 from https://now.org/

Nearing, S., & Nearing, N. (1912). *Women and social progress: A discussion of the biologic, domestic, industrial, and social possibilities of American Women.* New York: Macmillan.

Roser, M., & Ortiz-Espina, E. (2018). *Literacy.* Retrieved November 12, 2018 from https://ourworldindata.org/literacy

Save the Children. (2018). *Save the children annual review 2017.* New York/London: Save the Children.

Science. (2018). *Famous women scientists: The art of genius.* Retrieved November 20, 2018 from https://www.famousscientists.org/10-famous-women-scientists/

Striking Women. (2017). *Women after the war year.* Retrieved November 13, 2018 from http://striking-women.org/module/women-and-work/post-world-war-ii-1946-1970

Tiliouine, H., & Estes, R. J. (Eds.). (2016). *The state of social progress of Islamic societies: social, economic, political, and ideological challenges.* Cham, Switzerland: Springer.

UN Women. (2000). *Five-year Review of the implementation of the Beijing Declaration and Platform for Action (Beijing + 5) held in the General Assembly, 5–9 June 2000*. New York: UN Women.

UN Women. (2018a). *Women and the sustainable development goals (SDGs)*. New York: UN Women. Retrieved November 18, 2018 from http://www.unwomen.org/en/news/in-focus/women-and-the-sdgs

UN Women. (2018b). *Turning promises into action: Gender equality in the 2030 agenda for sustainable development*. New York: UN Women.

United Nations (UN). (1995). *List of documents considered at the FWCW*. Retrieved November 8, 2018 from http://www.un.org/esa/gopher-data/conf/fwcw/pim/doclist

United Nations (UN). (2015). *Millennium development goals 2015 and beyond*. Retrieved November 5, 2018 from http://www.un.org/millenniumgoals/gender.shtml

United Nations (UN). (2018). *Sustainable development goals: Knowledge platform*. Retrieved November 1, 2018 from https://sustainabledevelopment.un.org/

United Nations Development Programme (UNDP-HDR). (2005). Towards the rise of women in the Arab World. Cairo, Egypt: UNDP, Regional Bureau for Arab States (RBAS).

United Nations Development Programme (UNDP). (2018). *Human development report, 2018: Human development indices and indicators*. New York: UNDP.

United Nations Educational, Scientific, and Cultural Organization (UNESCO). (2018). *Annual statistical report, 2018*. Paris: UNESCO.

United Nations Inter-Agency Group for Child Mortality Estimation (UN IGME). (2018). The under-five mortality rate has fallen by more than half since 1990. Retrieved November, 11, 2018 from https://data.unicef.org/topic/child-survival/under-five-mortality/.

United Nations Population Division. (2017). *World population prospects: Key findings and advance tables, 2017 revision*. New York: UN Population Division, Department of Economic and Social Affairs (UNDESA).

Vagianos, A. (2016). Women. *HuffPost*, September 27. Retrieved November 4, 2018 from https://www.huffingtonpost.com/entry/rights-women-have-gained-since-earning-the-right-to-vote_us_57e9ed33e4b0c2407cd93434-201

Verloo, M. (2018). *Varieties of opposition to gender equality in Europe*. London/New York: Taylor & Francis and Routledge.

Wilensky, H. L., & Lebeaux, C. N. (1965). *Industrial society and social welfare*. New York: Free Press.

World Health Organization (WHO). (2017). *Annual statistical report* (p. 2017). Geneva, Switzerland: WHO.

World Health Organization (WHO). (2018a). *MDG 3: Promote gender equality and empower women*. Geneva, Switzerland: WHO. Retrieved November 5, 2018 from http://www.who.int/topics/millennium_development_goals/gender/en/

World Health Organization (WHO). (2018b). *WHO fact sheet: Sanitation*. Retrieved November 21, 2018 from http://www.who.int/news-room/fact-sheets/detail/sanitation

World Health Organization (WHO). (2018c). *WHO fact sheet: Maternal mortality*. Retrieved November 20, 2018 from http://www.who.int/news-room/fact-sheets/detail/maternal-mortality

World Health Organization, UNICEF, United Nations Population Fund, and The World Bank (WHO et al.). (2015). *Trends in maternal mortality: 1990 to 2015*. Geneva, Switzerland: WHO.

Chapter 9
Putting Poverty into a Museum

The famous Bangladeshi economist Muhammad Yunus (Bengali: মুহাম্মদ ইউনূস) began his career as a commercial banker serving mostly well-off individuals, small businesses, and corporations. Following several years of working in the commercial sector, however, he felt little satisfaction with his job as a banker to the economically well off. He turned his attention instead to the credit needs of the poor, especially to the needs of rural women struggling to establish small enterprises and to the urban poor, including the street beggars living and working in all major cities in Bangladesh. Yunus recognized that the most limiting characteristic of the poor was their inability to obtain credit at reasonable rates from commercial banks to initiate businesses or other enterprises of their own. After all, who is going to lend even a few Takas (0.88 Taka = 1 USD) to a blind man selling pencils or beverages from a communal cup on the streets of Dhaka? Indeed, who would be willing to invest in the credit needs of an impoverished woman who wanted to establish small gardens in which she and her friends could grow fruits or vegetables for sale to neighbors or local markets.

Yunus answered the question very simply, "I will." Drawing on his own resources and those of like-minded small businessmen, Yunus worked for several years to establish what is now known as the *Grameen Bank*, or "peoples bank," which is fully committed to providing small loans to individuals and groups of individuals to start or sustain their own small businesses or other commercial enterprises (http://www.grameen-info.org/). In exchange for the service, and consistent with Muslim values, the bank required that the borrowers, mostly poor women, to return only the principal amount of their loan on a timely basis in addition to a very small rate of interest consistent with the purpose to which the loan was put, e.g., to support advanced education versus business development versus general support. The income generated from the interest payments was used to cover the fewer than 3% of borrowers who failed to repay their loans or to hire representative members of the very people that the bank was set up to serve.

© Springer Nature Switzerland AG 2019
R. J. Estes, *The Social Progress of Nations Revisited, 1970–2020*, Social Indicators Research Series 78, https://doi.org/10.1007/978-3-030-15907-8_9

Yunus's goal, like the man himself, was a simple one, i.e., to lift large numbers of non-credit worthy people out of extreme poverty and, in time, "to put poverty itself in a museum." This was a goal that he was able to achieve not only in desperately poor rural Bangladesh but also in several dozen other countries that adapted the group-collective methods of the Grameen Bank to assist their poor with the goal of increasing their economic self-sufficiency. Wrote Yunus in 2007,

> All human beings have the inner capacity not only to care for themselves but also to contribute to increasing the well-being of the world. Some get the chance to explore their potential to some degree. But many never get any opportunity to unwrap this wonderful gift they were born with. They die with their gifts unexplored, and the world is deprived of all they could have done…. It is possible to eliminate poverty from our world because it is not natural to human beings—it is artificially imposed on them. Let's dedicate ourselves to bringing an end to it soon and putting poverty in the museums once and for all (p. 233).

Yunus and the staff of the Grameen Bank went on to gain international recognition for the innovativeness of their approach to poverty alleviation. In 2006, he and the World Bank were recognized for their achievements in using a group approach to extending credit to deeply impoverished people: They received the *Nobel Prize for Peace* "for their efforts through microcredit to create economic and social development from below."

Yunus's innovations, which he continues to promote with great success even today, impact the lives of tens of millions of poor people living in all regions of the world, including large segments of the poor living in economically advanced countries with social systems that support group-oriented approaches to loan making (Baradaran, 2017; Fitzpatrick & Lagory, 2010). Yunus went on to receive many international honors, including some rarely given to non-citizens, the American *Presidential Medal of Freedom* in 2009 and the American *Congressional Gold Medal* in 2010.

This chapter explores a variety of topics related to global poverty and approaches to poverty alleviation with a special focus on the major sectors and actors that are seeking to incorporate the extreme poor into the mainstream of society (Estes, 2010, 2012a, 2012b, 2015a, 2015c; Estes & Sirgy, 2017, 2018). The pursuit of social and economic justice for all peoples of the world is at the heart of this chapter (Rawls, 1971; Sen, 2011). More particularly, the chapter explores (a) the varied conceptions of poverty worldwide, including a brief discussion of "income poverty" versus the "culture of poverty" (International Monetary Fund, 2018; World Bank, 2018); (b) the distribution of income poverty by major world regions from 1970 to the present (Organization for Economic Cooperation and Development, 2018a, 2018b, 2018c); (c) the contribution of the state, the market sector, families, and civil society organizations to the resolution of both income poverty and the "culture" of poverty (Enjolras & Sivesind, 2009; Estes & Zhou, 2014); (d) the unique insights offered in identifying and more fully understanding the elusive drivers of individual and collective poverty using concepts embedded in the *Weighted Index of Social Progress* (Estes, 2007b, 2007c. 2010; Estes & Sirgy, 2018); and (e) some of the additional strategies that are designed to truly place income poverty into museums.

Poverty

In its simplest meaning, poverty is defined as the state of one who lacks a usual or socially acceptable amount of money or material possessions to satisfy his own daily needs or those of others who depend on him or her (Estes, 1999; Estes & Sirgy, 2017, 2018). The definition does, of course, refer to "income" or financial poverty and not to the more complex concept of the "culture" of poverty, which places emphasis on environmental, attitudinal, and societal forces that inhibit the capacity of people to achieve at least a minimal level of self-sufficiency within the context of the norms and traditions of the broader society. In both cases, issues associated with poor or inadequate education, poor or failing health, permanent and acute disabilities, recurrent joblessness, social discrimination, weak family ties, and other factors contribute to recurrent experiences of both income and social poverty (World Bank, 2018).

People often feel trapped in a culture of intergenerational poverty that, without a secure income social safety net, makes it difficult for many of the extreme poor to participate in the life of the community as contributive members (Day, 2009; Esping-Anderson, 1990, 1999). This situation is particularly acute among the aged, persons with serious disabilities, and children and youth who, because of age, are unable to provide fully for their own income security needs (Tiliouine & Estes, 2016; World Bank, 2018). Societies characterized by weak systems of social and income support for vulnerable populations add to the complexity of poverty alleviation approaches that are severely hampered in their efforts because of the need for basic economic support (International Social Security Association, 2018).

A Lingering Reality

Poverty has, of course, been with all societies since the beginning of civilization. Then, as now, poverty has been concentrated among age-dependent populations, those with serious disabilities, homeless persons, solitary widows, and families that experience recurrent joblessness among their key income earners. These conditions are especially serious in nations characterized by weak social infrastructures in combination with the inability of nearly all impoverished people to save some portion of their meager earnings on a regular basis (International Social Security Association, 2018). Indentured servitude often resulted in poverty at the end of the contracted labor period as did slavery: The enslaved had no possibility to accumulate savings, however small (C.W. & A.J.K.D., 2013). The situation improved only somewhat with the dramatic migration of working age men and women and, in time, their children and grandparents to urban industrial settings where jobs were at least available if not plentiful (Fitzpatrick & Lagory, 2010; Frank, 2007). This pattern has repeated itself in virtually all countries since the opening decades of the *Industrial Revolution* (1760–1840) and continues to be reflected in the often life and death choices that people in poor and conflict-ridden countries must make daily to try to gain entry as refugees into more economically advanced countries (Naldini, 2003). Unsafe seas, hostile receptions, no sponsors or jobs, and no personal financial resources have not been enough to reduce the numbers of people seeking to improve their economic circumstances by seeking either political or economic refugee status, or both, in often unwelcoming nations (UNHCR, 2018).

The Income Trap

It is important to note as well that few poor people wish to be poor. Most are trapped in a combination of complex interpersonal and social processes that keep them poor, even as others around them experience financial success. This level of relative deprivation is unwanted, especially as those affected by it perceive no way of significantly altering their income status (especially disadvantaged ethnic, racial, and religious minorities). Many of the poor, however willing, rarely can pull themselves up "by their own bootstraps," given the socioeconomic situations in which most find themselves (U.S. Census Bureau, 2010; World Bank, 2016a, 2016b, 2016c, 2016d, 2017b). After all, how does one pull oneself up by his or her own bootstraps? The picture of attempting to do so totally defies the laws of gravity!

The latter situation is especially true for the aged, children and youth, and persons with severe physical and/or emotional disabilities. Child and youth, however, have new educational opportunities available to them and in all societies are the major gateways for social mobility. For a small percentage of persons with severe disabilities, new opportunities for jobs using adaptive technologies have become available with the result that many who are blind can now read using braille and others who cannot walk or talk are able to perform seated office jobs using technologies that require only the use of their minds and arms.

External assistance, in combination with personal efforts on the part of the poor as fully as possible, has proven to be the only effective means for helping the most economically vulnerable among us to move out of poverty into a reasonable level of self-sufficiency (UN Millennium Development Goals, 2015). This assistance traditionally has taken the form of cash and technical assistance initiatives, but, increasingly, as illustrated in the efforts of Muhammad Yunus, can be even more effective when the poor themselves in partnership with major business and social enterprises become the central actors in lifting themselves out of poverty through their own means, however limited those mean may be. Political and economic migrants also are disproportionately represented among the poor as are refugees living in national or internationally sponsored places of safe haven.

Table 9.1 Poverty at the international poverty line of $1.90/day (in 2011 purchasing power parity) (World Bank, 2018)

Region	Headcount ratio (%)		No. poor (millions)	
	2013	2015	2013	2015
East Asia and Pacific	3.6	2.3	73.1	47.2
Europe and Central Asia	1.6	1.5	7.7	7.1
Latin America and the Caribbean	4.6	4.1	28.0	25.9
Middle East and North Africa	2.6	5.0	9.5	18.6
South Asia	16.2	12.4	274.5	216.4
Sub-Saharan Africa	42.5	41.1	405.1	413.3
World Total	**11.2**	**10.0**	**804.2**	**735.9**

Contemporary Trends in World Poverty

Table 9.1 identifies the number of poor people in the world as of 2013 and 2015 (World Bank, 2018). The figure reports the distribution of global poverty for major world regions using *purchasing power parity* as the uniform unit of measurement.[1] The figure also includes both headcount and actual numbers of the poor for each of the two comparison years. Using the World Bank's current standard of incomes averaging below USD 1.90 to identify the poor, several critical patterns are apparent from a critical analysis of the distribution of world poverty just reported by the World Bank and summarized in Table 9.1:

- Poverty is unevenly distributed throughout the world, albeit the rates are steadily declining in all but the Middle East and North Africa region, where poverty levels increased from 2.6% in 2013 to 5.0% of the region's population in 2015 or from 9.5 million people in 2013 to 18.6 million in 2015.
- In addition to those in the Middle East and North African region (4.0%), poverty rates were the *highest* in 2015 among the countries of the sub-Saharan Africa (41.1%) and South Asia (12.4%).
- Poverty rates during the same year were the *lowest* among the nations of Europe and Central Asia (1.5%), East Asia and the Pacific (2.3%), and Latin America and the Caribbean (4.1%).
- Major shifts also have occurred in the number of extreme poor since the outset of this study in 1970 and have declined even further in the few years that have passed between 2011, 2013, and 2015, from 804.2 million people worldwide in 2013 to 735.9 million in 2015.
- The percentage of people living in extreme poverty globally fell to a new low of 10% in 2015—the latest number available—down from 11% in 2013, reflecting *steady but slowing progress*, World Bank data show.

---

[1] *Purchasing power parity* is an economic theory that compares different countries' currencies through a "basket of goods" approach. According to this concept, two currencies are in equilibrium or at par when a basket of goods (considering the exchange rate) is priced the same in both countries. Closely related to purchasing power parity is the *law of one price*, which is an economic theory that predicts that after accounting for differences in interest rates and exchange rates, the cost of something in country X should be the same as that in country Y in real terms (Hall, 2018).

- The number of people living on less than $1.90 a day fell during this period by 68 million to 736 million.
- Significant reductions in the incidence of poverty since 2011 have and are continuing to occur among the group of socially least developed countries of Africa, Asia, and Latin America, with the most significant declines taking place in the poorest countries of developing Africa. The economic situations of these regions, countries, and populations are discussed more fully in Chaps. 4–6.

Poverty rates are expected to decline even more rapidly as the United Nations *Sustainable Development Goals* (SDG) campaign, which is centrally focused on poverty reduction, is fully implemented in the most economically vulnerable nations of developing sub-Saharan Africa, South Asia, and selected countries of Latin America and the Caribbean. However, currently and hopefully for only a short time, the reduction in global poverty has slowed since 2015 in response to the economic sluggishness of the world's largest trading economies (International Monetary Fund, 2018; United Nations Development Programme, 2014; World Bank, 2017a). These same countries are major military and political allies of selected groups of socially least developed countries. They also have been the center of major recurrent

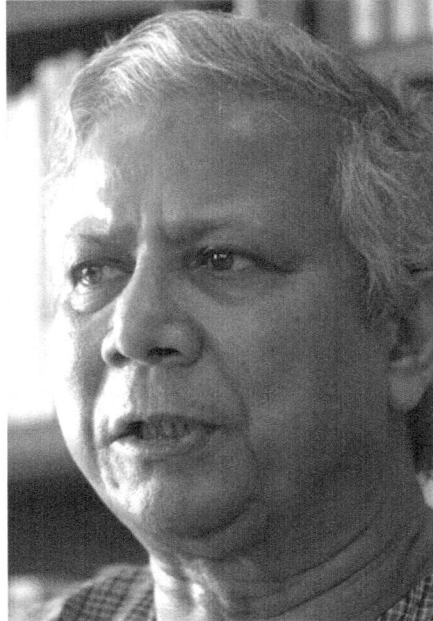

Fig. 9.1 Dr. Muhammad Yunus, Nobel Peace Prize winner, 2006. Photo by Tanveer Islam, Texas A&M University. (https://commons.wikimedia.org/wiki/File:Muhammad_Yunus.jpg. This file is licensed under the Creative Commons Attribution 3.0 Unported license)

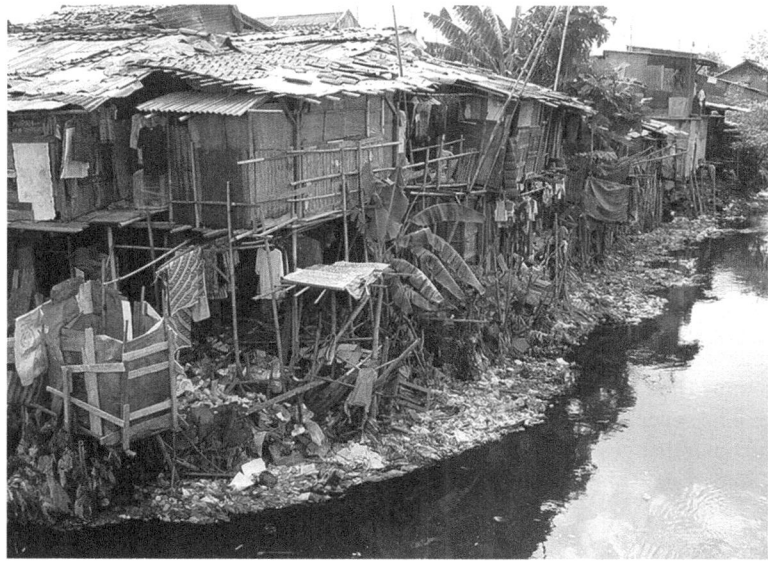

Fig. 9.2 Slums built on swamp land near a garbage dump in East Cipinang, Jakarta Indonesia. Photo by Jonathan McIntosh. (https://commons.wikimedia.org/wiki/File:Jakarta_slumhome_2. jpg. This file is licensed under the Creative Commons Attribution 2.0 Generic license)

military conflicts and prolonged intraregional wars (Stockholm International Peace Research Institute, 2018). This trend is not expected to continue over the long term (Figs. 9.1 and 9.2).

The World Bank has pointed to the need for even higher levels of international investments in poverty alleviation efforts to remain on its planned course of action to reduce the harsh economic challenges that confront the populations of many nations. These investments can take many forms but cannot simply be grants-in-aid or gifts made to or as foreign direct investment, cooperative trade agreements such as the North American Free Trade Agreement and those organized by the Association of Southeast Asian Nations and other approaches to the most economically impoverished nations. The key to what is needed, from the World Bank's perspective (and that of other partners in the Sustainable Development Goals [SDG]), is broad-based *investment* in the social, political, economic, and technological systems of developing countries. Improved educational systems, better and more effective health services, improved housing and sanitation systems, and incentives for external businesses to invest in the economic life of developing countries are especially critical to reducing the incidence of income poverty in nearly all developing nations. Less corrupt governments and businesses are necessary to achieve these objectives as are more participatory forms of governance at all levels of political organization (Freedom House, 2018; Transparency International, 2018). And, as Dr. Yunus taught us through his example, women and women's development must be central to these new initiatives if centuries of gender-defined economic and social disparities are to be eliminated.

The preceding outcomes are central objectives articulated in the SDG's current 15-year campaign of development assistance to the world's poorest and socially least developed countries. This campaign is now underway and most signatories to the SDGs are working actively to fulfill their commitments. Increased levels of political conservatism in the United States and Europe combined with the emergence of a larger number of autocratic political regimes in selected developing countries (e.g., Iran, Iraq, Syria, Yemen) have, however, prevented even the best intended international development assistance organizations from fully achieving their objectives (Transparency International, 2018). These problems will likely linger for some time until their leaders recognize the central role of participatory governance and open global markets in promoting national development through peaceful interchanges and cooperative alliances with their citizens and those of nearby and distant nations (International Monetary Fund, 2018; World Business Council, 2017).

Income Disparities and Global Poverty

Another approach to understanding the extent of national and global poverty is to examine the degree of income (and wealth) disparities that characterize nations. The data related to income disparity are more difficult to ascertain but, to the extent available, offer entirely new insights in more fully understanding the unique needs of national populations that are economically both more and less advanced than others (Estes, 2012a, 2012b). Income disparities exist within all societies including in the most economically egalitarian nations of Northern Europe, including in welfare advanced Scandinavia (Ascoli & Ranci, 2002; Esping-Anderson, 1990, 1999; Schramm-Nielsen, 2002). Disparity in income and wealth distribution is a global issue that requires attention by all major actors in the development sector, especially as these disparities contribute to reinforcement of poverty among that large majority of the population that, as Collier (2007) has reported, remains trapped at the bottom of the wealth pyramid (Clark & Senik, 2017; Graham, 2012; Helliwell, Layard & Sachs, 2017).

The Gap in Global Wealth (and Income) Distribution

This section explores the extent of income disparities in the world as a whole and in selected groups of income- and wealth-generating nations (Estes, 2010, 2015c; Estes & Sirgy, 2017, 2018; Glatzer, 2002; Layard, 2017; Thompson, 2012). The global wealth gap data reported in Fig. 9.3 magnify the dramatic discrepancies that exist among the four dominant wealth groups identified with the result that, today, 3.3 billion across the globe (71% of the global population) have access to less than

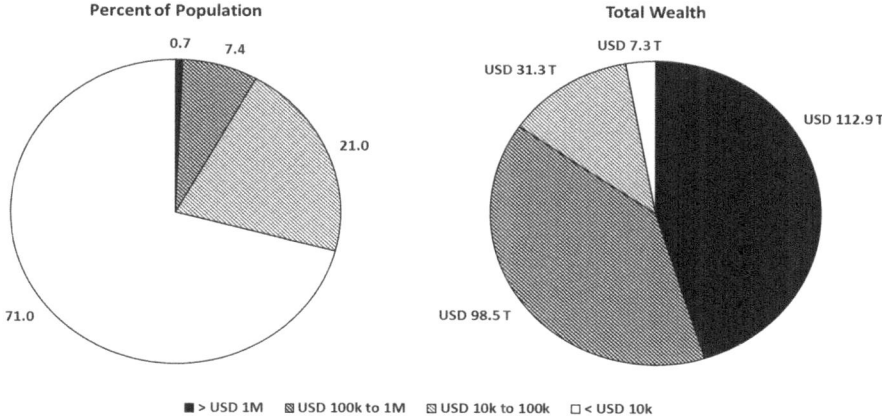

Fig. 9.3 World and distribution by percentage of global population, 2000–2014. (Prepared by David Walker based using data based on Davies, Lluberas, & Shorrocks, 2017)

$10,000 and, of that, fewer than 80% have incomes or wealth equivalent to more than USD 5000. On the other end, just 34 million people globally have resources of more than USD one million *but* the top 0.7% own outright more than 45% of all the wealth generated globally in any given year—in 2015, USD 113 trillion. The flow of wealth annually to the already rich represents an astonishing 84.6% of the world's total wealth (Henneberg, 2017; Organization for Economic Cooperation and Development, 2018a; World Bank, 2017a, 2017b).

The data presented in Fig. 9.3 were prepared by the international banking house *Credit Suisse* (2017), but the data summarized in the figure vary among other economic and social scholars. The well-known French economist Thomas Piketty notes that "wealth is so concentrated that a large segment of society is virtually unaware of its existence" (2017: 259). This is a troubling statement and speaks to the sense of economic isolation that many poor experience with respect to their participation in local and national markets. There is very little opportunity for them to achieve a more prominent position given the highly disadvantaged economic circumstances under which they live. Thus, even among scholars working within very differing conceptual and empirical frameworks agreement exists that, in all but the most socially progressive societies, the maldistribution of wealth and income remains essentially the same, i.e., more than half of a country's wealth tends to be concentrated among just 1–2% of the national population whereas 70–90% of a country's population have access to less than 5% of a country's total economic and fiscal resources (International Monetary Fund 2018; World Bank. 2017b).

These two patterns have changed little since the end of the Second World War and likely will continue to exist well into the future. Attainment of the 17 goals of the SDGs, however, will result in increasing levels of economic parity between the groups but the goal of full economic equality between the various groups of social "haves" and "have nots" will require a series of such campaigns over an extended

Table 9.2 Top 25 performing countries on the WISP18, 1990–2017/18 (N = 25)

WISP00	WISP10/11	WISP17/18	Country	WSPRNK00	WISP10/11RNK	RKWSP17/18
107	72	99	**Denmark**	2	1	1
100	71	98	**Germany**	6	4	2
100	70	97	**Austria**	7	5	3
91	65	97	**Japan**	18	17	4
107	71	95	**Sweden**	1	3	5
98	67	95	**Italy**	9	12	6
101	66	95	**Finland**	4	13	7
98	68	95	**Iceland**	8	8	8
97	68	94	**Belgium**	10	9	9
104	72	94	**Norway**	3	2	10
95	67	94	**Netherlands**	13	11	11
93	66	93	**New Zealand**	17	15	12
90	64	93	**Portugal**	20	21	13
74	59	93	**Lithuania**	38	37	14
96	65	92	**United Kingdom**	11	19	15
94	67	92	**France**	14	10	16
89	62	92	**Bulgaria**	23	28	17
94	65	92	**Ireland**	15	20	18
88	66	92	**Czech Rep**	24	14	19
89	68	92	**Australia**	22	7	20
81	57	91	**Estonia**	31	44	21
96	65	91	**Spain**	12	18	22
70	62	91	**Croatia**	42	27	23
90	65	91	**Greece**	21	16	24
86	64	90	**Canada**	26	24	25

period. Even then, a certain percentage of the population is likely to remain income poor but, hopefully, the drivers that sustain the "culture of poverty," especially those associated with intergenerational poverty, likely will be significantly diminished (Alber et al., 2004; Blome, Keck & Alber, 2009).

Highest Income and Most Socially Developed Countries

The countries with the highest average levels of per capita *gross national income* (GNI) levels and the Weighted Index of Social Progress (WISP) scores in 2018 (the proxy variable used for subjective well-being in this report) are listed by rank order in Tables 9.2 and 9.3. In addition to ordering the countries by the most recent WISP scores, WISP scores also are presented for these countries for each decade beginning with 1980. WISP rank order positions for these countries for the same decade

Table 9.3 Bottom 25 performing countries on the WISP18, 1990–2017/18 (N = 25)

WISP00	WISP10/11	WISP17/18	Country	WSPRNK00	WISP10/11RNK	RKWSP17/18
2	32	41	Cen African Rep*	151	152	162
−4	26	47	Chad*	154	156	161
−10	25	48	Sierra Leone*	159	159	160
8	35	48	Yemen*	145	141	159
1	17	48	Somalia*	152	161	158
−4	37	48	Nigeria	156	137	157
7	37	49	Uganda*	146	135	156
13	35	49	Sudan*	138	142	155
14	35	50	Niger*	133	143	154
−19	17	51	Afghanistan*	162	162	153
−12	38	51	Ethiopia*	160	134	152
24	37	51	Zimbabwe	119	136	151
12	35	52	Cote D'Ivoire	143	145	150
−10	26	52	Angola*	158	158	149
13	39	52	Mali*	137	130	148
22	39	54	Zambia*	125	126	147
20	42	54	Tanzania* Rep.	127	115	146
15	36	54	Cameroon	132	138	145
−2	26	54	Congo, DR*	153	157	144
3	40	54	Burkina Faso*	150	125	143
−15	29	55	Eritrea*	161	153	142
14	34	55	Togo*	135	147	141
4	33	55	Mozambique*	148	149	140
−4	32	56	Guinea*	155	151	139
13	34	56	Gambia* The	139	146	138

are summarized in the tables, which provide a fuller perspective of the overall development levels of the two groups of nations presented in the tables.

Gini income equality scores, historically a major measure of national wealth inequality, are inferred by the rank order positions of each nations and provide an even fuller understanding of the rate of development progress that is taking place within and between the richest and poorest countries for all 38 years reported on in Tables 9.2 and 9.3 using the 40-item WISP scores as the basis of analysis of WISP scores for each of the years and decades reported in the tables (Estes, 2015b, 2015c). Thus, Tables 9.2 and 9.3 confirm the relationship that exists between and within the net wealth levels accumulated by countries with already high levels of per capita income, an economic reality that has proven very difficult for many middle- and low-income countries to overcome (Baradaran, 2017; Lozado, 2017; Thompson, 2012).

The per capita GNI income scores reported in the two GNI tables are very clear and identify those economically advanced countries with the highest (Table 9.2) and lowest (Table 9.3) average per capita income levels. Most of these countries in the first table are in Europe, especially northern Europe, plus selected countries in North America, East Asia, and the Middle East.

Average GNI scores for the clusters of nations included in the tables and the larger WISP database range from a high of USD 103,630, USD 92,200, and USD 76,270 for Norway, Qatar, and Macau, respectively. The average GNI estimate for all 25 countries included in Table 9.2 for 2017 is USD 54,024 (Burton, 2017a). By contrast, average Gini coefficient scores ranged from a highly favorable 21.5 for Finland and a highly unfavorable Gini score of 53.7 for Hong Kong with a group average of 31.9 for 2016/17/18. Thus, GNI levels among the world's highest earning nations are very favorable albeit with the result that wealth redistribution outcomes are highly skewed in favor of already wealthy corporations, families, and individuals (CIA, 2018; *Economy Watch*, 2018).

The net wealth patterns of several countries included in Table 9.2 are governed by either direct or constitutional monarchy political systems (Serafin, 2009). These monarchies have accumulated vast sums of wealth, although in countries such as the United Kingdom many of the most precious resources previously owned by the monarchy now belong entirely to the state. As a result, many countries use the accumulated wealth of their monarchies as sources of the tangible resources to support their printed currencies, the latter of which have no intrinsic value other than the paper and ink used to print them. Accumulated over decades, indeed centuries, the personal and state-controlled wealth of many royal families often is astounding and provides the basis around which their macroeconomic systems are organized (Serafin, 2009; Woods, 2018).

In another sector, scores on the WISP may be considered "proxy variables" for assessing the extent of *subjective* well-being of an entire society's population. The WISP itself consists only of objective indicators, but each of its now 40 indicators represents a potential opportunity for and, in some cases, a roadblock to achieving progressively more advanced levels of subjective well-being for people at both ends of WISP's continuum (Estes, 2007a, 2010; Estes, 2019–SIR). WISP scores are global, regional, and national in their construction and permit important differences between each national population group to manifest themselves on a scale that has a theoretical range of 0 to 100 for each period studied. The WISP or variations of it also have been used at the subnational level to monitor the social progress and well-being of smaller agglomerations of people (Estes & Sirgy, 2017, 2018).

High-income countries with the most favorable WISP scores for the period 2000–2011 are Sweden (WISP rank = 1/162), Denmark (WISP rank = 1/162), and Norway (WISP rank = 3/162); these countries also frequently appear on the list of the world's happiest countries and, owing to their aggressive taxation policies, also are among the nations with the most favorable levels of wealth distribution (Layard, 2017; Organization for Economic Cooperation and Development, 2018a). The same pattern appears for all the data reported in Table 9.2 and reflects a broad range of societal policies focused on promoting the broadest possible distribution of wealth and income within their societies. These countries also are committed to having tightly woven social safety nets; at the same time, they contribute the highest percentage of their GDP to international development assistance to the world's poorest countries (Organization for Economic Cooperation and Development, 2018a).

These Scandinavian nations are both leaders within Europe and, as result of their commitment to peace through development, they have served as role models of a new paradigm[2] for assisting other nations in formulating their domestic and international development assistance policies (Organization for Economic Cooperation and Development, 2015a, 2015b, 2017a; 2018b, 2018c). The nations of Scandinavia arrived at their advanced social policy decisions following decades, in some cases centuries, of brutal warfare between neighboring societies. Most also experienced the ravages of Nazi occupation during WWII, which, among many other lessons, taught them the importance of peace, social development, and social welfare. Of importance as well are the high levels of happiness and life satisfaction that are reported repeatedly for these nations (Helliwell, Layard, and Sachs, 2017; Layard, 2017; Veenhoven, 2019; World Values Survey, 2015). Their comparatively small size, their shared cultural values and norms, and their national and regional commitments to one another have added considerably to the high standard of living enjoyed by the nations of Scandinavia. They also share their deeply felt realization that peace can only be achieved through development, including a more equitable distribution of national wealth among all the citizens of their countries. Recent diversity-related social conflicts associated with large-scale immigration to these countries (Schramm-Nielsen, 2002), have, at least for the moment, disrupted this social contract. In time, these conflicts, too, are expected to be minimized.

Lowest Income and Socially Least Developed Countries

The world's 25 lowest income and wealth accumulating countries are identified in Table 9.3 (Burton, 2017b). Table 9.3 is structured in the same way as Table 9.2 in that it orders economically low-performing countries primarily based on their GNI level for 2015. The table also reports Gini coefficients[3] for the most recent year available as well as rank position on the WISP for 2018 relative to the overall social performances of 162 countries that contain approximately 95% of the world's total population (Organization for Economic Cooperation and Development, 2018b).

As reported in Table 9.3, the countries with the lowest levels of GNI and, therefore of WISP scores and patterns of subjective well-being since 1990, include Malawi (WISP rank = 117/162), Burundi (WISP rank = 147/162), Central African Republic (WISP rank = 153/162), Liberia (WISP rank = 161/162), and the Democratic Republic of Congo (WISP rank = 154/162). Although many of the

---

[2] See Kuhn (1996) for a fuller discussion of the range of revolutionary paradigms that drive the social policies of nations.

[3] The Gini index or Gini coefficient is a statistical measure of distribution developed by the Italian statistician Corrado Gini in 1912. It is often used as a gauge of economic inequality, measuring income distribution or, less commonly, wealth distribution among a population. The coefficient ranges from 0 (or 0%) to 1 (or 100%), with 0 representing perfect equality and 1 representing perfect inequality. Values over 1 are theoretically possible due to negative income or wealth (*Investopedia*, 2018).

economies of these countries are not completely money-driven (but depend more on barter for economic exchanges), all 25 countries identified in Table 9.3 are desperately poor and lack many of the most essential resources needed to meet even the most basic needs of their growing populations (Galasso, 2013; Piketty, 2015). This process of profound and deepening poverty has been underway for many decades and has accelerated during the past 10-year period for several of these nations even as overall levels of social development in sub-Saharan Africa have increased (Estes, 2015a; World Bank, 2017c). This pattern is not an altogether surprising one since it mirrors patterns that exists among virtually all economically disadvantaged countries of developing Africa, Asia, and, to a lesser extent, Latin America and the Caribbean (Estes & Tiliouine, 2014; World Bank, 2016b, 2017b).

Most of the nations included in Table 9.3 are in sub-Saharan Africa and, as with the top 25 income-earning or wealthy countries, considerable variation exists with respect to the overall pattern of social development of these countries (Møller and Roberts, 2017). Most the world's poorest nations are characterized by widespread poverty, low levels of education, inadequate health systems, and weak to nonexistent social welfare systems. The bulk of their trade is intranational and, when outside of the country, primarily involves unrefined natural resources, low- to semi-skilled labor, and, increasingly, contract labor arrangements with more economically advanced nations in North Africa and West Asia (World Bank, 1999, 2016c, 2017a).

The bottom 25 of the world's income earning nations are located among the poorest countries of the developing Americas, Haiti, and two of Asia's poorest countries, Afghanistan and Nepal, albeit many others could be added to an extended list (World Bank, 2016b). All these countries have been on the list of the world's lowest income earning nations for many decades and, in the case of Afghanistan-Iraq-Syria, war and recurrent civil strife have deprived these countries not only of their own resources but also of those of international development assistance organizations as well (Stockholm International Peace Research Institute, 2018). All 25 of the world's lowest income earners are countries designated by the United Nations for preferential development assistance (e.g., UN Millennium Development Goals, 2015). Even so, the pace of social and economic development in all 25 of the currently lowest economically performing countries continues to lag behind the level of social progress being achieved by many of the world's developing nations (United Nations Development Programme, 2016). As has been the reality for several decades, these countries will continue to require proactive development assistance and even more favorable economic partnerships with the world's top and middle performing countries. These more aggressive actions are needed to reduce the high levels of poverty and low development in other sectors that continue to trap successive generations of young people in the social pathologies that have entrapped their parents and earlier generations.

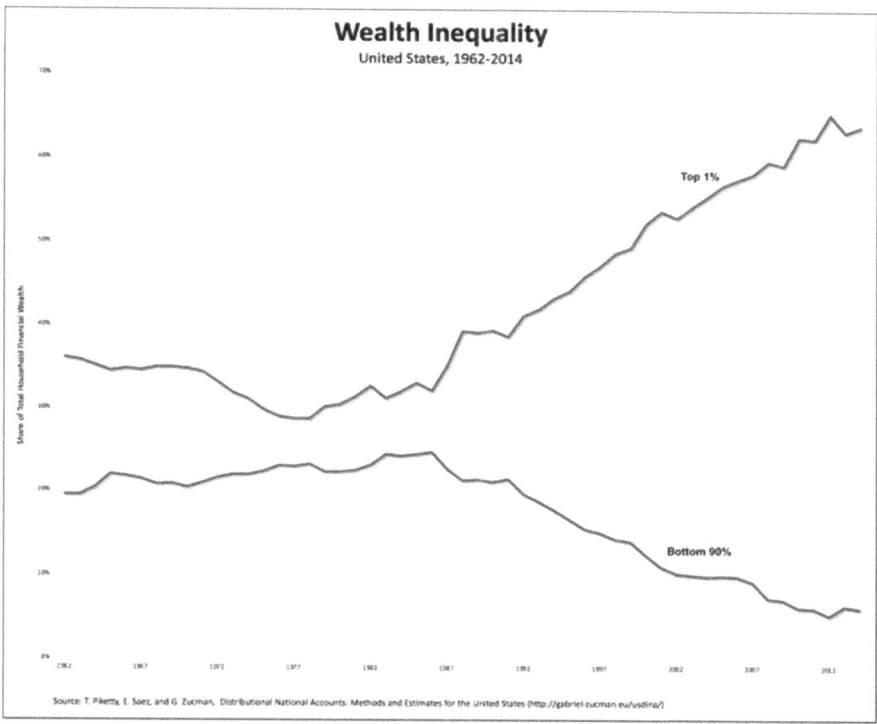

Fig. 9.4 Wealth inequality: United States, 1962–2014 (Piketty, Saez, & Zucman, 2018)

Wealth and Income Inequality: The Conundrum

The Widening Gap in Income and Wealth Gap Illustrated

The global wealth gap is most apparent within selected economically advanced nations. The gap is especially extreme in the highest income- and wealth-producing countries, albeit poverty rates also are high in many of these countries. We have discussed many of the dominant features of these nations, but for illustrative purposes, it is useful to paint some broad-brush strokes concerning these patterns. Figure 9.4 provides an illustration of the extreme income and wealth gap that exists in the United States, the country with the world's largest and most abundant economy. The data reflected in Fig. 9.4 portray the dramatic nature of the gap as well as the accelerated pace of economic inequality that has been increasing over recent decades. For policy specialists, these data are especially stark given the very high levels of national wealth available to the United States to resolve its economic inequality challenges combined with its failure to do so. Angela Monaghan, writing in *The Guardian*, noted that "not since the Great Depression has wealth inequality in the US been so acute" (Monaghan, 2014). The macroeconomic environment, as reported throughout the chapter, has not improved very much since the early 1980s.

One of the great challenges of this century will be to narrow the currently widening gap between the world's richest and poorest countries (Schrieberg, 2018; Vanham, 2015; World Bank, 2017a). This gap has continued to widen despite unparalleled levels of economic growth, declining poverty rates, and high levels of social and economic cooperation between nations, especially between those of the poorest countries of developing Africa, Asia, Latin America, and the Caribbean (Møller & Roberts, 2017; Schrieberg, 2018). Nevertheless, these impressive increases in national growth have not "trickled" down to the lowest income groups in either economically well-off or developing countries (Collier, 2007; UK Essays, 2013; Vanham, 2015). Further, the pattern of income distribution of Northern Europe and America as well as East Asia and Oceania remains highly concentrated. To date, public policies related to economic redistribution, including progressive income taxes, have not proven effective for bringing about the sought after economic redistributions to the lowest income classes—this despite the reality that the inequality between the world's well off and impoverished regions and nations continues to increase (Schrieberg, 2018; Vacas-Soriano & Fernández-Macías, 2017).

Part of the income gap reported for the world's rich and poor nations has had a profound impact on the *subjective* well-being of the populations of these countries, especially those at the lower end of the socioeconomic ladder. This experience also is pronounced among the highly vulnerable members of the middle class of these nations who are deeply in debt because of borrowing for expensive homes, payment of college fees for their age-eligible children (including for many Europeans with their generous free or subsidized tuition for higher education and health schemes), uninsured ill-health care, and various types of consumer debt but especially for home mortgages and automobiles, loans for financial gifts to children, home improvements, and vacations financed through borrowing. This gradual, in some countries, rapid, sliding downward of the middle class has considerably weakened their capacity to compete effectively with more economically secure nations (Fox, 2012; Frank, 2007; Krugman, 2003; Piketty, 2015, 2017; Stiglitz, 2013).

Growth in the wealth gap both within and between nations is not a new or even recent phenomenon (Collier, 2007; Organization for Economic Cooperation and Development, 2017a; World Bank, 1999, 2016b, 2017b). Indeed, the phenomenon has been occurring throughout most of recorded history but only now, has it reached a level that seriously interferes with the capacity of both rich and poor countries to strive for a *reasonable degree of economic parity* and, with it, social justice (Piketty, 2017; Sen, 2011; World Bank, 2017a). Comparatively little evidence can be found to show that, owing to the breadth of the wealth gap, economic parity can ever be achieved—despite robust public approaches to wealth redistribution that already are in place via progressive income and estate tax schemes associated with the gross income of individuals, or following their deaths, on their taxable estates (Organization for Economic Cooperation and Development, 2017b; World Bank, 1999, 2017a). Taken together, these critical drivers of wealth redistribution designed to promote wealth equality appear inadequate given the magnitude of the wealth gap that already exists and is continuing to increase (Estes, 2012b, 2015c; World Bank, 2016b, 2017b).

The Uneven Distribution of Income Poverty

Much of what drives public policy initiatives in promoting greater equality between income groups is the fact that low income, poverty, and structural rigidity with few opportunities for social mobility do not come naturally to modern nations, especially in the distribution of the abundant natural and human capital resources that characterize most nations…even those at the bottom of the income ladder (Estes, 2012a, 2012b). Indeed, low- and middle-income people typically work long hours, produce a wide range of goods, make many financial sacrifices to provide for the needs of their family member, and, contribute significant resources to the well-being of others in their communities (Italian National Institute of Statistics, 2017; Organization for Economic Cooperation and Development, 2017b). These families also borrow money to finance the educational career opportunities available to their children and provide social and economic support for aged, injured, and disabled members of both their immediate families and extended kinship systems. Most also support the religious organizations to which they belong and contribute to local and international charities. Now, as in the past, members of low- and middle-income groups also provide support for a broad range of philanthropic entities from which they receive no direct benefits.

Among the poor, these activities have been mirrored in the predominately agricultural communities in which they live, even in the absence of sufficient quantities of potable water and effective means for eliminating solid and liquid waste—a troublesome pattern that exists for many poor people worldwide. The gap between the very poor and the very rich, as well as those classified as part of the socioeconomic "middle class," is one that continues to widen (Baradaran, 2017; Henneberg, 2017).

Poverty combined with a shrinking of the middle class in Europe (Alber et al., 2004; Collins & Bendner, 2016; Vacas-Soriano & Fernández-Macías, 2017) and North America is a major driver of the wealth gap that accentuates the complex cultural norms, inadequate educational levels, uneven access to quality health care in combination with the low skills that many poor people bring to the labor force of their countries. The situation is especially complex among refugees who enter more economically advanced nations (either legally or illegally) and who possess few of the skills needed to make themselves economically competitive (UNHCR, 2018). This situation has reached historically high levels among the advantaged member states of the Organization for Economic Cooperation and Development, which depend on persons at the low end of the wealth continuum to perform services that members of the dominant population either no longer wish to perform (mostly low-skilled jobs involving manual labor) or where the national net population replacement rates are very low on average (< 2.0 births per household) such that the admittance of disproportionate numbers of migrants has become an economic necessity to sustain their economies and elderly-focused social welfare systems (International Social Security Association, 2018).

The contemporary situation involving the flow of migrants from developing to economically advanced countries is summed up by an article that appeared in a recent edition of the *New Scientist* (Editor, 2016).

As birth rates plummet in the developed world, migrants are keeping our economies afloat. They account for half of the increase in the US workforce since 2005, and 70 per cent in Europe. Even so, the number of people of working age supporting each retiree over 65 is falling. In 2000, this "dependency ratio" was 4:1 across the European Union. Today it is 3.5:1. And even with current levels of migration it is set to fall to 2 by 2050.

Employers benefit from the wealth surpluses generated by low- and middle-income workers as well as from the high, usually excessive, profits associated with the employment of workers who generated very high levels of wealth for their employers. This is especially the case in work settings where few benefits, in the absence of effective social safety nets, are paid to workers who become ill, injured, or disabled or lose their jobs entirely (International Social Security Association, 2018). Such workers, owing to their dependence on paid employment, are subject to high levels of economic exploitation even as the benefits of their low-wage labor flow from their communities to societies located in the richer nations located north of the equator. The difficulties associated with these situations are made more complex in the world's poorest countries that have very weak or entirely absent social welfare systems designed to insure at least minimum levels of financial support for population groups that are not able to provide fully for their income requirements, e.g., children and youth, the aged, and persons with severe disabilities (ILO, 2019).

As outlined by Estes & Zhou (2014), effective systems of social support for workers at all levels of society require the active reinforcement of four core sectors that make up the social systems of every society, i.e., *the market*—including businesses (Cawson, 1982; Day, 2009; Estes, 2012a), *the state*—at all levels of political organization (United Nations Development Programme, 1997), *the family*—including extended kinship systems (Blome, Keck, & Alber 2009), and *non-governmental organizations* (NGOs)—ranging from international to locally based NGOs (Ascoli & Ranci, 2002; Enjolras & Sivesind, 2009; NCCS, 2004; Salaman, 2012).

Fig. 9.5 Poverty alleviation stakeholders: The core institutions and civil society organizations (Estes & Zhou, 2014; Evers & Wintersberger, 1988)

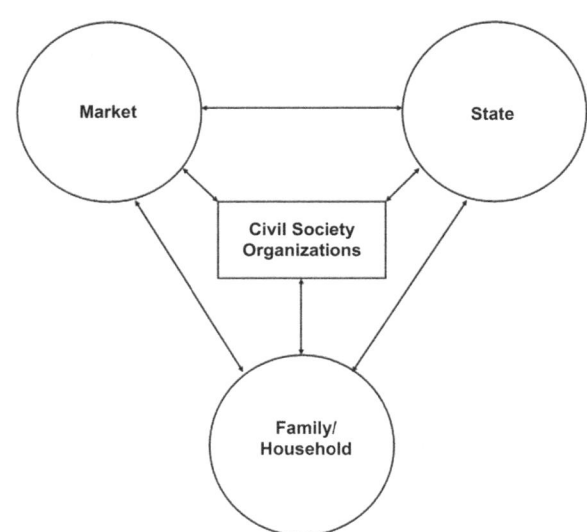

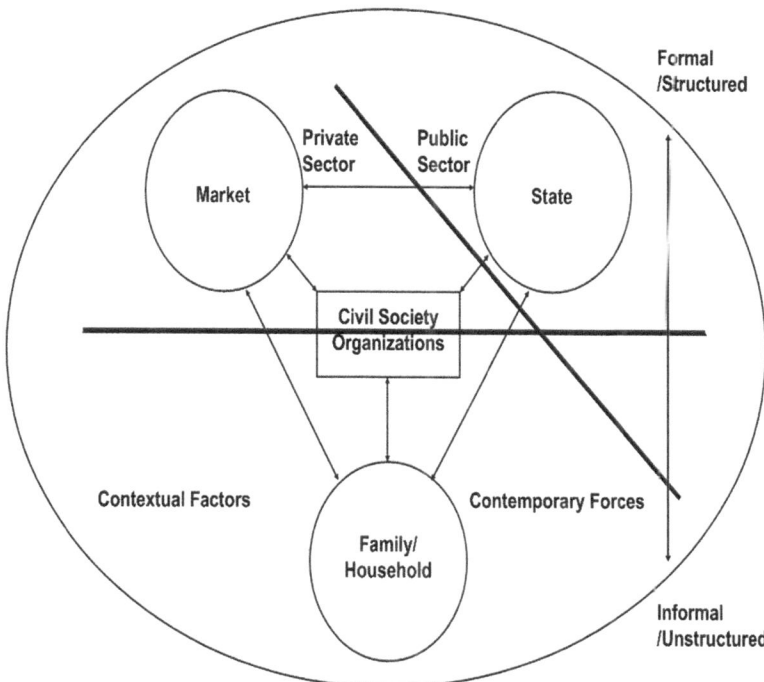

Fig. 9.6 Interactions between the major stakeholders in poverty alleviation. (Estes & Zhou, 2014)

Figures 9.5 and 9.6 illustrate the highly varied public-private relationships that exist between these key state and non-state actors and that emphasize all members of society within a social, political, demographic, and ecological context (Estes & Zhou, 2014). The figures also address the degree of formality of each sector as well as the reality that most of the contributors to the well-being of people, whether they are rich or poor or middle-income, are located primarily in the *private* sector. Only the governmental sector is *public* in origin, and its support systems are the many publicly funded NGOs that depend heavily or entirely on public financial resources to perform their functions. This pattern is more intriguing in that the three private sectors depend heavily on private philanthropy (composed primarily of the economically "well-off") to implement their mission in cooperation with local, national, and international levels of government. Progressive tax systems are at the center of the process and depend exclusively on tax revenues and fees generated from wealthy persons, businesses, and moderate to high-level wage earners to carry out its far-reaching public mandates—including the creation of at least a minimally secure social safety net for the benefit of all citizens (International Social Security Association, 2018; Salaman, 2012).

Stakeholders in Poverty Alleviation

The role of government as the provider of choice in social welfare has expanded considerably since the launch of the *Millennium Development Campaign* (MDC) in 2005.[4] The recently adopted 17 SDGs that followed the conclusion of the 8-goal MDC in 2015 reinforced the contribution of governments in working with the private sector in all regions of the world (United Nations, 2015). Their combined efforts have accentuated the importance of collaboration between various policy stakeholders in achieving objectives that no one actor can achieve alone. The major public and private actors in social development more generally and in poverty alleviation more specifically have been identified by Estes and & Zhou (2014) in graphic form. These stakeholders and their complex policy-oriented interactions are identified below.

Figure 9.5, for example, identifies the four major stakeholders in local, regional, national, and international development across the world. The figure is built on an earlier model conceptualized by Evers & Wintersberger (1988) identifies the major stakeholders needed to promote poverty alleviation, but the size of the oval assigned to each stakeholders in the figure are equal in size when, in fact, the level of contribution made by each stakeholder, especially that of the state sector, varies considerably and, thus, the size of the ovals should be adjusted accordingly. But the current depiction serves our present purposes and no further adjustments are needed given that the purpose of the figure is to both identify the four stakeholders and to show the highly dynamic interrelationships that exist between them. As depicted in Estes & Zhou (2014), in Fig. 9.5 effective systems of social support for families at all levels of society require the active participation and mutual reinforcement of all four major stakeholders found in every society, i.e., *the market* (including businesses and employers) (Habisch & Jonker, 2005), *the state*—at all levels of political organization, *the family* (including extended kinship systems), and NGOs[5] (ranging from international to locally based NGOs). All four of society's major policy stakeholders make a significant contribution toward both sustaining and alleviating poverty (Blome, Keck, & Alber, 2009; Cawson, 1982; Habisch & Jonker, 2005; Thompson, 2012). This is the situation in all societies of the world, both those that are economically advanced and those that are economically developing countries, including the poorest and least socially developed countries (Estes, 2015a).

---

[4] The eight *Millennium Development Goals* were established by the United Nations in 2005 for the purpose of (1) eradicating extreme poverty and hunger; (2) achieving universal primary school education; (3) promoting gender equality and the empowerment of women; (4) reducing child mortality; (5) improving maternal health; (6) combating HIV/AIDS, malaria, and other diseases; (7) ensuring environmental sustainability; and (8) establishing a global partnership for development (United Nations 2010; United Nations Development Programme, 2016).

[5] "Civil society organizations often are referred to as non-governmental organizations, private voluntary organizations, or as the third or independent sector. This chapter uses the umbrella term "civil society organizations" to include all private, voluntary organizations that are established and largely financed by people themselves to carry out some public benefit activity that they either do not want government to undertake (e.g., family planning services) or which government for a variety of reasons cannot or should not undertake (e.g., support for religions and the performance of religious services).

Contextual Factors Influencing Stakeholders in Their Poverty Alleviation Efforts

Figure 9.6 illustrates the highly varied public-private relationships that exist between the major policy stakeholders of every society (Gourevitch, 2008) and places the contribution of each stakeholder within its appropriate social, political, demographic, and ecological context. Figure 9.6 also addresses the degree of formality of each sector as well as the reality that most of the contributors to the well-being of people, whether they are rich or poor or middle-income, are located primarily in the *private* sectors. *Only the governmental sector is public in origin and support systems and, to an extent, so, too, are the many publicly funded non-governmental organizations that depend heavily or entirely on public financial resources to perform their functions.* This pattern is more intriguing in that the three private sectors depend heavily on private philanthropy (composed primarily of the economically "well-off") to implement their missions. The government, as the representative of the people, depends exclusively on tax revenues and fees generated from wealthy persons, businesses, and moderate to high-level wage earners to carry out its far-reaching public mandates (including the creation of a secure social safety net for the benefit of all citizens) (Italian National Institute of Statistics, 2017).

Discussion and Conclusion

This chapter has sought to offer a fresh perspective on the theory and methodology of comparative poverty and poverty analysis. More particularly, I have sought to reconceptualize an earlier model of the "welfare mix" from the vantage point of the major objectives associated with poverty alleviation as well as the central "policy stakeholders" who give direction to these initiatives. The underlying goals of the scholars associated with this area of policy development are multiple, but all are focused on the central goal of reducing both income inequality and the culture of poverty in all major regions of the world (Powell, & Barrientos, 2004; United Nations Development Programme, 2017b; World Bank, 2016c).

The author believes that a fuller understanding of the genesis, nature, structure, and dynamics of contemporary poverty alleviation efforts can best be understood through an examination of the interactions that occur over time between and within the four core welfare institutions and their complex networks of interstitial organizations.

Putting Poverty into Museums

The innovative poverty alleviation conceptual framework and stakeholder model identified by Estes & Zhou (2014) in this chapter incorporates an analysis of each of society's micro and macro social, political, economic and welfare institutions as well as the major factors that impact these systems. This latter set of policy responses differs dramatically across societies whereas the four core institutions and their four most critical policy challenges remain constant.

Further, the two figures used to illustrate the interrelationships (Figs. 9.5 and 9.6) and the nature of chronic poverty in the United States (Fig. 9.4) present a highly varied pattern of poverty and of potential solutions to poverty resolution that inform the major stakeholders in poverty alleviation as well as a wide range of actions that they can undertake to resolve the issues. As presented, the relationships among the stakeholders are multidimensional as are the types of fiscal and technical assistance interventions needed to reduce the extent of poverty in the world's poorest nations (Estes, 1999; World Bank, 2018). None of these courses of actions alone, though, can be undertaken immediately nor will the responses to them be rapid. Time, talent, resources, and perspiration over an extended period are needed to bring about the economic transformations that are needed to reduce poverty. Active engagement by all the societal stakeholders in bringing about social change is needed as is the full participation of people themselves in the efforts needed to bring about fundamental changes required to lift themselves out of poverty. These multilateral efforts are needed urgently if we are to succeed in putting extreme poverty in museums in our own lifetimes. Nothing short of this global level of socioeconomic, technological, and related sectors of development can be expected to achieve such a global goal that impacts on the quality of life and well-being of hundreds of millions of people living in social developing and even in selected economically advanced nations worldwide (Estes & Sirgy, 2017).

Full implementation of the UN's *Sustainable Development Goals* (2015–2030), which are built on the earlier decade of global achievements realized under the rubric of the MDC (2005–2015), is expected to be the major driver of poverty alleviation in the poorest developing countries of Africa, Asia, and Latin America (as well as in selected middle income socially advanced countries in Europe, North America, and the large number of countries that form the Middle East and North Africa region). These efforts are expected to be highly successful and, building on past international accomplishments, are expected to raise tens of millions of people out of extreme financial poverty, especially in China and India (United Nations Development Programme, 2017b; World Bank, 2017a, 2017b).

All the expected preceding sociopolitical and economic challenges are especially evident in developing and least developed countries (Estes, 2015a; United Nations, 2010; World Bank, 2017a, 2017b), but they also constitute the major policy challenges that confront economically advanced countries (Weingast & Wittman, 2006; Estes, 2010; United Nations Development Programme, 2010). A thoughtful review of each nation's contextual and contemporary social challenges is essential for arriving at an adequate understanding of the responsibilities that are assigned to each of social welfare's major institutional actors. Thus, the model is especially useful in (1) describing the current state of welfare provision of particular societies at different points in their social histories; (2) describing and explaining the dynamics of public-private welfare provision designed to meet the changing public policy needs of nations over time; (3) suggesting likely future outcomes associated with different approaches to policy implementation; (4) assisting in the development of more efficient and effective policies designed to respond more fully to national and international human needs; and (5) enabling scholars to gain a richer appreciation of the complex dynamics of cross-national welfare development across time and geopolitical regions.

Steps Toward Progress in Global Poverty Alleviation

Consistent with the poverty alleviation goals and objectives identified throughout the chapter, as well as the stakeholders who have been identified to lead the effort, the world's nations have made a major commitment to continue strengthening the economic capacity of impoverished developing countries (International Monetary Fund, 2017; World Bank, 2014, 2016a). The world's more economically mature societies continue to make ever higher investments in the economies of developing countries, and these investments are beginning to yield impressive outcomes, especially in reducing global poverty rates. This type of assistance is exactly that required by developing nations to bring about increased levels of equality within their borders. Further, the launching of the new United Nations SDGs will serve as a major stimulus in helping the economies of developing countries expand even more rapidly (Myers, 2016; United Nations Development Programme, 2017b; World Bank, 2017a, 2017b).

In addition to the model and actors identified above, four important principles have been reaffirmed by both the MDC and SDG campaigns of the United Nations in cooperation with large numbers of international private and public sector partners: (a) poverty alleviation requires the involvement and active engagement of all the leading social, political, and economic stakeholders that make up the public life of every society; (b) poverty alleviation, especially at the national and global levels, requires careful planning, adequate funding to implement these plans, and careful monitoring of the extent to which the plan's goals and objectives are being met over time; (c) the poor must participate actively with major societal stakeholders in helping to shape the plans, processes, and outcomes associated with each of the major approaches required to achieve permanent poverty resolution; and (d) poverty alleviations is not just about money, though money (rather its absence) is a big part of poverty but, involves focusing on major improvements in the health, education, social welfare, and technological sectors in order to be fully successful in reducing the incidence of poverty at all levels of political organization.

Further, and of central importance to effective action, effective poverty reduction approaches must place emphasis on the systematic engagement of the four major stakeholders who are needed to bring about fundamental changes of any magnitude in virtually all societies of the world: (a) the *government*, or the state; (b) the *market*, or the economy; (c) *families and extended kinship systems*; and, (d) civil society organizations, including international development assistance organizations, national charitable organizations, religious bodies, individual philanthropists, and the like.

Because of the complexity of the situation, all four underlying principles and society's four leading stakeholders must take an active role in helping people move out of intergenerational poverty and toward progressively higher levels of economic self-sufficiency. The problem of personal, national, and global income (and even cultural) poverty cannot be solved without careful attention to all eight underlying drivers that sustain both individual and global poverty.

Other global actors also contribute to the growth of developing nations and, in turn, to the elimination of extreme poverty in all its forms but especially through development assistance provided by major international NGOs. Business leaders contribute significantly and often can create preferential trade relationships with and between many of the world's socially least developed countries. The combined activities of these aid organizations and business leaders have proven to be essential elements in unraveling the recurrent puzzle of multigenerational poverty (Shah, 2014; United Nations Development Programme, 2017a; World Bank, 2013, 2016c).

I conclude the chapter with the following quote from Thomas Piketty, an economist who is committed to the promotion of social justice through more equitable patterns of economic growth and economic well-being. Piketty wrote in one of his earliest books, *Capital in the Twenty-First Century* (2013),

> Social scientific research is and always will be tentative and imperfect. It does not claim to transform economics, sociology, and history into exact sciences. But by patiently searching for facts and patterns and calmly analyzing the economic, social, and political mechanisms that might explain them, it can inform democratic debate and focus attention on the right questions. It can help to redefine the terms of debate, unmask certain preconceived or fraudulent notions, and subject all positions to constant critical scrutiny. In my view, this is the role that intellectuals, including social scientists, should play, as citizens like any other but with the good fortune to have more time than others to devote themselves to study (and even to be paid for it—a signal privilege (p. 101).

Thus, the recently adopted approaches to poverty alleviation at the global level make use of financial and sociocultural approaches to the elimination of poverty in all its manifestations. These approaches include subsidized employment opportunities for the poor, bilateral and multilateral aid designed to bring quality health and education services to the poor, international contract labor opportunities, *foreign direct investment* in the economies of developing nations as well as *official development assistance* provided by rich countries to economically poorer nations (Sachs, 2006; Stiglitz, 2010; World Bank, 2016c). Each approach has its own wisdom and levels of effectiveness, especially when tied to major progress in bringing about fundamental political reform (Wikipedia, 2018).

Finally, despite the guarded economic prospects that characterize rates of economic growth for many nations, investors and business enterprises need to remain optimistic that they can contribute toward a more positive future for all the world's poor. These more promising prospects for the near-term will result in new and important innovations in the productive processes of societies everywhere. Only in this way can we, as a world community, reduce the levels of global poverty and, at the same time, advance the economic status of our own countries and that of others. I also have concluded that money alone is not sufficient to solve the problem of intergenerational poverty in which decades of poverty have socialized the children of poor families into believing that no positive choices are open to them to advance their future (United Nations Development Programme, 2017a). This is an enormously complex problem to overcome but it must succeed if the world community is to move forward in promoting increasing levels of equity and equality for all its citizens (whatever their early background). Education, health care, housing and sanitation, and employment are the sectors in which the most dramatic social changes are needed. Ultimately, these form the key framework for poverty alleviation at all levels of social organization.

References

Alber, J., Alesina, A., & Glaeser, E. L. (2004). *Fighting poverty in the US and Europe: A world of difference*. New York: Oxford University Press.

Ascoli, U., & Ranci, C. (Eds.). (2002). *Dilemmas of the welfare mix: The new structure of welfare in an era of privatization*. New York: Kluwer Academic/Plenum Publishers.

Baradaran, M. (2017). *The color of money: Black banks and the racial wealth gap*. Cambridge, MA: Belknap Press.

Blome, A., Keck, W., & Alber, J. (2009). *Family and the welfare state in Europe: Intergenerational relations in ageing societies*. Cheltenham, UK: Edward Elgar Publishing.

Burton, J. (2017a, April 25). 25 Highest income earning countries. *World Atlas; Economics*. Retrieved March 23, 2018 from https://www.worldatlas.com/articles/the-highest-incomes-in-the-world.html

Burton, J. (2017b, April 25). Countries with the lowest income in the world. *World Atlas: Economics*. Retrieved March 23, 2018 from https://www.worldatlas.com/articles/countries-with-the-lowest-income-in-the-world.html

C.W. & A.J.K.D. (2013, September 27). Did slavery make economic sense? *The Economist*. Retrieved December 1, 2018 from https://www.economist.com/free-exchange/2013/09/27/did-slavery-make-economic-sense

Cawson, A. (1982). *Corporatism and welfare: Social policy and state intervention in Britain*. London: Heinemann.

Central Intelligence Agency (CIA). (2018). *The world factbook, 2018*. Washington, DC: Department of State. Retrieved March 20, 2018 from https://www.cia.gov/library/publications/the-world-factbook/

Clark, A., & Senik, C. (2017). *Happiness and economic growth: Lessons from developing countries*. Oxford: Oxford University Press.

Collier, P. (2007). *The bottom billion: Why the poorest countries are failing and what can be done about it*. New York: Oxford University Press.

Collins, M., & Bendinger, B. (2016). *The rise of inequality & the decline of the middle class*. London: First Flight Books.

Credit Suisse. (2017), *Annual report, 2017*. Retrieved March 20, 2018 from http://publications.credit-suisse.com/index.cfm/publikationen-shop/annual-report/annual-report-2017/

Davies, J., Lluberas, R., & Shorrocks, A. (2017). Estimating the level and distribution of global wealth, 2000–2014. *Review of Income and Wealth, 63*(4). Retrieved May 25, 2018 from https://onlinelibrary.wiley.com/doi/pdf/10.1111/roiw.12318/

Day, P. J. (2009). *A new history of social welfare* (6th ed.). Boston/New York: Allyn and Bacon.

Economy Watch. (2018). *Economy, poverty, and GINI coefficients*. Retrieved March 25, 2018 from http://www.economywatch.com/economic-statistics/.

Editor. (2016, April 6). The truth about migration: Rich countries need immigrants. *New Scientist*. Retrieved April 17, 2018 from https://www.newscientist.com/article/ mg23030681-100-the-truth-about-migration-rich-countries-need-immigrants/

Enjolras, B., & Sivesind, K. H. (Eds.). (2009). Civil society in comparative perspective. *A special issue of Comparative Social Research, 26*, 1–293.

Esping-Anderson, G. (1990). *The three worlds of welfare capitalism*. Cambridge, UK: Polity Press.

Esping-Anderson, G. (1999). *Social foundations of postindustrial economics*. Oxford, UK: Oxford University Press.

Estes, R. J. (1999). "Poverties" and "wealth": Competing definitions and alternative approaches to measurement. *Social Development Issues, 21*(2), 11–21.

Estes, R. J. (2007a). *Advancing quality of life in a turbulent world*. Dordrecht, The Netherlands/ Berlin, Germany: Springer.

Estes, R. J. (2007b). Asia and the new century: Challenges and opportunities. *Social Indicators Research, 82*(3), 375–410.

Estes, R. J. (2007c). Development challenges and opportunities confronting economies in transition. *Social Indicators Research, 83*(3), 375–411.

Estes, R. J. (2010). The world social situation: Development challenges at the outset of a new century. *Social Indicators Research, 98*, 363–402.

Estes, R. J. (2012a). Economies in transition: Continuing challenges to quality of life. In K. Land, A. C. Michalos, & M. Joseph Sirgy (Eds.), *Handbook of quality of life research* (pp. 433–457). Cham, Switzerland: Springer.

Estes, R. J. (2012b). Failed and failing states: Is quality of life possible? In K. Land, A. C. Michalos, & M. Joseph Sirgy (Eds.), *Handbook of quality of life research* (pp. 555–580). Cham, Switzerland: Springer.

Estes, R. J. (2015a). Development trends among the world's socially least developed countries: Reasons for cautious optimism. In B. Spooner (Ed.), *Globalization: The crucial phase*. Philadelphia: University of Pennsylvania Press.

Estes, R. J. (2015b). Global change and quality of life indicators. In F. Maggino (Ed.), *A life devoted to quality of life festschrift in honor of Alex C. Michalos* (pp. 173–194). Cham, Switzerland: Springer.

Estes, R. J. (2015c). Trends in world social development: The search for global well-being. In W. Glatzer (Ed.), *The global handbook of well-being: from the wealth of nations to the human well-being of nations*. Cham, Switzerland: Springer.

Estes, R. J., & Sirgy, M. J. (2017). *The pursuit of well-being: The untold global history*. Dordrecht, The Netherlands/Berlin, Germany: Springer.

Estes, R. J., & Sirgy, M. J. (2018). *Advances in well-being: Toward a better world for all*. London: Rowman and Littlefield.

Estes, R. J., & Tiliouine, H. (2014). Islamic development trends: From collective wishes to concerted actions. *Social Indicators Research, 116*(1), 67–114.

Estes, R. J. & Zhou, H. M. (2014, December 4). A conceptual approach to the creation of public–private partnerships in social welfare. *International Journal of Social Welfare*. 348–363.

Evers, A., & Wintersberger, H. (1988). *Shifts in the welfare mix: Their impact on work, social services and welfare policies*. Vienna, Austria: European Centre for Social Welfare.

Fitzpatrick, K., & Lagory, M. (2010). *Unhealthy cities: Poverty, race, and place in America* (2nd ed.). London: Routledge.

Fox, J. (2012). The economics of well-being. *Harvard Business Review, 90*(1–2), 78–83.

Frank, R. H. (2007). *Falling behind: How rising inequality harms the middle class*. Berkeley, CA: University of California Press.

Galasso, V. N. (2013). *The drivers of economic inequality: A primer.* Washington, DC: Oxfam USA. Retrieved April 3, 2017, from https://www.oxfamamerica.org/static/media/files/oxfam-drivers-of-economic-inequality.pdf

Glatzer, W. (Ed.). (2002). *Rich and poor: Disparities, perceptions, commitments.* Dordrecht, The Netherlands: Springer.

Graham, C. (2012). *Happiness around the world: The paradox of happy peasants and miserable millionaires.* New York: Oxford University Press.

Habisch, A., & Jonker, J. (Eds.). (2005). *Corporate social responsibility across Europe.* Berlin, Germany: Springer.

Hall, M. (2018, October 22). What is purchasing power parity (PPP)? *Investopedia.* https://www.investopedia.com/updates/purchasing-power-parity-ppp/

Helliwell, J., Layard, R., & Sachs, J. (2017). *World happiness report, 2017.* New York: Sustainable Development Solutions Network.

Henneberg, S. (2017). *The wealth gaps.* Farmington Hills, MI: Greenhaven Publishing.

House, F. (2018). *Freedom in the world, 2018.* New York: Freedom House.

International Labour Organization (ILO). (2019). *Statistics and data bases.* Geneva, Switzerland: ILO. Retrieved June 6, 2019 from https://www.ilo.org/global/statistics-and-databases/lang--en/index.htm

International Monetary Fund (IMF). (2017). *Comparative world economic outlook, 2018.* Retrieved April 4, 2017, from http://world-economic-outlook.findthedata.com/

International Monetary Fund (IMF). (2018). *Managing debt vulnerabilities in low-income and developing countries.* Washington, DC: IMF. Retrieved March 23, 2018 from http://www.imf.org/external/index.htm

International Social Security Association (ISSA). (2018). *Social security programs throughout the world.* Geneva, Switzerland: ISSA.

Investopedia. (2018). *Gini index.* Retrieved November 29, 2018 from https://www.investopedia.com/terms/g/gini-index.asp.

Italian National Institute of Statistics. (2017). *The 12 dimensions of well-being.* Rome: Italian National Institute of Statistics. Retrieved December 3, 2018 from http://www.istat.it/en/well-being-and-sustainability/well-being-measures/12-dimensions-of-well-being

Krugman, P. (2003). *The great unraveling: Losing our way in the new century.* New York: W.W. Norton.

Kuhn, T. (1996). *The structure of scientific revolutions* (3rd ed.). Chicago: University of Chicago Press.

Layard, R. (2017). *Making personal happiness and well-being a goal of public policy.* London: London School of Economics. Retrieved December 2, 2018 from http://www.lse.ac.uk/researchAndExpertise/researchImpact/caseStudies/layard-happiness-well-being-public-policy.aspx

Møller, V., & Roberts, B. (2017). New beginnings in an ancient region: Well-being in Sub-Saharan Africa. In R. J. Estes & M. J. Sirgy (Eds.), *The pursuit of human well-being: The untold global history* (pp. 161–215). Cham, Switzerland: Springer.

Monaghan, A. (2014, November 13). US wealth inequality - top 0.1% worth as much as the bottom 90%. *The Guardian.* Retrieved January 25, 2018 from https://www.theguardian.com/business/2014/nov/13/us-wealth-inequality-top-01-worth-as-much-as-the-bottom-90.

Myers, J. (2016). *Which are the world's fastest-growing economies?* Geneva, Switzerland: World Economic Forum. Retrieved July 1, 2017, from https://www.weforum.org/agenda/2016/04/worlds-fastest-growing-economies/

Naldini, M. (2003). *The family in the Mediterranean welfare states.* London: Cass Publishers.

Organization for Economic Cooperation and Development (OECD). (2015a). *Net official development assistance by country as a percentage of gross national income in 2015.* Retrieved April 15, 2017, from https://en.wikipedia.org/wiki/List_of_development_aid_country_donors

Organization for Economic Cooperation and Development (OECD). (2015b). *Net official development assistance by country as a percentage of gross national income in 2015*. Retrieved April 15, 2017, from https://en.wikipedia.org/wiki/List_of_development_aid_country_donors

Organization for Economic Cooperation and Development (OECD). (2017a). *Development aid rises again in 2016 but flows to poorest countries dip*. Paris: Organization for Economic Cooperation and Development. Retrieved July 2, 2017, from http://www.oecd.org/development/stats/development-aid-rises-again-in-2016-but-flows-to-poorest-countries-dip.htm

Organization for Economic Cooperation and Development (OECD). (2017b). *Economy: Developing countries set to account for nearly 60% of world GDP by 2030, according to new estimates*. Paris: Organization for Economic Cooperation and Development.

Organization for Economic Cooperation and Development (OECD). (2018a). *Data: Official development assistance*. Retrieved March 1, 2018 from https://data.oecd.org/oda/net-oda.htm.

Organization for Economic Cooperation and Development (OECD). (2018b). *Data: General*. Retrieved March 1, 2018 from https://data.oecd.org/.

Organization for Economic Cooperation and Development (OECD). (2018c). *Data: General*. Retrieved March 1, 2018 from https://data.oecd.org/.

Piketty, T. (2015). *The economics of inequality*. (A. Goldhammer, trans.). Cambridge, UK: Harvard University Press.

Piketty, T. (2017). *Capital in the twenty-first century*. (A. Goldhammer, Trans.). Cambridge, UK: Belknap Press.

Piketty, T., Saez, E., & Zucman, G. (2018). Distributional national accounts: Methods and estimates for the United States. *Quarterly Journal of Economics, 133*(2), 553–609. Retrieved March 2, 2018 from http://gabriel-zucman.eu/usdina/

Powell, M., & Barrientos, A. (2004). Welfare regimes and the welfare mix. *European Journal of Political Research, 43*(1), 83–105.

Rawls, J. (1971). *A theory of justice* (2nd ed.). Cambridge MA: Harvard University Belknap Press.

Sachs, J. (2006). *The end of poverty: Economic possibilities for our time*. London/New York: Penguin Books.

Salaman, L. M. (2012). *Americas nonprofit sector* (3rd ed.). New York: Foundation Center.

Schramm-Nielsen, J. (2002, May). Conflict in Scandinavia. *SSRN Electronic Journal*. https://doi.org/10.2139/ssrn.305153

Schrieberg, D. (2018, March 11). World Bank warning: Europe's poor are slipping further behind, fueling region's populism. *Forbes*. Retrieved March 24, 2018 from https://www.forbes.com/sites/davidschrieberg1/2018/03/11/world-bank-warning-europes-poor-are-slipping-further-behind-fueling-regions-populism/#533411426526.

Sen, A. (2011). *The idea of justice*. Cambridge, UK: Harvard University Press.

Serafin, T. (2009, June 17). The world's richest royals. *Forbes*.

Shah, A. (2014, September 28). Causes of poverty. *Global Issues*. Retrieved March 8, 2017, from http://www.globalissues.org/issue/2/causes-of-poverty

Stiglitz, J. E. (2010). *The Stiglitz report: Reforming the international monetary and financial systems in the wake of the global crisis*. New York/London: The New Press. ISBN 9781595585202.

Stiglitz, J. E. (2013). *The price of inequality: How today's divided society endangers our future*. New York: W.W. Norton Books.

Stockholm International Peace Research Institute (SIPRI). (2018). *List of armed conflicts, 2018*. Stockholm: SIPRI.

Thompson, D. (2012). The 10 things economics can tell us about happiness, *Atlantic*. Retrieved May 31, 2012 from https://www.theatlantic.com/business/archive/2012/05/the-10-things-economics-can-tell-us-about-happiness/257947/

Tiliouine, H., & Estes, R. J. (2016). *The state of social progress of Islamic societies: Social, economic, political, and ideological challenges*. Cham, Switzerland: Springer.

Transparency International. (2018). *Corruptions perceptions index*. Berlin, Germany: Transparency International.

UK Essays. (2013). *The impact of globalization on Income inequality*. Retrieved from http://www.ukessays.com/essays/economics/impact-of-globalization-on-income-inequality-economics-essay.php?vref=1

United Nations. (2010). *The millennium development goals report, 2010*. Retrieved October 12, 2018 from http://www.un.org/millenniumgoals/pdf/MDG%20Report%202010%20En%20r15%20-low%20res%2020100615%20-.pdf

United Nations. (2015). *Sustainable development goals: Knowledge platform*. New York: United Nations. Retrieved June 7, 2019 from https://sustainabledevelopment.un.org/post2015/summit

United Nations Development Programme (UNDP). (1997). *The shrinking state: Governance and sustainable human development*. New York: Oxford University Press.

United Nations Development Programme (UNDP). (2010). *Human development report, 2010: the real wealth of nations: pathways to human development*. Retrieved November 8, 2018 from http://hdr.undp.org/en/reports/global/hdr2010/

United Nations Development Programme (UNDP). (2014). *World human development report: Sustaining human progress—Reducing vulnerabilities and building resilience, 2014*. New York: UNDP.

United Nations Development Programme (UNDP). (2016). *World human development report, 2016: Human development for everyone*. New York: UNDP.

United Nations Development Programme (UNDP). (2017a). *Human development report, 2017: Human development for everyone*. New York: United Nations Development Programme.

United Nations Development Programme (UNDP). (2017b). *The sustainable development goals*. Retrieved January 10, 2017, from http://www.un.org/sustainabledevelopment/sustainable-development-goals/

United Nations High Commissioner for Refugees (UNHCR). (2018). *UNHCR data base*. Retrieved December 2, 2018 from http://popstats.unhcr.org/en/overview#_ga=2.164876031.1309627063.1543764150-991633591.1543764150

United States. Census Bureau. 2010. *Poverty*. Retrieved December 2, 2018 from http://www.census.gov/hhes/www/poverty/about/overview/index.html

Vacas-Soriano, C., & Fernández-Macías, E. (2017, June 23). *Europe's shrinking middle class*. https://www.eurofound.europa.eu/publications/blog/europes-shrinking-middle-class

Vanham, P. (2015). *5 Trends for the future of economic growth*. Geneva, Switzerland: World Economic Forum. Retrieved July 3, 2017 from https://www.scribd.com/document/307808653/5-Trends-for-the-Future-of-Economic-Growth-Agenda-The-World-Economic-Forum

Veenhoven, R. (2019). *World happiness database of Erasmus University of Rotterdam*. Rotterdam, The Netherlands: Eramus University. Retrieved June 9, 2019 from https://worlddatabaseofhappiness.eur.nl/

Weingast, B. R., & Wittman, D. A. (Eds.). (2006). *The Oxford handbook of political economy*. New York/Oxford UK: Oxford University Press.

Wikipedia. (2018). Theories of poverty. (2017, May 28). In *Wikipedia, the free encyclopedia*. Retrieved December 2, 2018, from https://en.wikipedia.org/w/index.php?title=Theories_of_poverty&oldid=782617400

Woods, L. (2018, April 24). How the British royal family spends their wealth: The British royal family has expensive tastes. *Bank Rates*. Retrieved April 25, 2018.

World Bank. (1999). *World development report, 1999: Global economic disparities*. Washington, DC: World Bank Group.

World Bank. (2010). *World development report, 2010: Development and climate change*. New York: Oxford University Press.

World Bank. (2013, June 4). World Bank aims to eliminate extreme poverty by 2030. *The Huffington Post*. Retrieved April 15, 2017, from http://www.huffingtonpost.com/2013/04/02/world-bank-extreme-poverty_n_2999287.html

World Bank. (2014). *Ending poverty requires more than growth, says WBG.* Retrieved December 1, 2018 from http://www.worldbank.org/en/news/press-release/2014/04/10/ending-poverty-requires-more-than-growth-says-wbg

World Bank. (2016a). *Latin America and the Caribbean overview.* Washington, DC: World Bank Group.

World Bank. (2016b). *Migration and remittances: Recent developments and outlook (Migration and Development Brief, No. 26).* Washington, DC: World Bank Group.

World Bank. (2016c). *Poverty and shared prosperity, 2016.* Washington, DC: World Bank Group.

World Bank. (2016d). *World development report, 2016.* Washington, DC: World Bank Group.

World Bank. (2017a). *Global economic prospects, 2017: Weak investment in uncertain times.* Washington, DC: World Bank.

World Bank. (2017b). *Poverty: Overview.* Washington, DC: World Bank.

World Bank. (2017c). *World development indicators.* Washington, DC: World Bank Group.

World Bank. (2018). Decline of global extreme poverty continues but has slowed. *Press release, September 19.* Retrieved November 28, 2018 from http://www.worldbank.org/en/news/press-release/2018/09/19/decline-of-global-extreme-poverty-continues-but-has-slowed-world-bank

World Business Council for Social Development (WBCSD). (2017). How we drive sustainable development. [Organization web site]. *Homepage.* Retrieved April 15, 2017, from http://www.wbcsd.org/

World Values Survey (WVS). (2015). *World values survey: wave 7.* (Database). Retrieved July 3, 2017, from http://www.worldvaluessurvey.org/WVSContents.jsp

Yunus, M. (2007). *Creating a world without poverty: Social business and the future of capitalism.* New York: Public Affairs.

Part VII

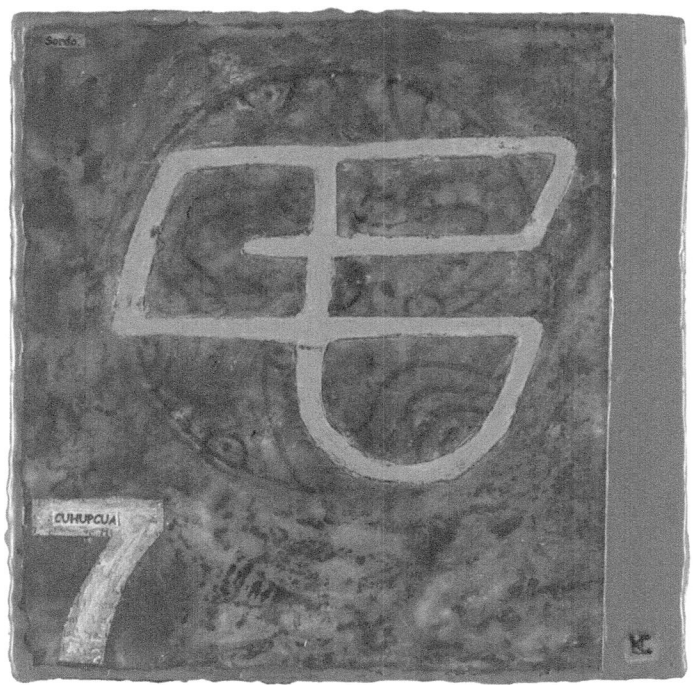

Image 7: © Lylia Ferero Carr: Muysca, Cuhupcua

Chapter 10
Discussion and Conclusions

At the beginning of this book, I stated that the world had arrived at a critical turning point, i.e., at a time in our shared histories when critical decisions needed to be made concerning the future of nations and that of the larger community of nations of which we are all part. The situation remains the same today despite five decades of progress of advancing the changing capacity of nations to meet not only the basic needs of their steadily increasing populations but their more advanced needs as well, especially in the social and economic security sectors. The situation is especially critical within nations identified in Chap. 6 and elsewhere in the book as "least developed" or "socially least developed countries" for which the basic needs of large numbers of their population go unmet, especially in response to diversity-related social conflict or warfare with neighboring states.

The reality is that many of the world's socially least developed countries have not yet been able to fully meet the basic health, education, social welfare, housing, transportation, environmental, or economic needs of their people. But they are on the way to doing so, and more sustained progress is expected over the near-term. Financial poverty is all too common within many of these countries and, in most cases, there are inadequate levels of public assistance at all levels of governments to provide for the basic income security needs of their citizens who are the least able to provide for their own basic needs without the assistance of governments and major nongovernmental organizations, i.e., those of children and youth, the advanced elderly, homeless persons, persons struggling with serious emotional or physical disabilities, persons who are solitary survivors, or those who otherwise do not have or contribute directly their own fiscal and other material well-being. Cities in many of the poorest of these countries typically experience high levels of air and water pollution, comparatively low levels of sanitation and, inadequate systems for disposing of liquid and solid waste disposal, despite recent progress in all these critical sectors worldwide. As a result, visitors to these countries are at significant risk of being exposed to transmittable infectious and other communicable diseases and must, therefore, exercise considerable caution with respect to the beverages

© Springer Nature Switzerland AG 2019
R. J. Estes, *The Social Progress of Nations Revisited, 1970–2020*, Social
Indicators Research Series 78, https://doi.org/10.1007/978-3-030-15907-8_10

they drink and the foods they eat, even when such necessities emerge from the gleaming and carefully supervised kitchens in guest houses and multistar hotels. Emergency medical services for both local and international visitors often are difficult to secure and, when available, are expensive, limited, and highly transactional with little continuity of care. Few patient records are available, including history of exposure to communicable and infectious diseases.

In-patient hospital care in the majority of the least socially developing countries also is extremely limited, even at significant out-of-pocket costs, as are reliable systems of communication and transportation given the extreme demands that are placed on essential services in highly dense urban populations. Technology and technological innovation in many of these societies also are quite limited except for expensive "out of the box" technologies (e.g., computers, smartphones, iPads) that are available for purchase by more affluent consumers including people engaged in for-profit businesses, tourists, and other international visitors with access to stable hard currencies.

Even so, most of the world's populations live under social conditions that are greatly improved compared with those of their parents or to themselves when they were children. Food in the world's economically advanced societies tends to be plentiful; quality and continuity of health care are accessible to most people, especially urban dwellers; water and air pollution largely have come under control; more housing units are available; and spacious, clean, and safe public transportation is characteristically available to all at an affordable cost; the increased regulations of financial and related institutions are better managed; and the disposal of solid and liquid waste is generally effective and often is recycled for use in generating new sources of energy. In short, advances in well-being and the quality of life in the world's most economically advanced nations have improved remarkably over the 50-year period since this analysis began. Prospects for even more rapid advances in all aspects of well-being for the future in these nations are even more optimistic than those that existed in the past and are expected to improve steadily over the near term (especially to the year 2050), particularly within the most economically developed nations of Africa, Asia, Europe, Latin America, North America, as well as for the more advantaged island nations of the Pacific and other world regions including Tahiti and other more affluent nations located in the Polynesian chain. These advances in well-being and quality of life have been dramatic and their impacts on quality of life for economically well-off populations over at least the recent past (since the end of World War II) have been both significant and impactful and almost certainly are expected to continue into other sectors of social, political, economic, technological, and environmental development for many decades into the future.

Well-Being Now and Over the Near Term: Progress, Progress, and More Progress

The process of change over the past century has been impressive and is continuing even as this still young century continues to unfold. I conclude this chapter with a moving quote from the former South Korean Secretary-General of the United Nations, Ban Ki-Moon, who, in 2013, eloquently summarized the contributions made by the G-20 group of nations[1] in advancing human well-being since the end of the Second World War. Said Ban Ki-Moon in Saint Petersburg, Russia (United Nations Secretary-General, 2013),

> Sustainable development is the pathway to the future we want for all. It offers a framework to generate economic growth, achieve social justice, exercise environmental stewardship and strengthen governance....
>
> At the same time, we need to set a more ambitious agenda beyond 2015 (when the Millennium Development Campaign [2005–2015] would end).
>
> The new agenda should place sustainable development at its core and make the eradication of poverty its top priority.
>
> The new agenda will need a renewed, broad-based global partnership, particularly to mobilize finance and technology.
>
> The new agenda will need to be supported by a single post-2015 UN development framework containing a single set of goals applicable to all countries but adaptable to different national realities.
>
> Financing needs for sustainable development are enormous. ODA and domestic resources remain crucial. But I also welcome the G20's focus on long-term investment financing, including the regulatory environment, incentives and risk-sharing to leverage private resources with public funds.
>
> The new agenda must be tuned to the leading challenges we face, including the need for decent jobs, inclusive growth, improved governance, peace, and action on climate change.
>
> The G-20 should lead by example.

Fortunately, the 192 member states of the General Assembly of the United Nations in 1993 developed a follow-up plan of action to sustain the rapid pace of social development among the socially least developed of the world's poorest nations. The new plan of global action brought together all the world's major stakeholders in international development and was referred to as the 17 *Sustainable Development Goals* that both built on and enlarged the range of development objectives to which the world has committed itself (United Nations Development Programme, 2018a, 2018b; Zondi & Mthembu, 2017)[2]. The *Sustainable Development*

---

[1] The 20 members of the G-20 are Argentina, Australia, Brazil, Canada, China, France, Germany, India, Indonesia, Italy, Japan, Korea, Mexico, Russia, Saudi Arabia, South Africa, Turkey, United Kingdom, United States, and the multistate European Union.

[2] The 17 *Sustainable Development Goals* emphasize no poverty; zero hunger; good health and well-being; quality education; clean water and sanitation; affordable and clean energy; decent work and economic growth; industry, innovation, infrastructure; reduced inequalities; sustainable cities and communities; responsible consumption and production; climate action; life below water; life on land; peace, justice and strong institutions; partnerships for the goals (United Nations Development Programme, 2018a, 2018b).

Goals, like the *Millennium Development Goals* that preceded them, hold every promise of advancing still further the significant social gains that already have been attained by the world's developing and least developed societies (Estes & Sirgy, 2018; United Nations Development Programme, 2018a, 2018b; World Bank, 2018).

At the outset of a new century, the need is apparent for new, more dramatic initiatives that will transform *all* the world's nations into more caring and socially productive societies (Estes & Zhou, 2014; International Social Security Association, 2018; World Bank, 2018). At a minimum, these initiatives must be informed by a renewed commitment to the three goals on which the world's leaders already agree: (1) the elimination of absolute poverty everywhere; (2) enhanced popular participation at all levels of political organization; and (3) a more equitable sharing of the planet's abundant resources. The pursuit of these goals is achievable in the context of the major accomplishments that nations around the world already are achieving.

The social changes implied by these goals are complex, and they have not, nor will they, yield easily to simple or quick solutions to the lingering challenges confronting humanity. Rather, sustained financial and human capital investments will be required over the long term to reverse the social, political, and economic conditions that have trapped such a large portion of the world's population in grinding poverty. At the heart of these efforts to change, though, must be a commitment to strengthening the capacity of local people to provide for their basic social and material needs within the realities of their own environment. No other approach to social development can hope to help the world's poorest countries appreciably reduce the deeply entrenched patterns of mal-development that have held their populations hostage for more than five decades.

Promoting a More Optimistic Future

Suggesting a worldwide working agenda for the future is both a challenging and humbling undertaking. The challenge is even greater in that the intention is focused on accelerating the pace of advances in quality of life and well-being for all the world's nations, especially given the extraordinary diversity that exists both within and between nations. Even so, having completed a study of the magnitude reported in this book warrants that priorities be assigned to at least some well-being objectives that will advance the human condition. Therefore, I have identified ten of what I regard as the most important advances that must be focused upon if, we the people, are to further improve both the objective and subjective conditions under which we live out our all too brief lives.

1. The elimination of *absolute poverty* remains the single greatest challenge confronting humanity. This is the case despite the tremendous progress that has been made worldwide in lifting hundreds of millions of people out of poverty since 2000, especially in East and South Asia (Estes & Sirgy, 2018; United Nations Development Programme, 2018a; World Bank, 2018).

(a) The challenge is especially significant among the remote rural communities of developing Africa, Asia, and Latin American where access to necessities such as potable water, fire wood, and adequate housing remains a challenge that consumes more than a third of the working hours of women and girls.

(b) In a conversation this author had with the Danish Foreign Minister, *Uffe Ellemann-Jensen* (10 September 1982–25 January 1993), he stated that "poverty is just too expensive a problem for us to afford." And right he was, as evidenced by the extraordinary levels of spending invested in the poor in all societies that have not taken seriously the challenge of poverty alleviation and, as a result, have deepened the complex social problems that sustain poverty, ill health, poor education, and other related social issues.

(c) Indeed, poverty is a social problem that is too expensive for any society, especially given its close association with high rates of school dropouts, imprisonment, broken families, drug abuse, and the other realities associated with it. Thus, the elimination of abject poverty remains front and center among the challenges that must be met head on if nations and the global community are to move forward.

2. The centuries of structural inequalities between *women* and men have long passed, and every effort must be made to provide women with the same educational, health, social, political, scientific, and other benefits that men have long enjoyed.

(a) Significant progress has been achieved in advancing the status of women even as women continue to lag significantly behind men in most sectors that promote a reasonable standard of quality of life and well-being (UN Women 2018).

(b) These efforts must be aggressive and far-reaching and, ultimately, must be successful if men and women alike are to free themselves from the limitations created by the all-pervasive inequalities that confront women and girls and, in doing so, deprive societies of the rich human resources they need to attain progressively higher levels of well-being.

(c) And these initiatives must be applied to girls as well who quickly will develop into women in their societies.

(d) This is not a win-lose strategy between men, boys, girls, and women but a strategy to advance the social well-being of both genders as co-equal partners and the well-being of society as a whole.

(e) Thus, men and boys have major roles to carry out in helping to promote the social status of women and, in the process, of themselves. Men cannot place this responsibility on women alone nor can they expect local or national governments to take responsibility for changing the attitudes and biases that limit social, political, and economic opportunities for men and women alike.

3. Societies need to restructure their *social support systems* to provide at least minimum levels of income security for their most financially vulnerable citi-

zens, including children and youth, the elderly, persons with severe physical and emotional disabilities, those who live on the margins of society, the poor, agricultural workers living in remote rural communities, and others with limited education and skills.

(a) These forms of social provisions require close public–private partnerships, including the stakeholders in the corporate sector, employers, nongovernmental organizations, and others who share a commitment to improving the quality of life of their citizens and residents.

(b) Special attention must be given to the varied contributions made to family economic insecurity by the following stakeholders who contribute to social well-being, i.e., the state or government, the economy or market, families and households, and nongovernmental organizations organized at all levels of political structure.

4. Health and access to high levels of *health care* are fundamental to the attainment of well-being everywhere in the world. The most socially successful nations spend approximately 6%–7% of their gross domestic product on health care, but to achieve parity with more socially advanced nations, developing and socially least developed nations may need to allocate at least twice their gross domestic product to providing quality health care at all levels of the political organization.

(a) Public investments in preventive health care often produce the greatest yields, i.e., immunization, decentralized neighborhood health centers, visiting nurses, and major investments in pre- and postnatal care.

(b) Adequate housing also is closely associated with advances in health well-being. So, too, is the safe and efficient elimination of liquid and solid waste, two vectors that are directly responsibility for the transmission of community-specific infectious and communicable diseases. Gains in one area reinforce gains in other related sectors; thus, the effort to improve individual and community health is dependent on social progress in other sectors of quality of life.

5. Nearly everywhere in the world formal *education* is key to social, political, and economic success.

(a) Education also is a critical factor in technological innovation and, in the end, serves as a gateway to the selection of political leaders. Advanced educational backgrounds are somewhat less related to the criteria required for leadership in business except for high technology, pharmaceutical, and related knowledge-driven enterprises.

(b) Societies everywhere need to strengthen their secondary and postsecondary approaches to education and, where possible, to reorient them towards a wide range of research and development priorities (Shaikin & Estes, 2018). Only in this way can previously less developed countries move into leadership positions vis-à-vis the already technologically advanced countries that are members of the Organization for Economic Cooperation and Development (2018).

6. Participatory systems of *political governance* in combination with open market economies have proven to be one of the great successes in promoting quality of life and well-being in virtually all regions of the world. These systems are responsible for exponential levels of economic growth, higher than average levels of per capita gross domestic product, and, in the physical sphere, increased public accountability on the part of public officials to their constituencies. Though variations in this general model are likely to persist well into the future, democracies and free markets have yielded the single greatest improvements in human well-being since the end of World War II.

7. Everywhere, even in selected democratic societies, the *public media* have come under attack by pro-authoritarian political regimes (Cillizza, 2017; Ngosa, 2017). These attacks persist despite the incredibly positive effects that free and unencumbered media contribute to democratic political and open market economic systems. They also provide a corrective force for the abuses of authoritarian regimes to enact policies, regulations, and even laws that countermand the very principles on which democratic institutions are based.

   (a) Every effort must be made to promote freedom of the press and media throughout the world, given the unique functions that are assigned to them to monitor and expose corruption wherever it may exist. This function is critical to the structure of free societies and makes possible the flourishment of political and economic systems on which democratic societies everywhere depend.

   (b) Persons and institutions in the public sector that seek to weaken the oversight responsibilities assigned to the public media must be held legally accountable for this profane violation of the public trust. New international oversight bodies and national laws need to be put in place that effectively punish the attempts by public officials to prevent the public media from carrying out their mandated responsibilities.

8. The world's leading *international development assistance organizations* have come under severe attack in recent years, including the European Union, the International Monetary Fund, the North America Free Trade Organization, the Organization for Economic Cooperation and Development, the North Atlantic Trade Organization, the United Nations, the World Bank, and others.

   (a) These critiques, often with the goal of disempowering the organization in question, must be resisted with the same sense of fervor that led to their creation. These organizations have proven to be critical for advancing world peace and for promoting global socioeconomic development. And, they have been largely successful in achieving the goal that literally has enabled us to "turn guns into plowshares."

(b) Even so, these organizations are critical to the social, political, economic, military, and other functions on which free market participatory democratic systems depend.

9. Much progress has been made in protecting the planet, including its highly fragile *ecological systems*. But still more gains are needed if we are to succeed in fully protecting the planet. At a minimum, these protections must include the following:

(a) Continued control of carbon wastes that wreak havoc on the air, water, and related systems of nearly all the world's nations.
(b) Stricter rules on the use of combustion engines, with their wasteful dependence on fossil fuels, that can be less expensively energized using other energy sources, to cool and heat living spaces, and for use in transportation.
(c) The use of recycled products to generate energy, which has received considerable attention since the 1980s, with considerable success. Virtually all organic products can be recycled to generate energy, including solid and liquid waste, paper products, and garbage, to name a few.
(d) The use of natural gas, wind and solar power and strictly controlled nuclear energy to replace our current overdependence on oil and related petroleum products.

10. *Research and evaluation* are central components for assessing changes over time in the capacity of nations to advance their quality of life and well-being.

(a) Mechanisms for implementing this well-being priority are clearly identified in the United Nations Sustainable Development Campaign and its 17 fully operationalized goals.
(b) Comparable systems for assessing changes in national and global well-being also have been articulated by the Development Assistance Committee of the European-based Organization for Economic Cooperation and Development (2018), Freedom House (2018), the Aid Commission of the World Bank (2018), as well as many major international nongovernmental organizations (Save the Children, 2017; Transparency International, 2018).
(c) The commitment to on-going data-driven approaches to development planning and implementation at the global level is critical to effective action at the national, regional, and global levels.

This author, and the many others associated with the preparation of this book, look forward to continued progress in well-being and to steady increases in the quality of life and well-being of people everywhere across the planet. Enthusiastic implementation of the principles that inform the preceding action agenda will take us a long way toward the attainment of these objectives. The late and highly influential Portuguese educator and activist, Paulo Freire (1921–1997), writing in support of these principles in *The Pedagogy of the Oppressed* (Freire, 2014), taught us, "liberation is a praxis: the action and reflection of men and women upon their world to transform it" (p. 56).

Final Thoughts

Though intentionally written in a relatively brief format, the research reported in this volume reflects 50 years of research into the changing sociopolitical-economic capacity of nations to provide for at least the basic and intermediate needs of their steadily increasing populations, especially those of their most vulnerable population groups.

Space limitations have prevented me from going into depth on many topics that are of special interest to me but, even so, the broad strokes of development as a critical component of quality of life and well-being have been presented at multiple levels of analysis. I hope that I have done so with clarity. I also hope that I have succeeded in reaching the reader with many of the most critical lessons that have been learned concerning the most salient drivers of development, quality of life, and well-being over nearly half a century. The next steps toward building a more positive future for all of us, though, must be taken by you, the reader, and those, informed by knowledge and true passion, I leave you to take on your own.

The above sentiment is summed by the following quotation from the much celebrated and prolific nineteenth century Danish philosopher Søren Kierkegaard (1813–1855).

> **Life can only be understood backwards; but it must be lived forwards.**
> Kierkegaard (2006), *Fear and trembling*

Similar ideas also were expressed by other philosophers and theoretical social scientists writing during the same time period. But Kierkegaard was the most prolific writer on the subject. Struggling with the sense of living life through time, Kierkegaard taught us one of the most valuable principles of living life in the present while building on the past and anticipating the future. This is a lesson that each of us needs to learn and, in turn, once learned, informs our sense of preparing for the future using the past and present as frames of reference for living in the present—a key component of the concept of time-based human well-being.

References

Cilliza, C. (2017, February 19). Media, under attack from Trump, needs to return to the fundamentals. *Washington Post*. Retrieved September 12, 2018 from https://www.washingtonpost.com/politics/media-under-attack-from-trump-needs-to-return-to-the-fundamentals/2017/02/19/1396a2ee-f6b8-11e6-9b3e-ed886f4f4825_story.html?noredirect=on&utm_term=.59933d73ca8a

Estes, R. J., & Sirgy, M. J. (2018). *Advances in well-being: Towards a better world*. London: Rowman & Littlefield.

Estes, R. J., & Zhou, M. H. (2014). A conceptual approach to the creation of public–private partnerships in social welfare. *International Journal of Social Welfare, 24*(4), 348–363.

Freedom House. (2018). *Freedom throughout the world, 2018*. New York: Freedom House.

Freire, P. (2014). *Pedagogy of the oppressed* (30th Anniversary ed.). New York/London: Bloomsbury Publishing.

International Social Security Association. (2018). *Social security programs throughout the world, 2018*. Geneva: International Social Security Association.

Kierkegaard, S. (2006). *Fear and trembling*. New York: Penguin Books.

Ngosa, N. (2017, October 16). Media under attack—RSF. *The Mast*. Retrieved February 12, 2018 from https://www.themastonline.com/2017/10/16/media-under-attack-rsf/

Organization for Economic Cooperation and Development. (2018). *Receipts and distributions of the Development Assistance Committee, 2018*. Paris: Organization for Economic Cooperation and Development, Development Assistance Committee.

Save the Children. (2017). *2017 Annual report: Results for children*. Retrieved August 12, 2018 from https://www.savethechildren.org/us/about-us/resource-library/annual-report

Shaikin, D., & Estes, R. J. (2018). Advancing development in Kazakhstan: The contribution of R&D. *Social Development Issues, 40*(2), 36–55(20).

Transparency International. (2018). *Corruption throughout the world, 2018*. Berlin: Transparency International.

UN Women. (2018). *Turning promises into action: Gender equality in the 2030 sustainable development goals*. Retrieved August 11, 2018 from http://www.unwomen.org/en/digital-library/publications/2018/2/gender-equality-in-the-2030-agenda-for-sustainable-development-2018

United Nations Development Programme. (2018a). *Human development report, 2018*. New York: United Nations Development Programme.

United Nations Development Programme. (2018b). *Sustainable development goals, 2018*. New York: United Nations Development Programme—SDGs. https://sustainabledevelopment.un.org/?menu=1300

United Nations Secretary-General. (2013). *Secretary-General's remarks at a G20 working dinner on "Sustainable Development for All"*. [Delayed in transmission]. Retrieved September 13, 2018 from https://www.un.org/sg/en/content/sg/statement/2013-09-05/secretary-generals-remarks-g20-working-dinner-sustainable

World Bank. (2018). *World development report 2018: Learning to realize education's promise*. Washington, DC: World Bank.

Zondi, S., & Mthembu, P. (2017). *From MDGs to Sustainable Development Goals: The travails of international development*. Pretoria, South Africa: Institute for Global Dialogue (associated with the University of South Africa).

Part Backmatter

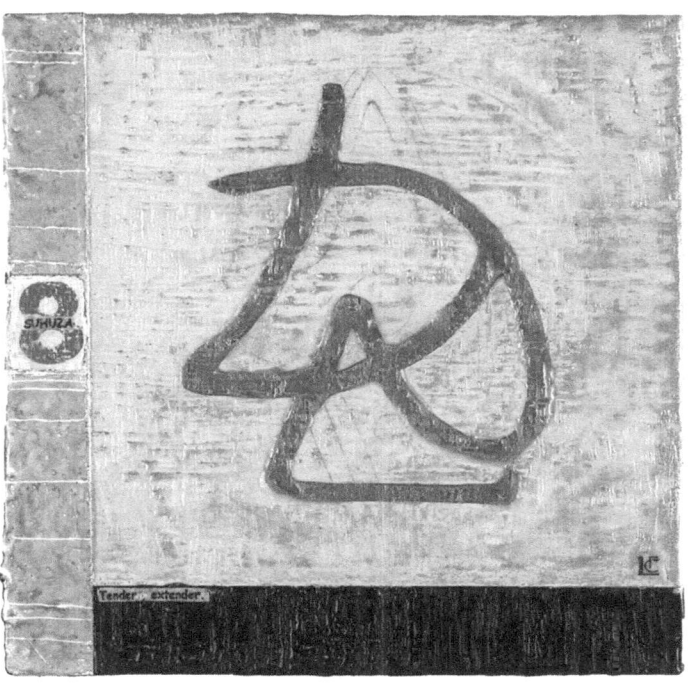

Image 8: © Lylia Ferero Carr: Muysca, Suhuza

Appendix A

Index and Subindex Computational Notes, 2016–2017 (ISP2018, WISP2018)

Index and Computational Notes

Index and subindex scores were computed in six steps:

1. Measures of central tendency and dispersion were computed for all indicators;
2. Raw indictor values were transformed into standardized units of measurement;
3. The signs of indicators negatively related to social development were reversed to correctly reflect their positive (or negative) contribution toward social progress;
4. Statistically unweighted subindex scores were computed;
5. Aggregated, but statistically unweighted, *Index of Social Progress* 18 (ISP2018) scores were computed; and then
6. *Weighted Index of Social Progress* 18 (WISP2018) scores were computed using statistical weights obtained through factor analysis.

Systat 13.2 (Systat, 2017) and Excel 2018 (Office 365) were used to carry out these procedures.

Step 1. Computation of Measures of Central Tendency and Dispersion

Raw score means, standard deviations, variance, and other measures of central tendency and dispersion were computed for each of the indicators that formed the ISP during the study's multiple time periods, i.e., 1970, 1980, 1990, 1994, 2000, 2005, 2010/2011, and 2016/2017.

Step 2. Raw Score Transformation into Standardized Units of Measurement

Indicator raw score values were transformed from variable units of measurement (e.g., rates, dollars, years, tons, scores on other standardized indexes) into standard-

© Springer Nature Switzerland AG 2019
R. J. Estes, *The Social Progress of Nations Revisited, 1970–2020*, Social Indicators Research Series 78, https://doi.org/10.1007/978-3-030-15907-8

ized "z-scores" using the following formula: ((x-M)/SD), where "x" is the original value of an individual case, M is the mean of the variable, and SD is the standard deviation.

Premised on the statistical assumptions of the normal distribution, the z-score transformation process assigned each variable a new group mean of "0" and a new group standard deviation of "1." The resulting z-score values assigned to individual countries through the standardization process represent the relative position of that country's raw score along the new standardized continuum, i.e., its score relative to that of all other countries. In effect, those countries with extreme positive or negative scores on a given indicator were assigned positive or negative z-score values that reflected their relative distance from the new group mean (as measured in standard deviation units) vis-a-vis that of other countries.

Step 3. Directionality of Indicators

The directional signs of some ISP indicators had to be changed so that net "gains" and "losses" on selected indicators could be properly reflected in composite index scores. In the *Health Subindex*, for example, three of the subindex's six indicators are inversely related to social progress in the health sector, i.e., *infant mortality rate* (−), *child mortality rate* (−), and *percent of population undernourished* (−). A lower score on these indicators measures a higher level of overall social progress; conversely, *higher levels of life expectation* (+), *physicians per 1000 population* (+), and *public expenditures as a percentage of GDP allocated to health and health care* (+) indicate higher levels of social progress. In all, performance on 17 of the ISP2018's 40 indicators is inversely related to overall level of social progress.

For computational purposes, the z-score values of all inversely stated ISP indicators were multiplied by a constant value of "-1."

Step 4. Computation of Standardized Subindex Scores

Three arithmetic steps were used to compute standardized, but statistically unweighted, subindex scores:

(a) the mathematical signs of negatively stated directional indicators were reversed in the manner just described;
(b) the unweighted z-score values of all subindex indicators were totaled; then,
(c) the sum of all indicator z-scores forming each subindex was divided by the number of indicators contained in that subindex (e.g., seven for the *Health Subindex*, five for the *Women Status Subindex*).

In effect, these procedures resulted in average raw subindex scores. The statistical impact of the averaging procedures was twofold: (1) They reduced the distortions associated with extremely positive or extremely negative performance on selected indicator values; and (2) the results provided a more representative picture of a country's performance on a given subindex than that provided by any single indicator. In the case of the *Welfare Effort Subindex z-*scores, the subindex score for each country was adjusted for the formal number of the five welfare programs that were in place as of 2017 (ranging from 0 to 5 programs). Countries without one or more formal welfare programs were assigned a modest z-score of 0.500 to their composite subindex score in recognition that all countries engage in some form of welfare effort even if their national welfare programs are less formal in nature and thus do not meet the international standards for national welfare programs established by the International Social Security Association (2017).

However, statistical averaging of indicator z-scores resulted in many numbers that proved to be too awkward to handle (e.g., average unstandardized scores for *years of average life expectancy* in the *health subindex* ranged from −2.188 [Central African Republic] to +1.418 [Japan]). Statistical constants were used to convert average subindex z-scores into more manageable numbers. In carrying out this procedure,

(d) composite subindex scores were multiplied by a constant value of +10; and, then,
(e) a constant value of +10 was added to each subindex score.

The subindex scores derived from these procedures resulted in standardized subindex scores that were both more understandable and easier to handle. Table A.1 illustrates the statistical transformation of raw scores into the statistically adjusted standardized z-scores (indicator z-score + 10) using 2018 *health subindex* data for India. The table also identifies the minimum, maximum, and average scores for each of the subindexes' six indicators for the world as a whole.

Step 5. Computation of Composite Index of Social Progress 18 Scores

ISP2018 scores were constructed through the simple addition of the standardized, but statistically unweighted, ten subindexes that make up the ISP.

Step 6. Weighted Index of Social Progress (WISP) Scores

Table A.1 Raw and standardized item scores on the health subindex, India 2016/17 (N = 1)

Health subindex indicators (N = 6)	India, raw score (N = 1)	India, z-score (N = 1)	World minimum (N = 162)	World maximum (N = 162)	World average (N = 162)
Years of average life expectancy (+)	68.3	−0.306	25.0	84.3	71.1
Infant mortality rate (−)	34.6	−0.493	1.6	88.5	24.0
Child mortality rate (−)	43.0	−0.356	2.1	132.5	31.9
Physicians per 1000 population (+)	0.8	−0.588	0.1	10.9	1.8
Percent of population undernourished (−)	14.5	−0.265	2.5	58.6	11.5
Public expenditures on health as percent of gross domestic product (+)	1.2	−1.157	0.8	10.6	4.0

A weighted version of the ISP was derived through an additional four statistical procedures.

(a) Both principal components and varimax factor analyses were conducted to identify the statistical relationships that exist between the 10 subindexes of the ISP, i.e., to identify the factor loadings for the ISP subindexes for use in creating the statistically weighted WISP.
(b) Standardized, but still statistically unweighted, ISP2018 subindex scores were then multiplied by the "loadings" that the factor analysis revealed to be most closely associated with that subindex.
(c) Weighted subindex scores were then summed by factor and, subsequently, the summated factor score was multiplied by the percent of variance that each factor contributed toward explaining the total ISP2018 variance.
(d) The statistically weighted factor scores were summed to obtain the total WISP2018 scores.

The following sections contain more complete descriptions of these computational steps.

Derivation of Index Statistical Weights Through Factor Analysis

Factor analysis was used to identify the system of statistical weights that best reflected the influence of each subindex on the study's unifying construct of "adequacy of national social provision." In carrying out the factor analysis, a principal components analysis with varimax rotation was undertaken (see Systat [2009] for a fuller explanation of the statistical assumptions used in carrying out this procedure).

As summarized in the rotated factor loadings reported below, this analysis confirmed the expected multidimensional nature of the ISP2018 and identified the four principal components of the ISP, i.e., those factors with eigenvalues of at least 0.70, which, separately, explained at least 10% of the variance contained in the ISP but which, when considered together, accounted for at least 75% of the total variance. As expected, the four principal components of the ISP2018 were found to be most closely associated with the following:

1. Changes over time in the adequacy of the national social provision (factor 1 = WISP1);
2. National resources (both environmental and the cultural diversity of the national population) (factor 2 = WISP2);
3. Expenditures on defense relative to world average military expenditures (factor 3 = WISP3);
4. Economic resources and stresses associated with their resources (factor 4 = WISP4).

Table A.2 WISP18 principal components factor analysis with varimax rotation (N = 162)

Rotated Loading Matrix (VARIMAX, Gamma = 1.000000)

	1	2	3	4
S_EDU18	0.730	0.048	0.187	0.144
S_HL18	0.895	0.081	0.109	0.250
S_WOM18	0.897	0.080	0.103	0.177
S_DEF18	0.207	0.017	0.965	0.101
S_ECON18	0.479	−0.132	0.039	0.753
S_DEMO18	0.885	0.032	0.052	0.248
S_ENV18	0.177	−0.842	0.036	0.412
S_CHAOS18	0.142	−0.074	0.076	0.916
S_DIV18	0.465	0.805	0.071	0.175
S_WEL18	0.548	0.002	0.221	0.488

"Variance" explained by rotated components

1	2	3	4
3.762	1.395	1.055	2.029

Percent of total variance explained

1	2	3	4
37.619	13.955	10.548	20.294

Taken together, these four factors, as reported in Table A.2, account for 82.4 percent of the total variance explained by the ISP2018.

Computing Weighted Index of Social Progress Scores

The final step in arriving at the WISP2018 scores was to combine the weighted subindex scores into a new composite index. Since each of the four factors accounted for a different amount of total ISP2018 variance, a new formula was constructed. Thus, and because factor 1 accounted for 37.6% of the total ISP2018 variance explained by the four factors, factor 1 was assigned a statistical weight of 45.6 in the final computation (i.e., 37.6% is 45.6% of the total variance explained by the four factors). Based on the percent of total variance explained through factor analysis, factor 2, in turn, was assigned a weight of 16.9%, factor 3 was assigned a weight of 12.8%, and factor 4 was assigned a weight of 24.5%. Table A.3 summarizes the factor loadings for each of the individual subindexes as well as the variance associated with each factor and its defining subindexes.

Table A.3 WISP18 factors
and factor loadings (N = 162)

Factor 18 (1) Adequacy of Social Provision (N = 5)
.90 * STN Health Status 2018 Subindex
` .90* STN Women's Status 2018 Subindex
.89 * STN Demographic Status 2018 Subindex
.73 * STN Education 2018 Subindex
.55 * STN Welfare Effort 2018 Subindex
Factor 18 (2) National Environment and Diversity Resources (N = 2)
.84 * STN Environmental Status 2018 Subindex
.81 * STN Cultural Diversity 2018 Subindex
Factor 18 (3) Defense and Military Expenditures (N = 1)
.97 * STN Defense Effort 2018 Subindex
Factor 18 (4) Economic Resources and Stress (N = 2)

STN = statistically standarized subindexes

Adjusted WISP2018 Scores

The statistical weighting procedures described above resulted in some of the lowest performing countries on the index having negative scores, whereas, at the same time, it was not easy to discern the highest performing countries on the WISP19. Thus, and given the author's preference for producing an index that ranged from 0 to 100, a constant value of +50 was added to all WISP2018 scores. This process resulted in adjusted numerical scores that were more readily understandable by a considerably larger audience. Thus, the final, but adjusted, WISP2018 scores were computed using the following values:

$$\text{WISP2018} = \left(\left(.456^* \text{factor} 1\right) + \left(.169^* \text{factor} 2\right) + \left(.128^* \text{factor} 3\right) + \left(.245^* \text{factor} 4\right) \right) + 50.$$

Pearson Correlation Coefficients

Table A.4 is a summary of Pearson correlation coefficients for the study's ten sub-indexes and the ISP2018.

Measures of Central Tendency and Dispersion

Finally, Table A.5 reports measures of central tendency and dispersion for all WISP2018 indicators, subindexes, and the composite WISP2018. These data are used throughout the major data-based chapters of this volume.

Table A.4 WISP18 Pearson correlation coefficient matrix by weighted subindex and composite indexes (N = 162)

Pearson Correlation Matrix

	S_HL18	S_EDU18	S_DEMO18	S_ECON18	S_WEL18	S_ENV18	S_WOM18	S_DIV18	S_CHAOS18	S_DEF18	ISP18	WSP18FNL
S_HL18	1.000											
S_EDU18	0.636	1.000										
S_DEMO18	0.846	0.579	1.000									
S_ECON18	0.595	0.458	0.580	1.000								
S_WEL18	0.598	0.433	0.629	0.543	1.000							
S_ENV18	0.182	0.134	0.227	0.493	0.314	1.000						
S_WOM18	0.866	0.622	0.813	0.565	0.517	0.147	1.000					
S_DIV18	0.511	0.397	0.480	0.261	0.360	−0.427	0.495	1.000				
S_CHAOS18	0.385	0.310	0.362	0.680	0.437	0.427	0.333	0.119	1.000			
S_DEF18	0.329	0.306	0.277	0.234	0.321	0.097	0.323	0.198	0.197	1.000		
ISP18	0.910	0.721	0.893	0.754	0.756	0.264	0.872	0.587	0.558	0.379	1.000	
WSP18FNL	0.936	0.731	0.918	0.701	0.721	0.222	0.906	0.573	0.497	0.365	0.993	1.000

Table A.5 WISP18 measures of central tendency and dispersion by weighted subindex and composite index scores (N = 162)

	S_HL18	S_EDU18	S_DEMO18	S_ECON18	S_WEL18	S_ENV18	S_WOM18	S_DIV18	S_CHAOS18	S_DEF18	ISP18	WSP18FNL
N of cases	162	162	162	162	162	162	162	162	162	162	162	162
Minimum	−13.638	−4.318	−6.731	−10.028	−11.366	6.208	−9.774	−7.800	−12.395	8.000	3.271	41.428
Maximum	28.888	23.996	28.947	24.291	26.712	15.157	23.777	21.400	18.669	11.706	186.895	99.014
Range	42.526	28.314	35.678	34.319	38.079	8.948	33.551	29.200	31.064	3.706	183.624	57.586
Median	11.212	10.152	9.231	10.092	8.301	9.983	11.846	11.450	10.087	10.579	96.440	73.362
Arithmetic mean	10.000	10.000	10.000	10.000	8.796	10.000	10.005	9.998	9.840	9.988	98.627	73.048
Standard deviation	8.180	6.141	9.241	6.118	7.974	1.884	7.797	7.329	4.859	1.009	45.459	14.311
Variance	66.919	37.710	85.396	37.427	63.579	3.548	60.797	53.712	23.612	1.018	2066.477	204.817
Skewness (G1)	−0.280	−0.275	0.105	−0.451	0.225	0.247	−0.614	−0.512	−1.460	−0.151	0.007	−0.106
Kurtosis (G2)	−0.578	−0.233	−1.056	0.268	−0.522	−0.554	−0.455	−0.562	4.273	−1.734	−0.979	−1.026

Selected References

International Social Security Association. (2017). *Social security programs through-out the world*. Geneva: International Social Security Association. Retrieved January 4, 2018 from https://www.issa.int/en/ssptw.

Systat. (2017). *Systat 13: Data*. [Product information]. Chicago: Systat Software International. Retrieved September 4, 2018 from https://systatsoftware.com/products/systat/

Appendix B

© Springer Nature Switzerland AG 2019   205
R. J. Estes, *The Social Progress of Nations Revisited, 1970–2020*, Social
Indicators Research Series 78, https://doi.org/10.1007/978-3-030-15907-8

Table B.1 Scores and percent changes on the Index of Social Progress by subindex, development grouping, country, and year, 1970–2018 (N=162)

Country	ISP	Educ	Health	Women	Defense	Econ	Demo	Environ	Chaos	Diversity	Welfare	WISP
Office of Economic Development and Other High-Income Developed Market Economies (N = 34)												
Australia												
1970	172.0	16.9	18.9	25.9	9.9	16.9	16.9	14.9	14.9	12.9	22.9	80.1
1980	176.0	19.0	19.0	15.0	15.0	18.0	18.0	7.0	26.0	18.0	21.0	82.0
1990	176.2	19.7	14.7	19.2	14.7	17.2	18.6	9.1	25.0	17.7	20.3	90.7
2000	167.3	22.7	18.7	19.5	13.4	16.9	18.5	4.8	20.8	9.8	22.2	89.4
2010	156.0	15.8	20.0	17.2	12.5	14.2	17.4	5.7	18.9	12.9	21.6	82.4
2018	167.7	17.1	20.8	19.5	11.1	18.1	17.0	15.2	16.3	12.9	19.8	92.1
%1970–2018	-2.5	1.2	10.0	-24.8	11.7	7.0	0.5	1.7	9.3	-0.1	-13.6	15.0
Austria												
1970	179.0	18.9	17.9	20.9	15.9	12.9	20.9	12.9	15.9	12.9	28.9	83.0
1980	197.0	19.0	21.0	16.0	17.0	18.0	21.0	11.0	26.0	19.0	28.0	90.0
1990	199.6	18.6	17.7	19.2	17.5	19.7	21.9	11.8	25.9	19.4	28.0	101.2
2000	199.7	19.2	19.4	16.6	15.9	19.0	24.7	17.7	20.2	18.9	28.1	99.6
2010	182.0	18.4	22.1	15.6	15.2	12.3	23.3	13.9	18.5	15.8	26.7	92.3
2018	176.6	16.5	23.1	19.6	11.2	18.0	22.3	10.9	13.3	15.8	25.8	96.9
%1970–2018	-1.4	-12.6	29.2	-6.1	-29.5	39.4	6.5	-15.9	-16.4	22.4	-10.7	16.7
Belgium												
1970	173.0	19.9	18.9	17.9	11.9	15.9	20.9	13.9	18.9	7.9	25.9	81.0
1980	190.0	19.0	24.0	19.0	13.0	19.0	21.0	14.0	26.0	9.0	27.0	89.0
1990	188.6	18.2	19.2	19.6	14.0	20.7	21.4	14.5	25.9	8.6	26.7	96.7
2000	186.5	20.4	20.7	19.5	14.2	20.0	25.7	12.7	17.9	6.8	28.6	96.8
2010	163.0	17.5	21.8	18.9	14.6	8.7	23.6	6.2	17.7	6.7	27.0	86.7

2018	166.9	17.4	20.6	20.0	11.2	17.2	20.3	12.9	14.6	6.7	26.1	94.1
%1970–2018	−3.5	−12.8	8.8	11.5	−5.8	7.9	−2.8	−7.4	−22.8	−15.3	0.7	16.2
Canada												
1970	157.0	23.9	18.9	17.9	12.9	18.9	17.9	5.9	16.9	5.9	16.9	76.0
1980	166.0	21.0	20.0	15.0	16.0	17.0	20.0	7.0	26.0	6.0	18.0	78.0
1990	177.5	24.8	19.2	19.3	16.0	22.0	19.3	8.4	25.9	5.7	16.9	93.3
2000	161.0	23.2	19.1	18.0	14.7	19.7	20.0	7.0	21.2	0.6	17.5	85.6
2010	144.0	15.8	19.6	16.8	14.6	15.3	19.2	3.4	19.0	0.7	19.4	77.0
2018	153.6	19.8	19.5	17.0	11.0	18.1	19.6	14.2	16.7	0.7	17.0	90.3
%1970–2018	−2.2	−17.3	3.2	−5.0	−14.7	−4.4	9.2	139.9	−1.1	−88.2	0.8	18.8
Czech Republic												
1995	169.7	17.4	17.3	17.7	12.9	15.8	18.6	18.2	16.9	11.9	23.0	84.4
2000	169.7	19.4	19.6	16.1	12.5	14.8	24.6	11.1	15.3	12.7	23.8	88.2
2010	162.0	17.1	20.6	14.7	12.5	16.4	23.7	10.1	16.2	8.2	22.7	84.7
2018	162.0	19.0	19.6	15.0	11.1	17.7	22.8	13.3	13.5	8.2	21.9	92.1
%1995–2018	−4.5	8.9	13.0	−15.1	−13.8	12.3	22.5	−27.2	−20.3	−30.9	−4.9	9.2
Denmark												
1970	196.0	23.0	19.9	21.9	12.9	14.9	21.9	16.9	14.9	19.9	28.9	91.0
1980	208.0	20.0	21.0	15.0	15.0	19.0	21.0	23.0	26.0	20.0	29.0	92.0
1990	218.8	22.0	19.1	19.0	15.5	23.7	22.4	23.1	25.9	19.6	28.7	108.1
2000	211.3	21.2	20.2	22.2	13.9	20.4	24.0	18.6	21.8	20.0	29.0	106.9
2010	190.0	21.5	20.6	20.0	12.5	13.3	21.6	12.7	19.5	20.6	27.3	98.0
2018	186.9	20.3	21.9	21.3	11.2	18.0	22.5	11.7	13.3	20.6	26.2	99.0
%1970–2018	−4.6	−11.6	9.8	−3.0	−13.1	20.1	2.8	30.9	−11.0	3.5	−9.4	8.8
Finland												
1970	167.0	20.9	17.9	22.9	15.9	10.9	21.9	5.9	12.9	17.9	18.9	80.0
1980	178.0	19.0	19.0	15.0	16.0	17.0	21.0	10.0	22.0	19.0	20.0	81.0

(continued)

Table B.1 (continued)

Country	ISP	Educ	Health	Women	Defense	Econ	Demo	Environ	Chaos	Diversity	Welfare	WISP
1990	189.2	21.3	18.8	20.2	16.7	19.2	20.7	10.1	23.4	18.8	20.0	97.2
2000	192.4	21.6	20.1	22.8	14.5	20.7	23.7	7.5	22.1	19.1	20.3	101.4
2010	173.0	19.4	19.3	20.7	13.7	14.8	22.8	7.2	19.5	17.6	18.0	91.2
2018	171.3	15.3	20.3	21.7	11.0	17.3	22.9	11.5	18.7	17.6	15.1	94.9
%1970–2018	2.6	–26.6	13.3	–5.3	–31.1	58.3	4.5	94.8	44.6	–1.7	–20.3	
France												
1970	175.0	18.9	18.9	15.9	9.0	16.9	18.9	14.9	18.9	14.9	26.9	81.0
1980	193.0	18.0	21.0	22.0	12.0	19.0	19.0	14.0	24.0	16.0	27.0	90.0
1990	192.4	20.0	18.1	20.1	12.4	20.7	20.2	14.8	23.6	15.7	26.7	98.4
2000	180.8	18.8	20.1	15.5	10.8	17.6	24.3	11.1	18.0	18.0	26.7	94.0
2010	166.0	18.6	22.4	14.9	10.4	10.9	22.0	4.7	17.9	18.6	25.6	89.1
2018	166.7	11.6	21.6	15.5	11.2	15.6	21.4	12.0	15.2	18.6	24.1	92.3
%1970–2018	–4.7	–38.6	14.3	–2.8	24.1	–7.8	13.3	–19.8	–19.7	24.7	–10.5	14.0
Germany												
1970	183.0	17.9	18.9	20.9	9.9	14.9	18.9	13.9	16.9	19.9	29.9	85.0
1980	201.0	24.0	21.0	18.0	13.0	20.0	22.0	13.0	24.0	18.0	29.0	94.0
1990	193.3	18.5	17.1	19.1	13.8	21.7	21.7	14.2	24.8	17.9	24.4	98.3
2000	195.1	21.7	19.6	20.1	13.9	18.4	25.9	16.4	18.6	11.1	29.4	99.8
2010	182.0	16.5	22.2	17.9	13.7	12.3	26.4	12.9	18.2	14.5	27.4	94.0
2018	179.7	14.4	22.0	22.4	10.7	18.4	25.8	12.1	12.7	14.5	26.7	98.0
%1970–2018	–1.8	–19.6	16.3	7.1	8.0	23.4	36.4	–13.0	–24.9	–27.2	–10.7	15.3
Greece												
1970	136.0	10.9	18.9	14.9	6.9	11.9	20.9	12.9	18.0	19.9	16.9	64.0
1980	164.0	12.0	22.0	15.0	9.0	16.0	20.0	10.0	22.0	20.0	18.0	76.0
1990	165.4	16.7	20.0	18.2	8.4	11.2	21.8	9.9	20.7	20.0	18.6	87.5
2000	164.5	19.5	20.3	15.0	4.4	16.5	26.5	6.7	14.5	21.9	19.1	89.6

2010	156.0	15.7	20.2	13.4	5.5	14.7	25.2	7.0	14.8	20.7	18.8	84.1
2018	150.1	10.9	21.3	15.7	8.6	11.3	24.6	7.8	12.7	20.7	16.6	90.7
%1970–2018	10.4	−0.3	12.9	5.3	24.4	−5.2	17.4	−39.4	−29.5	4.0	−2.1	41.7
Hong Kong SAR (Peoples Republic of China)												
1980	129.0	12.0	19.0	11.0	17.0	11.0	18.0	6.0	15.0	17.0	6.0	59.0
1990	140.2	14.0	15.5	18.8	18.7	12.0	17.9	5.0	15.6	16.9	6.0	71.3
2000	177.0	19.8	16.3	17.2	18.1	18.8	18.3	23.8	18.2	19.7	6.6	83.8
2010	156.0	15.6	19.7	13.5	18.0	12.5	19.6	14.1	14.6	18.4	9.4	76.2
2018	124.1	8.6	16.1	17.9	10.7	15.2	21.9	10.0	0.1	18.4	5.3	82.3
%1980–2018	−3.8	−28.5	−15.3	62.7	−37.3	37.8	21.7	66.7	−99.3	8.2	−11.7	39.4
Hungary												
1970	173.0	18.9	16.9	16.9	11.9	16.9	22.9	17.9	9.9	16.9	22.9	79.0
1980	165.0	17.0	19.0	18.0	11.0	17.0	20.0	21.0	3.0	15.0	23.0	75.0
1990	175.6	15.6	20.0	18.4	10.2	14.7	20.9	21.8	14.0	17.3	22.7	86.9
2000	175.0	20.6	19.1	15.4	13.9	14.4	26.2	9.6	16.6	16.1	22.9	91.0
2010	168.0	17.2	18.9	14.3	13.4	14.7	24.6	9.8	16.3	15.9	22.9	86.8
2018	155.1	14.8	17.1	14.4	10.7	14.0	23.9	10.9	11.6	15.9	21.7	90.1
% 1970–2018	−10.4	−21.7	0.9	−14.8	−9.9	−17.3	4.5	−38.9	17.2	−6.0	−5.4	14.1
Iceland												
1995	170.1	18.6	18.9	15.9	13.4	16.9	18.2	9.1	18.2	20.0	20.9	87.5
2000	194.6	22.0	20.6	21.1	18.1	21.5	18.4	12.7	21.5	19.3	19.6	98.4
2010	181.0	21.3	23.2	18.6	18.0	18.4	16.4	7.9	19.3	18.1	19.6	93.0
2018	171.8	22.1	21.1	20.1	11.1	20.1	15.6	10.6	15.6	18.1	17.4	94.5
%1995–2018	1.0	18.7	11.6	26.0	−16.8	19.2	−14.2	16.0	−14.3	−9.5	−16.8	8.0

(continued)

Table B.1 (continued)

Country	ISP	Educ	Health	Women	Defense	Econ	Demo	Environ	Chaos	Diversity	Welfare	WISP
Ireland												
1970	184.0	16.9	18.9	20.9	15.9	11.9	21.9	16.9	13.9	19.9	25.9	84.0
1980	187.0	18.0	22.0	15.0	16.0	16.0	17.0	12.0	26.0	20.0	27.0	85.0
1990	188.9	19.9	16.5	19.4	17.3	15.1	18.8	11.5	24.1	19.8	26.6	95.5
2000	180.9	20.5	18.2	15.6	16.1	22.8	18.9	5.2	19.9	16.8	26.7	93.7
2010	148.0	16.6	19.5	16.6	16.1	−0.5	14.5	5.7	18.0	16.0	25.5	76.4
2018	166.9	20.8	18.3	16.0	10.7	21.0	14.8	10.6	14.6	16.0	24.2	92.2
%1970–2018	−9.3	22.9	−3.1	−23.6	−32.9	76.0	−32.4	−37.5	4.9	−19.6	−6.8	9.8
Israel												
1970	84.0	18.9	18.9	13.9	40.0	18.9	13.9	14.9	12.9	11.9	7.9	55.0
1980	104.0	21.0	19.0	25.0	−37.0	6.0	14.0	13.0	22.0	9.0	11.0	63.0
1990	125.9	19.0	18.9	19.7	−10.4	9.9	15.8	12.4	19.7	11.0	10.1	73.3
2000	130.7	20.3	19.4	16.1	−4.2	17.3	9.8	11.3	16.1	14.3	10.6	72.2
2010	116.0	19.6	21.1	14.1	−11.5	11.7	11.0	11.3	14.1	12.3	12.6	67.7
2018	134.8	16.8	18.8	16.2	11.2	16.4	10.6	11.0	12.4	12.3	9.0	83.9
%1970–2018	60.4	−11.0	−0.7	16.7	72.1	−13.1	−23.8	−26.5	−3.9	3.3	14.2	52.5
Italy												
1970	176.0	17.9	18.9	14.9	11.9	12.9	19.9	15.9	14.9	20.9	26.9	81.0
1980	203.0	18.0	23.0	28.0	15.0	15.0	20.0	16.0	22.0	20.0	26.0	93.0
1990	193.5	17.0	17.5	18.9	15.8	17.2	21.6	14.9	25.0	20.0	25.6	97.2
2000	187.8	17.8	22.7	15.5	12.2	18.3	28.0	9.2	16.8	21.5	25.7	98.2
2010	169.0	16.8	22.0	14.0	12.2	12.5	25.8	6.2	16.2	19.7	23.0	89.1
2018	171.1	14.2	21.1	16.4	10.8	15.9	25.3	10.0	16.5	19.7	21.2	94.9
%1970–2018	−2.8	−20.6	11.5	9.7	−9.1	23.1	27.2	−36.9	10.5	−5.8	−21.3	17.2
Japan												
1970	155.0	15.9	18.9	14.9	16.9	16.9	17.9	1.9	16.9	20.9	12.9	73.0

1980	178.0	18.0	20.0	29.0	18.0	19.0	19.0	-3.0	24.0	20.0	16.0	86.0
1990	182.7	19.0	18.2	19.0	17.8	22.1	20.1	4.1	25.6	19.7	16.9	95.2
2000	177.0	20.8	16.9	13.6	15.3	20.1	26.7	8.2	18.4	19.6	17.6	91.5
2010	170.0	16.3	19.5	12.5	14.9	16.8	26.7	9.4	17.1	18.8	18.1	87.4
2018	170.6	14.0	28.9	14.3	8.7	17.6	28.9	10.1	13.6	18.8	15.6	96.6
%1970–2018	10.1	-11.7	52.8	-4.1	-48.4	4.3	61.6	427.6	-19.7	-10.1	21.0	32.3
Korea, Republic of (South Korea)												
1970	103.0	8.9	16.9	14.9	8.9	11.9	9.9	1.9	13.9	13.9	0.9	49.0
1980	117.0	11.0	17.0	13.0	8.0	15.0	15.0	5.0	10.0	18.0	4.0	55.0
1990	139.6	18.7	17.6	17.5	9.1	16.3	16.0	6.4	16.5	18.2	3.4	74.3
2000	136.7	21.7	15.3	14.6	10.3	18.7	15.9	8.7	14.7	13.7	3.1	71.3
2010	127.0	16.8	15.6	14.1	10.1	16.1	17.6	6.6	15.2	8.6	6.1	67.2
2018	131.7	16.9	17.0	17.7	10.6	15.8	19.3	11.7	10.0	8.6	4.1	84.7
%1970–2018	27.9	90.1	0.5	18.7	19.1	32.9	95.0	510.6	-28.1	-38.2	346.5	72.9
Luxembourg												
1995	182.2	15.4	18.1	17.5	15.7	19.7	19.1	14.5	18.2	18.4	25.5	90.7
2000	194.8	21.2	19.6	17.2	16.1	27.6	20.6	9.3	21.0	16.2	25.8	100.0
2010	169.0	14.2	20.7	17.1	15.5	20.6	19.3	4.2	18.7	14.1	24.8	88.4
2018	163.4	16.2	19.0	17.7	11.2	24.3	14.1	13.0	14.0	14.1	19.9	90.2
%1995–2018	-10.3	4.7	5.1	1.6	-29.1	23.6	-26.5	-10.5	-23.5	-23.4	-21.9	-0.5
Mexico												
1970	119.0	7.9	13.9	14.9	16.9	11.9	5.9	11.9	13.9	14.9	5.9	50.0
1980	116.0	12.0	15.0	13.0	19.0	9.0	7.0	6.0	15.0	12.0	8.0	51.0
1990	122.5	11.8	15.6	15.6	18.6	7.8	10.2	8.8	13.0	12.4	8.8	59.3
2000	122.6	15.2	15.1	15.6	16.7	8.4	8.0	9.0	13.1	13.6	7.8	59.9

(continued)

Table B.1 (continued)

Country	ISP	Educ	Health	Women	Defense	Econ	Demo	Environ	Chaos	Diversity	Welfare	WISP
2010	124.0	14.3	13.0	15.5	16.8	9.7	9.8	9.2	12.2	11.9	11.2	60.3
2018	123.1	21.6	13.8	15.1	8.7	11.5	9.5	8.9	11.1	11.9	11.0	81.7
%1970–2018	3.5	172.6	−0.8	1.5	−48.4	−3.7	60.6	−25.4	−20.0	−20.2	86.9	63.5
Netherlands												
1970	185.0	20.9	19.9	21.9	9.9	14.9	19.9	13.9	20.9	15.9	25.9	87.0
1980	188.0	21.0	21.0	15.0	14.0	20.0	21.0	13.0	26.0	14.0	26.0	87.0
1990	194.0	22.2	19.7	19.6	13.8	19.7	20.4	13.5	26.2	13.2	25.8	100.0
2000	179.3	20.7	20.0	20.7	13.6	19.0	22.1	7.8	21.1	10.1	24.2	94.8
2010	166.0	17.4	19.8	19.8	13.4	9.6	20.7	13.5	19.2	9.8	22.7	85.4
2018	165.6	15.4	22.1	21.1	11.0	18.9	21.4	13.2	15.8	9.8	16.8	93.6
%1970–2018	−10.5	−26.2	10.9	−3.6	10.5	27.0	7.6	−4.9	−24.4	−38.4	−35.2	7.6
New Zealand												
1970	176.0	16.9	18.9	27.9	13.9	9.9	16.9	13.9	16.9	13.9	25.9	82.0
1980	176.0	18.0	19.0	16.0	16.0	14.0	18.0	9.0	26.0	15.0	25.0	81.0
1990	179.1	20.1	16.7	18.9	15.7	15.7	18.6	8.6	25.0	14.9	24.9	92.5
2000	182.3	23.6	18.4	20.5	15.3	18.3	17.6	15.9	21.7	5.9	25.1	92.6
2010	167.0	19.0	19.4	18.7	14.9	14.4	16.9	13.1	19.5	10.5	20.9	85.1
2018	167.8	19.8	21.2	20.4	11.1	17.7	17.3	14.1	14.2	10.5	21.5	93.3
%1970–2018	−4.7	17.0	12.0	−26.8	−20.1	78.6	2.4	1.4	−16.0	−24.5	−17.2	13.8
Norway												
1970	184.0	21.9	19.9	23.9	9.9	15.9	20.9	6.9	18.9	19.9	24.9	89.0
1980	192.0	23.0	20.0	15.0	14.0	19.0	21.0	9.0	26.0	20.0	25.0	90.0
1990	198.7	21.2	18.6	19.5	13.8	24.6	21.8	9.0	25.2	20.1	24.9	103.4
2000	205.9	23.9	19.6	21.1	13.1	20.6	23.2	18.7	20.9	20.0	24.9	104.4
2010	179.0	21.2	22.0	19.7	12.8	15.7	20.7	3.7	19.0	19.8	24.2	95.8

2018	170.7	12.7	22.3	21.8	8.9	20.0	18.1	11.5	14.4	19.8	21.3	94.1
%1970–2018	−7.2	−42.1	11.8	−8.7	−10.4	25.8	−13.4	65.9	−23.9	−0.6	−14.6	5.7
Poland												
1970	167.0	18.9	17.9	20.9	6.9	17.9	19.9	15.9	10.9	17.9	18.9	78.0
1980	157.0	15.0	20.0	17.0	9.0	16.0	18.0	19.0	7.0	18.0	19.0	71.0
1990	159.6	15.6	19.4	19.2	8.8	10.9	17.5	19.6	11.3	18.2	19.1	79.5
2000	163.7	20.7	18.5	15.7	12.8	10.7	22.2	9.8	15.5	21.3	16.4	84.7
2010	161.0	17.6	17.2	13.8	12.2	11.8	22.2	12.6	15.4	20.5	17.9	81.9
2018	151.3	13.6	16.5	17.0	9.0	15.9	22.5	9.1	14.0	20.5	13.2	89.4
%1970–2018	−9.4	−27.9	−8.0	−18.5	30.1	−11.0	12.8	−42.9	28.1	14.5	−30.1	14.7
Portugal												
1970	133.0	7.9	16.9	10.9	1.9	10.9	19.9	13.9	14.9	20.9	13.9	62.0
1980	158.0	16.0	18.0	11.0	13.0	8.0	18.0	17.0	22.0	20.0	16.0	70.0
1990	173.1	14.6	19.8	18.1	13.8	13.4	20.1	15.3	21.1	20.0	16.9	86.9
2000	173.3	15.2	19.6	16.9	12.2	16.2	25.5	9.6	18.7	21.9	17.5	90.0
2010	164.0	17.0	21.0	16.4	11.0	10.5	23.0	8.3	17.2	19.7	19.8	86.4
2018	164.0	12.5	20.5	16.5	11.0	15.7	24.9	10.6	15.1	19.7	17.6	92.7
%1970–2018	23.3	58.5	21.0	50.8	476.8	44.1	24.8	−24.1	1.1	−5.8	26.5	49.5
Singapore												
1970	105.0	13.9	18.9	6.9	6.9	12.9	15.9	9.9	7.9	5.9	4.9	50.0
1980	127.0	12.0	20.0	12.0	9.0	22.0	20.0	11.0	9.0	7.0	5.0	60.0
1990	133.2	14.5	18.7	17.9	8.8	19.1	17.5	10.9	13.7	7.1	5.0	69.7
2000	115.6	16.4	18.3	15.7	4.7	21.1	9.9	1.3	13.3	8.7	6.1	64.5
2010	105.0	15.0	14.7	14.4	3.7	15.4	13.8	5.8	13.6	0.9	8.2	58.4
2018	111.3	6.6	14.4	18.2	9.4	16.8	14.0	14.3	8.0	0.9	8.5	77.6
%1970–2018	6.0	−52.2	−23.8	163.4	36.6	30.0	−12.1	44.6	1.8	−84.8	73.2	55.1

(continued)

Table B.1 (continued)

Country	ISP	Educ	Health	Women	Defense	Econ	Demo	Environ	Chaos	Diversity	Welfare	WISP
Slovak Republic												
1995	160.4	16.1	17.2	17.3	11.4	13.1	17.3	18.2	14.4	12.3	23.0	79.6
2000	171.1	20.3	19.5	16.6	13.1	12.8	21.1	15.4	15.1	13.3	23.8	86.7
2010	165.0	16.6	18.1	15.9	12.8	15.1	21.2	13.2	16.0	13.5	22.7	83.9
2018	149.8	9.6	18.2	19.1	10.9	16.6	21.0	10.1	13.5	13.5	17.4	89.2
%1995–2018	−6.6	−40.6	5.3	10.9	−4.7	26.7	21.3	−44.7	−6.4	9.9	−24.5	12.1
Spain												
1970	158.0	10.9	18.9	19.9	13.9	9.9	18.9	15.9	13.9	12.9	21.9	72.0
1980	176.0	13.0	21.0	15.0	15.0	17.0	19.0	17.0	22.0	13.0	22.0	78.0
1990	178.2	18.6	19.0	18.8	15.3	15.8	19.7	15.2	22.2	11.8	21.8	90.0
2000	183.8	17.8	19.8	20.4	14.5	16.5	26.8	10.1	18.3	15.3	24.3	95.7
2010	167.0	17.5	20.3	18.8	14.6	13.4	21.1	6.7	17.4	13.9	22.9	87.3
2018	156.1	9.5	20.5	21.1	11.1	15.6	21.2	11.3	16.3	13.9	15.6	91.0
%1970–2018	−1.2	−12.5	8.6	6.1	−20.5	57.0	12.0	−29.0	17.4	7.7	−28.8	26.4
Sweden												
1970	195.0	23.9	19.9	26.9	9.9	19.9	21.9	6.9	20.9	19.9	23.9	95.0
1980	194.0	23.0	20.0	17.0	14.0	19.0	22.0	10.0	26.0	19.0	25.0	91.0
1990	195.6	20.3	19.5	19.3	14.4	20.8	22.2	9.8	25.5	18.5	25.2	101.6
2000	203.1	23.2	20.5	24.8	12.2	20.0	25.7	10.6	21.3	19.2	25.5	107.2
2010	187.0	20.3	22.1	21.8	13.4	14.5	23.6	10.2	19.4	17.5	24.5	98.3
2018	172.7	12.9	21.9	23.8	9.0	18.4	20.6	13.1	13.5	17.5	22.0	95.0
%1970–2018	−11.4	−46.1	10.0	−11.6	−8.8	−7.5	−6.0	89.4	−35.4	−12.1	−7.9	0.0
Switzerland												
1970	164.0	16.9	19.9	9.9	12.9	15.9	20.9	14.9	19.9	11.9	19.9	75.0
1980	180.0	18.0	21.0	15.0	16.0	20.0	22.0	11.0	26.0	10.0	21.0	83.0

1990	186.4	17.9	19.7	19.0	15.7	24.5	21.6	10.7	26.6	9.8	20.8	96.3
2000	181.1	22.1	20.4	18.3	15.0	19.7	24.6	14.4	20.7	4.9	20.9	93.3
2010	165.0	17.3	21.5	17.0	14.9	7.9	22.2	15.4	19.2	8.6	21.0	83.9
2018	147.0	1.7	21.6	17.5	11.1	19.2	20.9	12.9	14.1	8.6	19.3	87.4
%1970–2018	−10.4	−89.8	8.6	76.5	−14.3	20.5	0.0	−13.5	−29.0	−27.8	−2.8	16.5
Taiwan (Republic of China)												
1980	96.0	11.0	18.0	27.0	32.0	13.0	15.0	11.0	9.0	17.0	7.0	58.0
1990	147.4	18.3	16.7	19.3	11.3	18.8	16.5	12.3	11.3	15.1	7.9	75.1
2000	147.1	21.1	15.8	14.6	10.3	18.3	16.4	8.4	17.2	15.0	9.9	76.8
2010	140.0	13.5	19.5	13.6	9.5	15.4	18.5	8.2	15.8	14.4	11.2	73.2
2018	117.8	6.9	0.9	14.3	8.6	18.3	20.7	12.2	10.0	14.4	11.4	76.8
%1980–2018	22.7	−37.0	−95.0	−47.0	127.0	40.9	38.2	10.7	11.1	−15.3	62.7	32.3
Turkey												
1970	102.0	9.9	5.9	12.9	7.9	7.9	7.9	11.9	13.9	16.9	5.9	44.0
1980	114.0	11.0	12.0	10.0	6.0	9.0	10.0	10.0	21.0	17.0	3.0	49.0
1990	113.8	10.3	12.0	10.5	11.5	10.2	10.6	11.0	13.4	17.2	7.1	55.0
2000	93.8	12.2	12.7	8.0	4.4	8.9	9.8	7.4	5.1	18.4	7.0	48.0
2010	107.0	10.7	14.9	9.0	9.5	10.8	9.7	8.9	7.4	17.9	8.5	52.9
2018	107.3	11.3	14.2	11.6	8.9	9.7	12.7	8.5	2.9	17.9	9.6	76.7
%1970–2018	5.2	14.5	140.3	−10.2	12.9	22.9	60.2	−28.9	−79.1	5.9	62.2	74.3
United Kingdom												
1970	186.0	18.9	18.9	20.9	6.9	11.9	19.9	15.9	32.9	12.9	25.9	87.0
1980	177.0	18.0	20.0	17.0	10.0	16.0	20.0	10.0	26.0	14.0	27.0	84.0
1990	184.5	17.6	18.1	19.9	11.1	19.2	20.2	12.9	25.5	13.6	26.5	95.6

(continued)

Table B.1 (continued)

Country	ISP	Educ	Health	Women	Defense	Econ	Demo	Environ	Chaos	Diversity	Welfare	WISP
2000	185.0	20.7	18.1	18.9	11.1	17.1	24.3	14.2	19.5	14.4	26.7	95.7
2010	167.0	17.9	19.7	17.0	9.8	8.5	22.8	12.5	18.7	14.2	25.4	87.0
2018	165.6	13.8	19.9	17.4	11.2	17.5	20.7	12.2	14.5	14.2	24.2	92.5
%1980–2018	−11.0	−26.9	5.4	−16.7	61.6	47.3	4.0	−23.6	−55.9	10.0	−6.8	6.3
United States												
1970	124.0	20.9	19.9	20.9	3.1	22.9	12.9	−20.1	21.9	12.9	13.9	72.0
1980	147.0	20.0	21.0	20.0	9.0	18.0	16.0	−12.0	26.0	16.0	13.0	77.0
1990	145.9	24.2	21.1	18.8	9.3	22.6	16.5	−22.6	26.0	16.2	13.7	90.2
2000	157.4	23.7	19.3	15.7	9.4	19.5	18.7	6.5	20.0	10.5	14.1	84.8
2010	139.0	17.5	19.5	15.3	5.5	14.7	17.1	5.1	16.6	13.6	14.4	76.2
2018	146.7	10.0	19.5	15.4	9.5	19.2	17.5	11.8	12.6	13.6	17.7	86.9
%1970–2018	18.3	−52.3	−2.3	−26.4	−204.9	−16.0	35.5	158.8	−42.5	5.3	26.9	20.7
Newly Independent States of the Former Soviet Union (N = 21)												
Albania												
1970	136.0	15.9	14.9	11.9	10.9	18.9	14.9	12.9	9.9	14.9	9.9	61.0
1980	116.0	16.0	15.0	12.0	5.0	13.0	16.0	14.0	−2.0	14.0	12.0	54.0
1990	110.0	17.3	17.9	16.5	10.0	8.5	12.7	13.1	2.2	14.3	−2.6	55.0
2000	131.2	14.0	16.1	9.7	14.7	15.1	16.2	9.4	11.0	17.1	7.8	64.8
2010	126.0	12.5	14.0	11.4	13.7	12.5	14.8	9.9	11.0	16.2	10.0	62.0
2018	124.4	19.2	12.9	11.0	10.8	10.0	18.3	10.4	9.5	16.2	6.2	81.2
%1970–2018	−8.5	20.9	−13.5	−7.7	−1.4	−47.2	22.8	−19.5	−4.2	8.7	−37.4	33.2
Armenia												
1995	135.8	13.1	15.9	14.2	11.2	11.1	13.0	10.4	6.0	20.1	20.7	67.5
2000	128.4	15.2	15.3	9.1	5.8	10.9	16.6	11.8	3.3	20.2	20.2	64.9
2010	143.0	12.9	12.5	12.0	9.8	13.6	21.4	12.0	8.6	21.4	18.5	71.4

2018	131.0	16.8	12.9	13.1	11.0	5.9	18.4	7.3	8.6	21.4	15.6	83.9
%1995–2018	−3.6	28.1	−18.8	−7.6	−2.0	−46.7	41.0	−30.0	43.0	6.3	−24.6	24.4
Azerbaijan												
1995	95.6	16.1	16.4	17.6	2.2	0.6	14.2	13.1	4.3	18.3	1.7	52.1
2000	118.6	17.6	15.2	14.3	10.6	16.7	12.5	9.2	1.5	18.7	2.5	59.5
2010	124.0	12.1	11.9	11.3	10.4	19.3	12.8	9.4	4.0	18.5	14.3	61.0
2018	110.0	16.7	10.7	14.1	10.9	3.9	11.0	7.2	5.5	18.5	11.4	77.9
%1995–2018	13.1	3.4	−53.6	−24.3	79.8	84.6	−28.8	−80.4	22.9	1.2	85.1	33.1
Belarus												
1995	137.2	19.0	16.1	19.4	16.2	1.2	18.1	15.5	8.2	10.3	15.5	67.6
2000	152.3	16.9	19.1	15.4	14.5	18.3	23.8	8.5	5.2	16.2	14.4	78.0
2010	157.0	18.3	18.6	18.0	14.3	17.1	24.9	8.7	4.6	15.8	17.1	81.2
2018	138.4	16.3	16.8	19.7	10.9	4.7	21.3	10.5	8.5	15.8	13.8	87.4
%1995–2018	0.8	−14.2	4.8	1.3	−32.6	290.9	17.7	−32.7	3.0	53.8	−10.6	29.2
Bulgaria												
1995	166.0	17.9	18.9	13.9	10.9	21.9	23.9	14.9	9.9	11.9	20.9	77.0
2000	167.3	16.5	18.1	19.9	9.7	12.9	29.0	8.7	14.2	16.3	22.0	89.1
2010	164.0	15.5	17.7	17.1	10.7	13.8	27.4	10.2	14.4	15.1	21.9	85.8
2018	159.7	15.6	17.0	16.8	11.1	13.9	26.5	10.6	13.4	15.1	19.8	92.3
%1995–2018	−3.8	−13.0	−10.2	20.5	1.5	−36.6	11.0	−29.0	35.2	26.8	−5.3	19.8
Croatia												
1995	126.7	15.1	17.9	19.1	4.8	9.6	18.9	16.4	6.3	15.3	12.8	68.7
2000	135.2	14.7	17.0	16.4	9.7	10.2	23.4	10.1	6.7	15.5	11.4	70.3
2010	156.0	15.1	18.4	15.9	13.1	12.9	25.7	9.1	13.4	18.8	13.1	80.5
2018	152.2	13.6	18.5	17.7	10.8	15.2	25.4	8.6	14.6	18.8	9.0	90.7
%1995–2018	20.2	−10.4	3.0	−7.4	125.4	58.4	34.0	−47.5	133.3	23.0	−29.8	32.0

(continued)

Table B.1 (continued)

Country	ISP	Educ	Health	Women	Defense	Econ	Demo	Environ	Chaos	Diversity	Welfare	WISP
Estonia												
1995	150.0	17.9	16.8	21.4	9.5	14.7	19.7	9.3	15.7	6.0	18.9	79.8
2000	152.9	16.2	14.3	17.2	13.6	13.2	28.1	7.2	16.9	7.4	18.8	80.7
2010	147.0	17.6	13.9	16.1	13.4	15.9	25.8	9.8	14.3	1.2	19.0	76.7
2018	153.6	18.7	17.9	17.0	11.0	16.5	25.1	12.7	16.4	1.2	17.2	91.5
%1995–2018	2.5	4.4	6.5	−20.7	15.5	12.4	27.2	36.6	4.3	−79.9	−9.2	14.6
Georgia												
1995	109.3	10.9	14.3	16.3	12.9	1.1	19.4	10.2	9.1	8.8	6.4	55.3
2000	124.9	16.5	16.2	11.3	15.6	9.1	23.8	9.6	8.0	9.4	5.5	63.2
2010	124.0	11.4	14.1	11.8	7.3	11.7	25.2	10.5	10.7	14.1	7.3	64.6
2018	121.4	16.9	14.3	16.2	8.0	10.2	20.0	9.4	9.5	14.1	2.8	82.6
%1995–2018	11.1	55.7	−0.3	−0.4	−37.9	814.3	3.0	−7.3	4.1	59.5	−55.9	49.2
Kazakhstan												
1995	98.3	12.5	14.8	18.0	10.2	6.1	15.6	12.4	7.1	1.9	3.5	50.3
2000	114.8	17.6	16.9	15.5	16.1	13.5	17.2	7.1	6.2	2.6	2.1	58.8
2010	105.0	15.4	13.4	11.1	14.6	15.4	15.5	5.0	6.3	5.8	2.8	53.6
2018	88.5	13.0	14.4	14.0	9.6	6.8	9.7	10.0	7.4	5.8	−2.4	72.9
%1995–2018	−10.0	4.3	−2.3	−22.1	−5.9	11.3	−37.6	−19.4	4.9	205.3	−168.9	44.9
Kyrgyz Republic												
1995	124.0	14.4	10.2	17.5	15.3	7.8	12.9	8.7	10.7	4.3	22.3	61.8
2000	122.4	17.4	14.5	13.6	12.8	9.4	10.4	10.0	6.2	6.0	22.2	61.0
2010	113.0	15.0	11.8	9.3	8.6	11.5	10.3	10.2	8.0	6.5	22.0	56.7
2018	106.0	15.6	12.1	11.1	9.6	6.3	7.1	9.2	8.6	6.5	19.9	76.4
%1995–2018	−14.5	8.1	18.5	−36.6	−36.8	−19.4	−44.7	5.6	−20.2	52.9	−10.7	23.6

Latvia												
1995	146.9	17.5	14.2	21.6	16.7	11.1	20.1	15.2	15.7	1.7	13.1	73.5
2000	149.7	15.9	17.3	14.9	15.3	13.6	27.9	12.8	14.8	3.9	13.3	76.5
2010	147.2	17.0	17.0	13.7	12.8	14.2	26.9	12.7	15.9	2.6	14.3	76.2
2018	136.3	14.9	16.0	16.3	8.6	15.1	27.2	13.4	11.0	2.6	11.5	86.8
%1995–2018	−7.2	−15.2	12.7	−24.7	−48.8	36.5	35.2	−12.0	−30.4	54.5	−12.3	18.1
Lithuania												
1995	155.7	14.9	17.6	20.5	17.4	11.5	17.8	20.3	16.9	5.3	13.5	75.4
2000	142.4	17.1	17.2	14.5	13.1	11.4	23.6	11.4	16.2	5.3	12.6	73.7
2010	165.0	17.5	19.2	14.8	14.3	14.9	25.1	10.7	15.9	14.9	18.0	85.1
2018	158.6	16.3	17.7	18.1	11.0	16.8	27.0	9.8	12.6	14.9	14.3	92.6
%1995–2018	1.9	9.8	0.8	−11.8	−36.9	45.3	51.5	−51.6	−25.2	181.9	6.2	22.8
Macedonia, Former Yugoslav Republic of												
1995	104.7	14.8	17.2	14.9	8.8	4.3	16.4	10.0	12.1	8.3	1.9	55.0
2000	123.7	15.7	17.0	11.9	12.2	10.0	18.2	9.3	10.1	9.0	10.2	63.3
2010	104.0	13.5	16.9	12.0	11.3	5.2	19.3	9.7	11.3	6.8	−2.6	53.5
2018	108.5	12.9	15.1	18.4	8.7	7.4	19.1	10.6	9.5	6.8	0.1	79.8
%1995–2018	3.7	−12.9	−12.0	23.5	−0.9	73.0	16.6	6.1	−21.4	−17.7	−96.8	45.0
Moldova												
1995	136.8	13.6	13.5	18.7	12.6	10.5	16.7	20.2	10.7	12.1	8.0	65.6
2000	131.7	15.1	17.0	16.0	17.0	7.5	19.9	8.8	11.3	12.3	6.8	66.5
2010	135.0	14.0	14.8	16.1	17.1	13.1	23.3	9.3	10.0	11.7	5.2	67.7
2018	116.7	15.5	11.6	15.7	10.7	10.9	21.9	8.2	10.0	11.7	0.4	81.4
%1995–2018	−14.7	14.5	−14.3	−16.0	−15.4	4.2	31.0	−59.5	−6.9	−3.4	−95.1	24.1

(continued)

Table B.1 (continued)

Country	ISP	Educ	Health	Women	Defense	Econ	Demo	Environ	Chaos	Diversity	Welfare	WISP
Romania												
1995	162.0	17.9	16.9	17.9	10.9	18.9	18.9	15.9	10.9	14.9	17.9	74.0
2000	148.8	17.3	13.1	13.9	12.2	9.9	24.5	9.4	13.3	15.3	19.8	76.6
2010	154.0	13.2	14.8	13.3	11.9	14.3	25.5	8.5	13.3	19.5	19.6	79.2
2018	144.7	9.1	15.7	13.5	8.9	16.1	23.6	8.8	13.0	19.5	16.4	87.1
%1995–2018	93.9	−49.5	−6.9	−24.5	−18.8	−14.7	24.8	−44.4	19.3	30.8	−8.2	17.7
Russian Federation												
1995	138.5	16.2	15.3	19.1	12.1	7.2	16.1	10.6	11.9	5.7	24.2	71.2
2000	124.4	16.5	18.3	11.7	6.9	11.9	23.7	6.3	−3.0	7.7	24.3	66.6
2010	126.0	15.0	16.9	12.6	5.5	13.1	24.3	7.2	2.1	5.4	23.6	67.9
2018	124.7	7.3	15.8	15.8	11.1	9.2	20.2	12.2	5.7	5.4	22.0	82.5
%1995–2018	−11.0	−122.4	2.6	−20.8	−8.9	21.0	20.5	12.8	−107.1	−5.8	−9.6	13.7
Slovenia												
1995	167.5	18.3	19.3	17.4	10.0	15.1	19.2	11.3	16.3	19.1	21.4	86.9
2000	166.1	16.7	18.4	14.3	14.7	16.2	23.7	8.5	16.4	15.8	21.4	85.5
2010	166.0	19.0	19.5	14.2	13.4	15.0	24.0	10.3	17.3	12.0	21.3	86.2
2018	154.8	10.1	19.3	15.2	11.1	17.2	24.3	11.2	14.8	12.0	19.5	90.2
%1995–2018	−7.6	−44.6	0.2	−12.7	11.1	14.0	26.3	−0.6	−9.3	−37.3	−9.2	3.8
Tajikistan												
1995	78.8	17.8	11.1	16.0	10.5	1.9	8.4	6.8	3.1	9.1	1.9	40.4
2000	106.8	17.1	10.2	11.2	14.7	13.9	6.8	9.6	4.3	14.3	4.5	50.5
2010	94.0	14.4	3.4	10.3	11.3	15.7	5.9	14.4	6.3	15.1	−2.6	42.2
2018	75.3	7.9	4.0	15.2	10.5	4.6	3.6	7.7	6.6	15.1	0.1	66.6
%1995–2018	−4.5	−55.5	−63.7	−4.8	0.6	141.1	−57.3	14.0	110.7	65.6	−96.8	64.8

Turkmenistan

1995	78.0	18.2	9.1	17.5	11.4	16.1	6.2	9.4	3.2	12.6	6.4	38.3
2000	106.0	16.9	14.6	17.4	7.5	15.1	3.7	8.3	3.1	14.1	5.5	54.0
2010	94.0	14.1	13.3	12.4	9.2	4.1	8.0	7.2	3.6	14.6	7.6	47.3
2018	76.5	1.4	6.1	14.6	10.7	4.3	7.0	7.6	3.3	14.6	7.0	67.3
%1995–2018	−1.9	−92.5	−32.5	−16.4	−6.6	−73.2	11.8	−19.8	0.9	16.3	9.7	75.9

Ukraine

1995	158.1	21.1	16.1	22.6	13.8	6.5	17.7	21.6	11.9	3.1	23.6	78.1
2000	130.8	11.6	17.8	16.5	8.0	12.2	25.6	7.0	8.6	1.8	21.6	70.7
2010	158.0	19.4	15.2	13.1	10.7	15.8	27.3	7.6	11.7	14.1	23.1	83.3
2018	134.8	5.9	17.2	13.6	11.1	9.6	23.2	9.6	10.7	14.1	19.8	85.1
%1995–2018	−14.7	−72.2	6.9	−39.9	−19.7	47.2	30.9	−55.7	−9.9	349.7	−15.9	9.1

Uzbekistan

1995	114.1	25.0	11.8	16.2	9.8	8.4	9.5	11.2	3.0	12.8	6.4	57.7
2000	105.6	17.8	16.2	13.1	13.4	6.5	6.4	8.1	4.0	14.7	5.5	52.1
2010	120.0	19.9	10.2	13.8	16.4	13.0	8.3	8.8	3.3	14.0	11.9	57.6
2018	93.6	6.6	11.4	15.2	10.8	4.0	8.5	7.8	6.9	14.0	8.5	73.1
%1995–2018	−17.9	−73.5	−3.4	−6.6	10.6	−52.3	−10.8	−30.2	126.0	9.1	34.0	26.7

Developing Countries (N = 67)

Algeria

1970	85.0	9.9	7.9	3.9	12.9	7.9	3.9	7.9	0.9	14.9	13.9	36.0
1980	86.0	12.0	6.0	5.0	14.0	6.0	5.0	9.0	1.0	15.0	13.0	36.0
1990	108.9	14.6	11.6	6.5	14.2	9.5	7.9	11.7	4.1	15.4	13.4	50.3
2000	88.9	9.4	13.2	7.1	8.3	6.6	6.2	8.7	−4.5	20.1	13.7	41.9
2010	107.0	11.1	11.5	9.6	9.2	11.6	8.2	8.2	2.7	19.7	14.8	51.8
2018	105.1	15.9	12.8	5.9	10.9	4.8	6.7	7.0	9.2	19.7	12.3	74.7
% 1970–2018	23.6	60.7	61.4	49.9	−15.6	−39.0	70.6	−11.5	909.8	32.1	−11.8	107.6

(continued)

Table B.1 (continued)

Country	ISP	Educ	Health	Women	Defense	Econ	Demo	Environ	Chaos	Diversity	Welfare	WISP
Argentina												
1970	136.0	14.9	14.9	17.9	13.9	6.9	17.9	14.9	5.9	14.9	12.9	61.0
1980	128.0	16.0	17.0	19.0	13.0	1.0	16.0	10.0	3.0	18.0	14.0	60.0
1990	146.2	15.1	16.7	18.8	17.1	-0.1	15.2	10.5	20.6	16.9	15.3	73.3
2000	135.3	19.0	15.1	20.1	14.5	-1.8	14.4	8.3	12.0	17.7	16.0	69.2
2010	150.0	14.3	17.1	19.4	14.9	8.8	14.3	9.9	12.7	19.5	18.7	75.1
2018	150.5	20.8	15.3	19.8	11.0	13.2	13.2	7.5	13.8	19.5	16.4	89.3
% 1970–2018	10.6	39.8	2.7	10.6	-21.0	90.8	-26.5	-49.9	132.9	30.8	27.2	46.4
Bahamas												
2000	112.0	12.6	13.8	16.3	10.0	13.1	9.3	6.6	15.7	9.9	4.8	58.0
2010	118.0	14.7	13.0	15.2	9.2	8.5	9.9	7.5	14.6	19.0	6.4	60.5
2018	124.7	10.8	13.5	14.5	9.0	15.0	13.6	9.2	13.7	19.0	6.4	80.4
% 2000–2018	11.3	-14.0	-2.3	-11.3	-9.6	14.6	45.3	40.2	-12.4	92.0	32.9	38.6
Bahrain												
1995	94.5	16.0	16.4	11.3	5.5	8.4	11.5	9.2	5.7	9.8	0.7	49.6
2000	78.9	10.2	15.0	12.7	6.9	13.9	5.4	-4.0	8.3	11.7	-1.3	44.4
2010	93.0	16.5	13.4	13.7	7.0	12.2	7.6	0.3	9.3	11.7	1.2	51.1
2018	91.1	14.7	14.5	12.6	9.6	8.0	5.6	11.4	6.6	11.7	-3.6	71.5
% 1995–2018	-3.7	-8.2	-11.4	11.7	74.9	-4.5	-51.7	24.6	14.7	18.9	-624.7	44.1
Belize												
2000	76.4	12.2	12.2	14.8	-4.5	12.7	5.4	7.9	14.6	1.7	0.5	44.1
2010	85.0	13.5	12.8	11.6	-6.6	8.8	4.1	21.0	13.6	3.9	2.5	43.9
2018	86.6	13.0	11.4	10.3	8.8	12.6	4.2	10.9	13.2	3.9	-1.8	69.9
% 2000–2018	13.4	6.4	-6.7	-29.9	-295.1	-0.3	-22.1	38.9	-9.2	126.6	-242.0	58.6

Bolivia												
1970	81.0	11.9	11.9	6.9	15.9	3.9	5.9	7.9	1.9	4.9	8.9	35.0
1980	91.0	11.0	4.0	12.0	14.0	8.0	6.0	10.0	15.0	2.0	7.0	37.0
1990	61.5	6.5	3.8	7.6	14.2	-9.3	5.1	9.2	13.6	2.1	8.7	26.8
2000	90.5	10.6	8.6	7.8	13.9	3.4	3.5	14.4	12.4	4.5	11.4	40.2
2010	101.0	16.0	8.7	10.9	13.1	5.7	4.3	14.6	11.0	3.8	12.9	46.8
2018	96.8	13.8	6.8	11.6	8.9	11.3	6.7	8.7	12.6	3.8	12.7	73.4
% 1970–2018	19.5	15.7	-43.0	68.3	-44.2	189.8	12.9	9.5	559.4	-22.6	42.6	109.6
Botswana												
1995	71.9	16.0	9.3	10.4	6.2	8.4	6.8	-10.1	15.7	7.3	2.0	44.3
2000	94.2	13.6	5.6	14.2	7.8	4.5	2.4	16.0	16.4	10.6	3.1	44.3
2010	105.0	18.1	5.6	11.8	8.9	5.6	9.3	17.0	14.7	11.6	2.3	50.0
2018	91.3	14.2	3.8	10.2	9.3	10.9	5.1	10.3	13.1	11.6	2.7	69.5
% 1995–2018	27.0	-11.3	-58.8	-2.1	50.4	30.1	-24.0	-202.2	-17.0	59.7	39.1	57.0
Brazil												
1970	123.0	13.9	13.9	17.9	12.9	2.9	6.9	6.9	9.9	19.9	16.9	56.0
1980	131.0	12.0	12.0	10.0	18.0	11.0	10.0	6.0	14.0	20.0	19.0	57.0
1990	132.0	7.4	9.7	16.5	18.2	7.8	9.6	7.9	15.7	20.0	19.1	63.0
2000	109.8	8.8	13.0	15.1	14.5	-5.4	10.5	10.2	12.5	11.1	19.6	53.3
2010	134.0	14.7	15.2	14.9	13.1	6.6	9.8	13.7	13.2	13.0	19.6	65.4
2018	137.9	21.8	13.7	12.5	11.0	11.2	13.1	10.2	13.7	13.0	17.6	84.6
% 1970–2018	12.1	56.6	-1.3	-30.1	-14.6	285.0	89.6	47.4	38.2	-34.7	4.3	51.1
Cameroon												
1970	60.0	4.9	1.1	9.9	13.9	6.9	6.9	9.9	10.9	8.1	4.9	23.0
1980	59.0	5.0	4.0	6.0	16.0	9.0	6.0	12.0	1.0	-8.0	7.0	22.0
1990	50.6	6.3	1.6	4.3	7.9	11.0	3.5	11.2	5.1	-8.5	8.0	21.4
2000	45.2	1.8	-0.7	3.2	14.5	4.2	1.9	10.9	4.4	-2.9	8.0	14.9

(continued)

Table B.1 (continued)

Country	ISP	Educ	Health	Women	Defense	Econ	Demo	Environ	Chaos	Diversity	Welfare	WISP
2010	45.0	-0.7	-1.5	0.6	14.0	9.0	2.8	11.7	5.6	-6.3	9.9	14.4
2018	39.6	8.5	-0.7	-2.0	10.8	5.0	-1.9	11.3	7.6	-6.3	7.3	54.3
% 1970–2018	-33.9	73.3	-162.1	-119.7	-22.5	-28.0	-127.6	13.8	-30.1	-177.8	49.0	136.2
Chile												
1970	135.0	12.9	13.9	15.9	13.9	4.9	12.9	4.9	15.9	17.9	20.9	62.0
1980	112.0	15.0	14.0	14.0	13.0	-9.0	16.0	6.0	7.0	14.0	22.0	54.0
1990	135.7	10.9	17.0	16.6	13.1	10.4	14.5	6.1	10.2	15.2	21.7	69.2
2000	149.0	16.7	16.3	14.5	8.9	6.5	11.8	15.4	17.8	19.3	21.8	74.5
2010	137.0	14.6	14.5	13.2	6.4	8.4	13.2	9.0	17.6	18.2	21.6	71.2
2018	151.4	18.7	14.4	13.9	11.1	15.2	14.8	9.9	15.6	18.2	19.7	87.5
% 1970–2018	12.2	44.5	3.3	-12.7	-20.4	210.3	14.6	101.9	-2.0	1.6	-5.8	41.2
China, People's Republic of												
1980	69.0	12.0	13.0	10.0	0.1	14.0	2.0	3.0	3.0	16.0	6.0	36.0
1990	96.5	9.2	16.8	12.5	11.7	17.8	0.5	1.0	4.9	15.8	6.4	48.5
2000	112.3	15.7	12.8	16.6	12.2	14.0	14.2	10.8	4.9	4.2	6.8	56.3
2010	89.0	10.7	11.7	13.2	11.9	14.0	15.2	-4.3	5.3	2.1	8.7	49.1
2018	97.7	11.9	14.6	15.3	9.0	6.4	16.5	10.3	3.9	2.1	7.8	76.9
% 1980–2018	41.6	-1.1	12.2	52.9	8867.8	-54.3	925.9	443.3	30.5	-86.9	29.8	113.5
Colombia												
1970	118.0	8.9	11.9	11.9	15.9	8.9	5.9	7.9	13.9	19.9	11.9	50.0
1980	131.0	12.0	13.0	13.0	17.0	11.0	10.0	7.0	21.0	14.0	11.0	57.0
1990	129.6	10.9	13.6	16.2	15.8	10.8	11.9	8.1	16.5	14.0	11.6	64.2
2000	109.3	12.3	13.2	16.2	11.7	2.4	7.5	12.1	6.4	13.6	13.9	52.8
2010	118.0	12.7	15.7	14.9	6.7	5.9	7.9	29.3	-2.1	12.1	15.0	52.4
2018	116.3	13.2	14.0	12.7	10.9	10.2	11.2	8.1	11.4	12.1	12.5	79.3

% 1970–2018	–1.4	48.1	17.4	6.7	–31.5	14.2	89.9	2.9	–17.9	–39.2	4.8	58.7
Congo, Republic of the (Brazzaville)												
1980	54.0	8.0	3.0	8.0	12.0	0.1	7.0	10.0	2.0	3.0	10.0	22.0
1990	59.9	12.7	9.5	2.4	11.3	4.8	3.6	8.8	0.2	–3.7	10.2	26.9
2000	54.7	4.7	–1.0	5.0	7.5	9.8	–0.9	10.1	6.7	2.6	10.1	22.4
2010	53.5	2.9	–0.8	1.4	13.7	6.2	–2.7	14.1	6.1	1.1	11.6	17.3
2018	49.0	9.6	2.5	1.4	9.0	–2.8	–0.2	9.9	8.0	1.1	10.6	58.5
% 1980–2018	–9.3	19.6	–18.0	–82.7	–25.3	–2885.8	–102.9	–1.2	499.8	–63.3	6.3	165.9
Costa Rica												
1970	137.0	19.9	14.9	13.9	15.9	9.9	6.9	10.9	16.9	19.9	6.9	60.0
1980	155.0	19.0	17.0	14.0	18.0	10.0	14.0	11.0	26.0	16.0	10.0	69.0
1990	150.9	13.8	18.3	18.5	18.6	7.8	13.9	10.9	21.8	16.2	11.1	74.9
2000	142.8	14.3	16.2	18.0	18.1	9.6	5.4	14.3	15.9	19.6	11.5	67.5
2010	154.0	15.9	16.5	22.7	18.0	10.0	8.4	15.5	16.1	18.3	12.4	74.1
2018	150.7	24.0	16.5	20.0	10.8	15.3	12.3	9.3	14.3	18.3	9.9	89.0
% 1970–2018	10.0	20.5	10.3	43.6	–31.9	54.9	78.5	–14.8	–15.6	–8.1	43.0	48.3
Cote d'Ivoire												
1970	68.0	4.9	0.9	3.9	15.9	10.9	5.9	13.9	8.9	4.1	5.9	24.0
1980	65.0	11.0	2.0	5.0	17.0	8.0	0.1	11.0	7.0	–6.0	9.0	24.0
1990	48.2	6.3	1.7	–0.9	17.5	8.0	0.8	9.6	1.8	–6.5	10.0	16.0
2000	40.6	–2.6	0.8	–1.6	15.3	4.7	2.0	11.4	8.0	–5.2	7.8	11.6
2010	32.0	–2.0	–0.6	–4.2	13.4	5.2	3.2	14.1	1.4	–7.6	9.3	6.4
2018	37.7	3.1	–3.7	–4.5	10.7	9.6	0.3	13.3	11.4	–7.6	5.1	51.8
% 1970–2018	–44.6	–37.4	–506.7	–215.0	–32.6	–12.1	–94.5	–4.5	27.8	–85.8	–14.1	115.8

(continued)

Table B.1 (continued)

Country	ISP	Educ	Health	Women	Defense	Econ	Demo	Environ	Chaos	Diversity	Welfare	WISP
Cuba												
1970	139.0	21.9	16.9	18.9	3.9	11.9	13.9	12.9	5.9	19.9	11.9	67.0
1980	122.0	21.0	19.0	16.0	7.0	11.0	18.0	13.0	1.0	7.0	9.0	59.0
1990	126.6	18.6	20.6	17.5	9.9	6.9	18.0	13.7	5.9	6.5	9.0	65.4
2000	121.6	12.8	19.6	20.2	6.9	11.3	18.7	8.0	3.3	12.0	8.8	65.0
2010	134.0	22.3	22.8	19.6	5.8	9.6	19.1	9.1	5.2	11.2	9.6	73.3
2018	130.4	13.4	26.1	20.3	9.2	2.1	21.5	10.0	3.1	11.2	13.4	88.0
% 1970–2018	−6.2	−38.6	54.2	7.6	136.3	−82.7	54.6	−22.6	−47.2	−43.7	12.3	31.3
Cyprus												
1995	147.0	15.6	19.0	13.9	5.7	16.7	17.0	18.2	18.2	12.4	10.3	74.8
2000	132.5	11.7	18.8	12.5	9.2	17.1	16.8	6.4	17.4	13.0	9.7	69.7
2010	136.0	19.0	16.4	12.4	13.7	12.2	15.9	8.1	15.7	11.9	10.9	69.9
2018	130.9	15.5	16.1	15.4	10.8	16.5	15.5	8.4	14.3	11.9	6.7	84.1
% 1995–2018	−10.9	−0.4	−15.1	10.7	88.6	−1.0	−9.1	−54.2	−21.7	−4.1	−34.8	12.3
Dominican Republic												
1970	112.0	5.9	14.9	13.9	12.9	9.9	3.9	10.9	12.9	19.9	5.9	47.0
1980	129.0	6.0	11.0	18.0	17.0	10.0	8.0	15.0	21.0	16.0	8.0	53.0
1990	123.0	7.1	8.4	16.5	17.1	9.3	10.3	12.9	16.8	16.4	8.1	57.2
2000	129.0	10.1	10.8	17.1	15.0	11.9	7.6	18.5	13.7	16.3	8.1	59.0
2010	117.0	7.4	9.5	17.2	16.4	6.9	6.7	15.3	12.8	15.7	9.0	53.0
2018	107.1	12.8	9.0	13.2	10.8	12.1	8.6	8.9	9.4	15.7	6.7	75.1
% 1970–2018	−4.3	116.8	−39.6	−5.1	−16.6	22.3	119.4	−18.7	−27.3	−21.1	13.3	59.8
Ecuador												
1970	108.0	10.9	10.9	15.9	13.9	10.9	5.9	1.9	11.9	13.9	10.9	49.0

1980	121.0	15.0	9.0	11.0	15.0	10.0	8.0	5.0	22.0	12.0	13.0	53.0
1990	114.8	12.3	8.2	14.2	16.7	7.5	8.9	3.9	16.8	12.5	13.6	56.9
2000	129.8	15.2	13.6	14.6	8.6	7.1	6.7	26.1	10.9	12.6	14.6	59.5
2010	117.0	7.8	12.9	16.0	10.1	8.1	8.4	15.3	10.4	13.4	14.8	55.9
2018	115.6	16.5	12.2	13.4	10.9	8.9	8.6	8.8	8.8	13.4	14.1	78.6
% 1970–2018	7.0	51.7	11.5	−15.7	−21.4	−18.8	45.4	360.7	−26.2	−3.7	29.0	60.4
Egypt												
1970	70.0	8.9	8.9	3.9	10.1	7.9	6.9	6.9	9.9	19.9	5.9	35.0
1980	81.0	8.0	11.0	4.0	0.1	6.0	9.0	9.0	9.0	17.0	8.0	37.0
1990	93.0	11.0	13.5	6.5	3.0	6.7	7.9	9.2	9.0	17.1	9.1	47.3
2000	102.3	8.9	14.1	6.1	11.7	13.8	6.3	8.8	6.0	17.4	9.4	48.3
2010	100.0	11.1	10.4	7.2	9.5	11.3	6.0	10.2	6.9	16.9	10.8	47.5
2018	83.2	10.5	9.6	6.2	9.1	5.7	2.4	7.5	4.8	16.9	10.6	68.1
% 1970–2018	18.9	17.6	7.9	58.8	−10.3	−28.1	−65.4	8.3	−51.4	−15.1	79.2	94.6
El Salvador												
1970	115.0	8.9	13.9	10.9	11.9	8.9	6.9	14.9	13.9	16.9	6.9	48.0
1980	109.0	5.0	10.0	6.0	14.0	11.0	8.0	16.0	12.0	17.0	9.0	73.0
1990	113.0	5.2	9.6	15.0	12.6	9.9	9.6	14.1	12.3	17.0	7.8	52.5
2000	111.0	8.9	12.7	13.9	16.1	7.7	6.3	8.7	12.9	17.7	6.1	52.6
2010	110.0	7.4	12.6	13.8	16.1	6.7	6.4	9.5	12.7	17.6	7.5	51.7
2018	114.6	14.6	12.2	11.8	10.7	11.1	12.8	8.4	9.6	17.6	5.7	78.1
% 1970–2018	−0.3	64.3	−12.6	8.1	−9.8	24.8	85.5	−43.7	−31.0	4.1	−17.1	62.7
Fiji												
1995	95.2	15.6	14.3	10.9	14.6	12.5	11.1	1.2	12.1	0.8	2.1	50.2
2000	71.6	5.8	8.5	9.5	13.9	3.1	8.5	8.9	11.2	1.8	0.4	33.0
2010	88.0	17.0	11.7	10.6	14.3	5.0	9.1	9.4	7.4	1.0	2.4	42.8

(continued)

Table B.1 (continued)

Country	ISP	Educ	Health	Women	Defense	Econ	Demo	Environ	Chaos	Diversity	Welfare	WISP
2018	83.3	11.0	10.1	7.9	10.6	9.9	10.3	11.2	10.1	1.0	1.1	69.5
% 1995–2018	−12.5	−29.7	−29.3	−27.2	−27.1	−20.5	−7.1	834.7	−16.1	21.5	−49.5	38.3
Gabon												
1995	67.0	3.5	3.3	3.5	13.1	9.0	5.4	9.0	9.6	1.0	10.4	28.6
2000	67.4	7.1	4.8	3.8	17.3	5.9	3.7	9.8	7.6	−2.0	9.5	27.5
2010	68.0	7.0	5.7	6.3	13.4	5.6	4.2	10.1	8.1	−3.3	11.0	29.8
2018	55.7	9.1	5.5	2.8	10.8	2.4	3.0	9.3	7.8	−3.3	8.2	61.5
% 1995–2018	−16.9	163.8	66.2	−21.4	−17.6	−73.2	−44.4	3.0	−18.6	−430.0	−20.7	114.8
Ghana												
1970	57.0	5.9	7.9	5.9	12.9	8.9	5.9	13.9	−1.1	−6.1	1.9	22.0
1980	56.0	4.0	4.0	2.0	19.0	2.0	3.0	12.0	12.0	−6.0	5.0	18.0
1990	48.8	5.2	2.7	0.9	18.0	7.7	3.5	11.0	0.1	−6.4	6.2	16.1
2000	63.5	4.5	5.8	3.9	15.3	6.9	2.5	11.1	12.7	−1.8	2.5	25.8
2010	72.0	4.9	3.9	3.6	15.8	10.7	2.9	13.9	14.1	−1.9	4.3	28.9
2018	69.4	11.0	3.2	4.5	11.2	13.3	0.8	11.3	14.3	−1.9	1.8	62.7
% 1970–2018	21.8	85.4	−60.0	−23.8	−13.0	49.3	−87.3	−18.8	1480.8	−68.8	−5.3	185.2
Guatemala												
1970	64.0	3.9	8.9	7.9	16.9	8.9	4.9	12.1	13.9	6.9	2.9	30.0
1980	67.0	3.0	8.0	3.0	17.0	12.0	7.0	−6.0	12.0	7.0	5.0	30.0
1990	70.5	1.8	8.3	9.2	15.7	10.1	6.9	−6.3	12.4	7.0	5.3	36.3
2000	81.0	2.4	10.3	8.0	15.9	7.1	1.3	15.7	10.1	5.2	5.1	32.8
2010	79.0	2.6	9.1	7.2	17.1	7.1	1.2	15.3	9.3	4.4	5.8	31.3
2018	72.2	6.9	7.8	6.6	11.0	9.3	3.7	9.7	8.4	4.4	4.4	65.0
% 1970–2018	12.8	76.9	−12.4	−16.8	−35.0	4.9	−25.2	180.0	−39.8	−36.3	51.1	116.7
Guyana												
1995	97.7	10.8	9.1	9.8	14.5	9.3	11.9	5.7	15.7	2.1	8.7	48.7

2000	113.5	15.4	9.1	14.7	13.4	5.8	12.8	14.0	14.4	5.8	8.2	55.1
2010	111.0	25.3	9.6	12.3	12.8	5.3	12.7	9.4	11.6	3.4	8.8	56.9
2018	118.0	21.5	7.1	16.6	10.8	10.9	10.5	11.6	11.1	3.4	14.4	79.5
% 1995–2018	20.7	99.4	−21.6	69.7	−25.9	17.1	−11.9	102.8	−29.5	61.2	66.4	63.1
Honduras												
1970	88.0	8.9	11.9	9.9	13.9	8.9	3.9	1.1	10.9	17.9	1.9	40.0
1980	80.0	8.0	8.0	8.0	12.0	4.0	5.0	1.0	10.0	18.0	5.0	35.0
1990	98.4	7.5	10.9	14.1	12.8	6.5	6.3	0.8	14.1	17.7	7.7	50.0
2000	94.6	6.5	11.5	14.9	16.4	4.0	1.2	5.2	11.2	19.6	4.1	44.3
2010	114.0	8.3	10.8	17.5	16.1	7.9	2.4	14.9	10.7	19.1	6.0	51.1
2018	85.5	9.8	9.9	6.3	8.6	8.8	5.2	7.9	8.1	19.1	1.8	68.5
% 1970–2018	−2.9	9.7	−16.6	−36.4	−37.9	−1.5	31.8	−615.9	−25.7	6.6	−6.5	71.2
India												
1970	54.0	3.9	4.9	7.9	11.9	4.9	10.1	6.9	14.9	0.9	6.9	19.0
1980	70.0	3.0	4.0	3.0	14.0	9.0	−2.0	3.0	22.0	6.0	8.0	27.0
1990	82.6	4.2	8.2	3.6	12.8	12.2	−1.2	14.0	14.3	6.3	8.3	34.6
2000	76.8	5.5	5.9	3.0	11.4	9.7	7.8	10.6	9.4	5.2	8.3	34.1
2010	69.0	6.7	4.8	4.9	9.5	13.9	7.8	1.5	2.7	4.4	12.7	33.9
2018	90.3	9.0	4.7	7.3	11.0	12.7	8.5	9.6	9.7	4.4	13.4	69.9
% 1970–2018	67.3	130.4	−3.7	−7.6	−7.5	158.9	184.3	38.7	−35.2	383.5	94.2	267.8
Indonesia												
1970	26.0	4.9	1.9	9.9	10.9	23.1	0.2	5.9	7.9	3.9	2.9	9.0
1980	95.0	9.0	7.0	23.0	13.0	10.0	7.0	9.0	9.0	4.0	6.0	42.0
1990	90.8	9.0	9.8	9.8	15.1	12.6	8.5	9.1	6.4	3.9	6.6	42.2
2000	97.8	12.0	9.6	7.9	15.0	10.5	9.4	13.1	9.1	4.7	6.5	44.7
2010	66.0	7.9	9.0	10.4	14.3	11.9	9.7	−15.8	8.9	3.7	5.4	39.1

(continued)

Table B.1 (continued)

Country	ISP	Educ	Health	Women	Defense	Econ	Demo	Environ	Chaos	Diversity	Welfare	WISP
2018	87.2	10.5	6.9	11.3	9.1	11.9	9.3	10.4	9.5	3.7	4.6	70.4
% 1970–2018	235.5	113.9	261.0	14.3	−16.4	151.3	4560.7	76.1	20.6	−5.4	56.9	682.1
Iran												
1970	65.0	4.9	7.9	1.9	4.9	13.9	4.9	5.1	12.9	7.9	9.9	32.0
1980	76.0	15.0	6.0	6.0	6.0	12.0	6.0	−5.0	7.0	11.0	12.0	38.0
1990	80.8	12.3	16.4	7.3	5.3	6.8	7.1	−0.9	4.4	11.0	10.9	44.6
2000	93.1	10.9	13.9	11.0	7.5	10.7	5.2	9.3	4.7	8.6	11.5	46.1
2010	87.0	13.0	11.2	10.5	0.4	11.2	8.7	4.2	5.4	9.5	13.2	48.0
2018	88.3	7.8	12.3	9.9	8.7	5.0	9.3	8.0	7.6	9.5	10.1	71.9
% 1970–2018	35.9	59.8	55.4	417.0	77.5	−63.9	90.3	257.5	−41.0	20.1	2.0	124.8
Iraq												
1970	62.0	12.9	13.9	3.1	10.1	10.9	5.9	9.9	0.9	13.9	5.9	32.0
1980	61.0	11.0	11.0	12.0	−21.0	13.0	4.0	12.0	−2.0	14.0	7.0	35.0
1990	43.8	11.2	13.5	6.3	−38.3	11.3	5.6	11.5	−0.1	13.8	9.1	35.3
2000	67.6	0.8	5.8	2.7	10.0	17.2	0.9	8.3	2.2	11.0	8.7	28.1
2010	34.0	5.9	8.7	7.7	9.2	5.4	−0.2	8.4	−18.8	10.4	−2.6	11.6
2018	56.3	8.1	5.8	11.0	10.8	5.0	−1.2	7.1	−3.6	10.4	2.8	61.7
% 1970–2018	−9.2	−37.1	−58.2	455.0	297.5	−53.8	−120.0	−28.0	−495.1	−25.2	−53.3	92.7
Jamaica												
1970	129.0	10.9	16.9	13.9	17.9	11.9	10.9	11.9	10.9	18.9	3.9	55.0
1980	141.0	16.0	18.0	22.0	17.0	3.0	12.0	13.0	21.0	16.0	4.0	62.0
1990	135.5	14.7	16.2	17.6	17.8	4.2	14.3	11.9	18.7	15.5	4.6	66.7
2000	114.0	12.1	14.7	16.9	10.0	7.5	12.9	7.4	12.5	15.3	4.6	58.9
2010	125.0	12.4	11.3	15.5	16.1	6.5	12.5	12.4	12.1	15.0	11.0	59.7
2018	116.9	9.3	10.9	13.1	11.1	10.1	13.7	9.3	14.7	15.0	9.8	78.2
% 1970–2018	−9.4	−15.1	−35.4	−5.8	−38.0	−15.4	25.5	−22.1	34.9	−20.7	149.7	42.2

Jordan												
1970	41.0	4.9	14.9	4.9	33.1	7.9	3.9	7.9	4.9	19.9	3.9	29.0
1980	62.0	13.0	11.0	21.0	-31.0	10.0	5.0	10.0	1.0	19.0	2.0	39.0
1990	91.1	18.5	15.8	11.4	-3.9	8.4	7.0	9.3	6.1	19.3	-0.7	50.2
2000	72.4	12.2	15.9	11.3	-8.4	10.5	-2.4	9.7	9.2	16.1	-1.7	40.5
2010	94.0	14.8	15.0	11.4	1.9	11.5	2.3	11.5	10.0	14.9	1.0	48.2
2018	89.8	8.1	18.2	12.6	11.0	5.0	2.2	7.9	8.9	14.9	1.0	71.7
% 1970–2018												
Kenya												
1970	68.0	6.9	10.9	1.9	15.9	12.9	4.9	7.9	8.9	-4.1	1.9	27.0
1980	63.0	13.0	6.0	5.0	11.0	7.0	2.0	10.0	10.0	-5.0	4.0	26.0
1990	57.6	6.6	7.5	8.7	15.3	8.7	1.4	9.4	1.3	-5.6	4.3	23.7
2000	36.2	5.7	0.4	3.9	13.1	-0.1	0.8	11.5	5.6	-8.9	4.2	11.8
2010	59.0	11.4	-0.3	6.4	12.8	4.4	0.5	12.8	9.1	-3.7	6.0	24.0
2018	58.5	8.0	9.6	2.3	10.6	3.5	1.2	12.9	8.6	-3.7	5.6	61.0
% 1970–2018	-14.0	16.2	-12.2	19.2	-33.7	-73.0	-76.2	63.0	-3.6	-9.5	192.9	125.8
Korea, People's Democratic Republic (North Korea)												
1980	70	6.0	17.0	17.0	17.0	13.0	12.0	7.0	-2.0	18.0	2.0	40.0
1990	70	11.0	19.0	14.0	-23.8	11.2	11.8	8.2	3.1	18.0	-2.6	47.2
2000	-11	16.2	5.8	15.7	-62.8	10.0	12.9	-32.5	3.8	13.0	6.8	34.6
2010	10	13.4	10.0	14.6	-70.1	8.7	13.8	5.2	4.7	11.7	-2.6	34.2
2018	74.5	13.3	9.7	9.9	8.9	-2.7	14.9	8.5	0.5	11.7	0.1	69.6
% 1980–2018	6.5	120.9	-42.9	-41.9	152.1	-121.0	23.9	20.8	125.0	-35.0	-96.9	74.0

(continued)

Table B.1 (continued)

Country	ISP	Educ	Health	Women	Defense	Econ	Demo	Environ	Chaos	Diversity	Welfare	WISP
Kuwait												
1995	91.3	13.3	17.4	12.5	12.6	17.3	13.5	9.0	8.2	12.0	0.7	54.7
2000	80.4	11.0	16.7	10.6	-4.8	14.4	14.9	-1.4	10.1	10.5	-1.7	49.9
2010	82.0	15.4	14.1	10.7	3.4	18.3	3.8	-5.3	10.4	9.6	1.2	47.9
2018	92.3	11.9	14.2	10.0	9.3	11.1	7.8	11.6	7.5	9.6	-0.7	71.5
% 1995–2018	1.0	-10.4	-18.3	-20.1	173.3	-36.3	-41.7	29.0	-9.3	-19.9	-202.4	30.6
Lebanon												
1970	117.0	14.9	15.9	9.9	11.9	9.9	13.9	9.9	12.9	10.9	5.9	53.0
1980	137.0	16.0	14.0	27.0	9.0	12.0	14.0	14.0	12.0	11.0	9.0	64.0
1990	77.6	12.4	5.3	11.2	-13.0	8.3	13.9	12.3	7.0	10.8	9.3	44.8
2000	103.2	9.7	15.9	11.3	8.0	10.1	7.3	7.1	8.1	16.5	9.2	52.1
2010	100.0	10.0	15.3	10.0	4.3	9.2	11.2	8.1	7.1	13.8	10.8	51.7
2018	117.7	11.8	14.9	10.4	10.9	8.1	18.5	9.4	10.5	13.8	9.4	79.9
% 1970–2018	0.6	-21.2	-6.6	4.9	-8.7	-18.5	33.3	-4.7	-18.5	26.5	59.7	50.8
Libya												
1970	47.0	11.9	3.1	1.1	3.1	13.9	4.9	5.9	1.1	16.9	1.9	21.0
1980	90.0	10.0	15.0	5.0	4.0	21.0	3.0	9.0	1.0	18.0	4.0	40.0
1990	83.8	19.1	13.8	2.9	-0.5	7.0	4.0	8.5	4.5	18.4	6.0	43.8
2000	93.7	10.3	13.3	8.4	7.2	9.4	6.0	6.7	4.8	21.2	6.3	46.3
2010	99.0	11.0	13.6	10.8	11.9	8.7	6.1	5.9	4.0	20.7	6.3	48.1
2018	106.8	10.5	12.2	9.3	10.7	20.8	6.4	6.2	2.6	20.7	7.3	74.4
% 1970–2018	127.2	-11.8	494.5	955.9	361.9	49.9	29.7	5.0	341.1	22.4	280.9	254.5
Malaysia												
1970	80.0	9.9	12.9	7.9	10.9	9.9	6.9	7.9	11.9	4.1	4.9	36.0
1980	102.0	14.0	16.0	9.0	11.0	13.0	12.0	12.0	13.0	-3.0	5.0	46.0

1990	104.8	14.4	13.7	15.0	12.0	15.6	10.5	11.4	9.8	-2.6	5.0	52.3
2000	97.6	14.2	13.5	14.8	12.8	13.7	5.8	8.6	9.3	-2.9	7.7	48.7
2010	102.0	15.4	12.8	13.3	10.7	10.9	6.2	15.0	11.1	-2.0	8.7	49.4
2018	88.4	9.8	13.1	11.5	8.9	12.6	9.1	11.5	7.9	-2.0	6.1	71.9
% 1970–2018	10.5	-1.4	1.4	45.3	-18.8	26.9	32.3	46.0	-33.8	51.1	23.9	99.6
Mauritius												
1980	133.0	16.0	16.0	14.0	19.0	12.0	10.0	21.0	15.0	1.0	8.0	56.0
1990	142.5	11.8	16.7	16.4	19.3	12.4	15.5	21.3	18.8	1.1	9.2	66.7
2000	125.1	15.6	15.0	9.7	17.5	12.0	13.7	11.5	15.9	4.8	9.4	60.8
2010	123.0	13.5	12.9	14.6	17.4	10.3	12.8	9.5	14.9	6.9	10.1	60.4
2018	111.1	11.3	10.6	3.8	8.6	14.9	15.7	12.3	17.2	6.9	9.7	75.4
% 1980–2018	-16.4	-29.7	-33.6	-72.5	-54.9	24.2	57.3	-41.2	14.9	590.0	21.4	34.6
Mongolia												
1980	71.0	10.0	14.0	10.0	1.0	7.0	12.0	4.0	2.0	14.0	2.0	37.0
1990	74.1	15.5	13.1	13.0	-1.2	9.4	7.9	3.1	2.2	13.7	-2.6	42.5
2000	118.2	14.4	8.0	14.7	11.1	11.1	7.9	12.1	12.9	19.3	6.8	57.0
2010	111.0	15.9	11.1	13.9	13.1	13.9	8.3	12.2	12.8	12.8	-2.6	53.8
2018	103.8	13.9	10.2	12.8	8.7	13.2	7.1	10.6	14.5	12.8	0.1	74.0
% 1980–2018	46.2	39.2	-27.2	28.0	774.1	87.9	-40.9	164.4	823.9	-8.6	103.1	99.9
Morocco												
1970	73.0	6.9	3.9	1.1	11.9	9.9	3.9	7.9	7.9	10.9	9.9	29.0
1980	88.0	7.0	8.0	3.0	6.0	6.0	5.0	13.0	13.0	16.0	11.0	36.0
1990	98.2	7.6	9.9	5.0	10.6	10.6	7.8	12.2	7.4	16.0	11.2	44.9
2000	81.1	1.6	11.1	3.8	6.4	4.5	6.5	8.9	8.9	18.3	11.1	38.1
2010	94.0	6.5	9.8	5.3	4.3	10.3	8.9	9.2	9.0	17.9	12.3	46.0
2018	96.1	9.8	9.7	4.1	9.3	7.9	9.8	7.2	10.2	17.9	9.7	71.9

(continued)

Table B.1 (continued)

Country	ISP	Educ	Health	Women	Defense	Econ	Demo	Environ	Chaos	Diversity	Welfare	WISP
% 1970–2018	31.6	41.3	147.4	531.3	−22.0	−20.1	149.6	−9.6	29.4	64.1	−2.5	147.9
Namibia												
1995	91.1	14.5	5.6	9.8	13.4	8.2	5.9	8.2	14.4	13.1	1.9	43.3
2000	77.2	12.6	3.3	13.7	8.9	4.3	1.8	14.6	14.7	0.7	2.6	35.6
2010	114.0	5.2	9.7	16.7	15.8	8.3	5.8	15.6	10.8	15.5	10.9	51.3
2018	82.8	6.6	4.4	11.6	10.8	8.4	2.1	8.9	13.8	10.6	5.6	67.2
% 1995–2018	−9.1	−54.7	−21.7	18.6	−19.2	3.2	−64.9	9.6	−4.1	−19.4	386.6	55.0
Nicaragua												
1970	81.0	6.9	11.9	9.9	15.9	7.9	2.9	8.1	10.9	17.9	3.9	38.0
1980	68.0	9.0	9.0	9.0	9.0	1.0	5.0	−3.0	9.0	15.0	7.0	33.0
1990	55.9	9.0	10.2	18.6	−10.8	−3.6	5.8	−2.9	7.4	15.2	7.1	38.6
2000	94.5	4.8	9.8	17.1	15.0	3.5	0.7	9.8	10.6	16.1	7.2	42.9
2010	114.0	5.2	9.7	16.7	15.8	8.3	5.8	15.6	10.8	15.5	10.9	51.3
2018	97.1	7.5	11.1	10.4	10.8	7.9	8.4	8.7	10.3	15.5	6.5	72.4
% 1970–2018	19.9	9.2	−7.0	5.3	−32.2	0.4	188.0	207.3	−5.4	−13.5	65.1	90.5
Nigeria												
1970	19.0	1.9	5.9	0.9	1.0	1.9	1.9	13.9	2.1	8.1	1.9	6.0
1980	72.0	8.0	2.0	4.0	14.0	9.0	3.0	16.0	21.0	−10.0	5.0	26.0
1990	43.0	1.4	3.1	0.6	17.8	4.3	0.5	15.7	4.0	−9.6	5.3	11.2
2000	44.4	3.7	−0.6	0.3	15.6	9.3	−0.1	10.2	6.4	−5.5	5.2	14.3
2010	33.0	0.7	−1.8	−1.2	15.8	11.2	−0.3	10.5	10.8	−7.1	4.1	4.3
2018	23.9	−0.6	−3.7	−5.1	10.8	6.3	−2.1	12.6	8.2	−7.1	4.7	48.1
% 1970–2018	26.0	−130.4	−162.0	−656.5	975.9	227.3	−211.6	−9.7	289.2	−187.7	148.3	702.0
Oman												
1995	57.7	9.7	16.4	3.2	16.3	12.8	5.0	9.3	5.7	11.3	0.7	35.7

2000	49.0	8.6	12.0	8.6	−9.0	11.7	−2.2	6.0	8.3	6.3	−1.3	29.3
2010	48.0	11.0	13.3	8.1	−18.2	10.9	6.3	4.1	8.3	5.3	0.2	35.3
2018	81.7	11.3	13.7	11.2	11.7	6.3	5.8	9.6	8.2	5.3	−1.3	69.8
% 1995–2018	41.7	17.1	−16.5	246.3	−28.2	−50.8	16.0	2.9	43.3	−53.0	−285.1	95.3
Pakistan												
1970	53.0	3.1	9.9	0.1	9.9	8.9	2.9	8.9	2.9	7.9	3.9	20.0
1980	50.0	−2.0	8.0	−2.0	10.0	7.0	3.0	9.0	1.0	10.0	5.0	18.0
1990	60.3	−0.9	6.2	−1.8	8.0	11.4	1.7	10.8	11.2	9.9	3.8	24.5
2000	54.8	3.6	5.6	−1.1	5.5	10.0	2.3	10.8	5.8	6.8	5.7	23.1
2010	49.0	−2.4	2.9	3.7	7.3	13.1	2.4	−0.5	5.8	9.2	7.1	22.8
2018	62.6	2.5	−0.8	4.3	9.4	8.2	4.9	9.4	6.9	9.2	8.6	60.6
% 1970–2018	18.1	−19.1	−108.5	4227.0	−5.6	−7.7	68.0	5.8	137.7	16.3	120.3	202.8
Panama												
1970	125.0	15.9	15.9	13.9	16.9	8.9	7.9	6.9	12.9	16.9	7.9	56.0
1980	125.0	16.0	15.0	14.0	17.0	6.0	13.0	10.0	9.0	15.0	10.0	56.0
1990	126.0	16.2	14.5	17.0	14.2	8.6	13.0	10.0	6.9	15.4	10.2	62.5
2000	130.4	14.7	14.9	14.0	14.7	8.1	9.2	16.2	15.1	13.2	10.3	62.0
2010	124.0	12.0	13.8	14.5	14.9	7.5	8.0	13.7	13.7	14.9	10.6	58.7
2018	117.2	10.0	14.4	13.8	9.0	15.0	9.4	8.6	10.7	14.9	11.3	78.7
% 1970–2018	−6.3	−37.1	−9.7	−0.8	−46.5	68.1	18.8	24.9	−17.0	−11.9	43.1	40.4
Papua-New Guinea												
1980	71.0	6.0	4.0	4.0	16.0	10.0	8.0	2.0	22.0	0.1	0.1	29.0
1990	60.6	4.5	6.4	0.1	16.9	9.2	8.3	1.6	13.3	−0.4	0.6	27.6
2000	41.0	1.4	2.1	2.0	15.9	5.6	1.9	9.0	13.0	−9.6	−0.2	14.3
2010	53.0	3.8	5.9	2.0	16.1	7.1	1.7	9.8	10.3	−6.3	2.0	20.2
2018	42.5	0.3	4.3	0.1	9.0	10.7	3.1	8.1	12.1	−6.3	0.9	57.2

(continued)

Table B.1 (continued)

Country	ISP	Educ	Health	Women	Defense	Econ	Demo	Environ	Chaos	Diversity	Welfare	WISP
% 1980–2018	−40.1	−94.2	8.3	−97.1	−43.5	7.0	−60.9	307.0	−44.8	−6400.0	774.3	97.4
Paraguay												
1970	113.0	10.9	14.9	9.9	13.9	8.9	6.9	9.9	9.9	17.9	8.9	49.0
1980	123.0	9.0	17.0	12.0	16.0	11.0	9.0	10.0	9.0	18.0	11.0	54.0
1990	117.1	6.8	12.6	13.2	17.8	10.1	9.1	12.9	4.5	18.3	11.8	52.8
2000	109.7	13.8	11.2	12.6	15.3	4.0	2.6	10.3	11.5	19.0	9.5	51.2
2010	112.0	11.5	10.9	13.7	15.8	5.8	3.8	10.5	10.7	19.5	9.7	51.9
2018	101.0	4.7	11.3	10.4	8.8	10.9	8.2	7.1	9.2	19.5	10.8	73.4
% 1970–2018	−10.6	−56.7	−23.9	4.8	−36.6	22.6	19.0	−28.5	−7.2	8.9	21.1	49.7
Peru												
1970	79.0	10.9	10.9	11.9	10.9	1.9	6.9	0.9	6.9	6.9	9.9	38.0
1980	77.0	11.0	9.0	9.0	9.0	3.0	9.0	0.1	10.0	5.0	11.0	37.0
1990	90.4	13.2	6.6	13.0	10.8	5.6	9.8	1.2	14.3	4.7	11.3	47.8
2000	104.9	15.6	11.8	13.0	10.0	3.9	8.0	9.6	10.9	10.7	11.4	52.5
2010	113.0	10.6	11.3	15.4	13.7	8.1	7.8	13.6	12.1	8.9	11.5	53.5
2018	106.3	7.2	11.8	16.6	8.7	10.9	10.0	9.7	9.6	8.9	12.9	76.4
% 1970–2018	34.6	−34.1	8.4	39.5	−19.9	469.7	44.9	967.3	39.0	28.8	29.8	101.2
Philippines												
1970	97.0	13.9	9.9	14.9	15.9	8.9	4.9	7.9	12.9	1.9	4.9	42.0
1980	93.0	11.0	12.0	9.0	16.0	11.0	10.0	8.0	9.0	−1.0	7.0	41.0
1990	104.5	14.6	12.2	14.9	17.3	6.3	8.3	9.3	15.1	−1.0	7.4	51.0
2000	103.2	17.5	11.5	14.2	14.7	8.6	4.6	10.3	8.8	9.3	3.6	49.4
2010	101.0	10.5	9.8	15.9	15.2	10.1	5.1	10.2	8.0	10.1	5.7	47.1
2018	87.6	7.6	6.3	12.5	8.8	12.0	5.4	10.7	9.4	10.1	4.7	68.9
% 1970–2018												

Qatar												
1995	90.1	12.4	16.2	9.5	9.5	13.9	12.6	9.0	4.6	4.4	1.9	45.6
2000	35.4	9.5	15.2	11.9	−9.8	14.9	6.3	−25.0	7.2	7.6	−2.4	36.2
2010	25.0	11.8	13.8	9.0	−12.4	13.8	−2.6	−22.3	9.3	6.9	−2.6	29.5
2018	86.3	6.4	12.5	12.9	11.5	17.3	6.9	10.6	8.2	6.9	−6.9	69.5
% 1995–2018	−4.2	−48.7	−22.5	35.9	21.1	24.1	−45.1	18.1	79.4	57.6	−462.8	52.4
Saudi Arabia												
1980	62.0	9.0	9.0	1.0	7.0	16.0	3.0	9.0	1.0	20.0	4.0	29.0
1990	92.6	9.3	14.5	7.6	−3.5	24.8	4.6	8.6	2.5	19.8	4.3	48.2
2000	60.4	8.1	16.5	7.6	−14.3	14.2	0.6	4.1	5.2	14.4	4.1	37.7
2010	82.0	13.6	12.7	8.0	−6.9	13.8	2.4	15.3	5.6	14.0	3.8	42.6
2018	84.8	10.2	14.1	9.2	10.8	6.0	7.0	7.9	5.7	14.0	−0.2	70.3
% 1980–2018	36.8	13.5	56.3	816.5	54.9	−62.5	134.4	−11.7	472.3	−30.0	−105.1	142.3
South Africa												
1970	120.0	9.9	7.9	20.9	13.9	12.9	7.9	18.9	12.9	5.1	18.9	51.0
1980	100.0	7.0	12.0	10.0	13.0	11.0	9.0	12.0	7.0	3.0	16.0	43.0
1990	93.9	9.6	11.5	5.9	12.9	8.5	9.3	11.3	6.1	2.7	16.0	43.8
2000	105.5	14.1	5.9	18.0	13.9	5.3	7.0	7.7	16.2	4.4	13.0	52.4
2010	102.0	12.9	7.6	16.7	13.4	5.1	7.9	7.3	14.5	4.1	12.3	50.7
2018	97.0	6.0	7.1	15.9	8.8	8.6	8.4	9.5	14.1	4.1	14.5	73.6
% 1970–2018	−19.2	−39.6	−10.2	−23.7	−36.9	−33.8	6.7	−49.9	8.9	−19.6	−23.1	44.3
Sri Lanka												
1970	118.0	10.9	14.9	15.9	16.9	10.9	11.9	11.9	11.9	5.9	5.9	51.0
1980	129.0	12.0	12.0	14.0	16.0	10.0	15.0	16.0	21.0	7.0	7.0	55.0
1990	114.6	11.8	15.3	16.9	12.4	9.2	14.3	11.9	11.6	7.3	4.1	57.3
2000	106.2	16.3	12.4	13.5	5.5	13.1	13.0	14.5	2.6	10.9	4.3	53.0
2010	106.0	14.2	9.7	11.7	10.1	10.9	14.7	11.1	7.3	10.0	6.0	52.4

(continued)

Table B.1 (continued)

Country	ISP	Educ	Health	Women	Defense	Econ	Demo	Environ	Chaos	Diversity	Welfare	WISP
2018	92.2	7.9	9.2	11.9	9.1	11.0	13.1	9.8	-3.1	10.0	13.2	72.4
% 1970–2018	-21.9	-27.9	-38.0	-25.2	-46.2	0.8	10.3	-17.7	-125.8	69.2	122.9	41.9
Suriname												
1995	79.7	10.6	11.7	9.3	11.9	8.9	12.5	9.6	13.2	6.2	1.9	39.8
2000	91.9	15.1	11.9	14.7	13.6	-3.7	13.2	5.2	15.3	-3.9	10.4	48.5
2010	93.0	13.7	11.1	18.1	13.1	8.3	11.4	8.9	13.2	-2.4	-2.6	47.4
2018	91.8	14.6	9.6	14.1	8.6	9.9	10.0	13.5	13.8	-2.4	0.1	72.4
% 1995–2018	15.3	37.7	-17.4	51.0	-27.5	10.6	-20.2	41.0	4.4	-138.7	-96.8	82.0
Swaziland												
1995	81.2	13.9	6.0	11.6	11.7	10.7	3.5	0.4	7.1	14.7	1.7	40.9
2000	85.3	10.7	5.7	8.1	13.6	5.0	4.2	14.2	8.8	14.9	-0.1	36.6
2010	75.0	7.2	2.1	13.6	12.5	2.0	5.1	10.2	6.4	13.8	2.1	33.1
2018	48.8	-0.2	2.5	5.0	9.0	0.8	2.2	8.0	6.6	13.8	1.0	57.7
% 1995–2018	-39.9	-101.3	-57.7	-57.0	-22.6	-92.5	-37.8	2010.8	-7.1	-6.2	-39.6	40.9
Syria												
1970	70.0	8.9	13.9	1.9	6.1	12.9	4.9	14.9	0.9	14.9	1.9	32.0
1980	81.0	10.0	15.0	8.0	-11.0	16.0	6.0	15.0	7.0	12.0	3.0	40.0
1990	76.9	10.5	16.2	7.7	-1.9	5.6	5.9	14.6	1.8	13.0	3.3	38.8
2000	76.1	10.9	13.7	8.0	2.7	11.8	1.6	7.8	5.1	11.9	2.5	38.6
2010	78.0	12.2	13.2	10.1	2.5	10.7	2.2	8.5	3.8	11.0	3.3	39.7
2018	46.9	3.7	9.2	10.6	9.7	-10.0	13.6	7.0	-11.8	11.0	3.9	63.1
% 1970–2018	-33.0	-58.1	-33.7	453.0	58.8	-177.7	177.7	-53.1	-1397.9	-26.2	104.4	97.1
Thailand												
1970	102.0	9.9	12.9	14.9	11.9	12.9	6.9	8.9	8.9	11.9	1.9	45.0
1980	123.0	12.0	11.0	12.0	12.0	15.0	11.0	17.0	14.0	15.0	4.0	52.0

1990	129.8	10.0	13.0	15.9	12.9	13.1	12.5	16.0	14.6	16.6	5.0	61.9
2000	112.3	14.2	11.8	14.3	13.6	10.9	11.2	13.6	12.6	10.3	-0.3	54.1
2010	108.0	11.6	10.4	14.3	14.6	12.6	13.4	10.7	6.9	9.7	3.9	52.1
2018	93.2	5.4	12.2	13.5	10.6	7.8	17.4	7.4	8.4	9.7	0.9	74.5
% 1970–2018	-8.6	-45.9	-5.2	-9.2	-11.2	-39.4	151.2	-17.3	-6.2	-18.6	-54.5	65.7
Trinidad &Tobago												
1970	122.0	13.9	15.9	14.9	17.9	8.9	14.9	10.9	10.9	8.9	3.9	54.0
1980	134.0	12.0	16.0	12.0	18.0	10.0	17.0	16.0	22.0	4.0	7.0	57.0
1990	133.6	13.6	15.6	16.9	17.8	6.6	14.1	11.7	24.3	5.4	7.5	66.5
2000	104.4	15.2	14.1	16.0	10.0	11.4	15.1	1.9	13.7	-3.4	10.5	57.7
2010	101.0	14.4	9.2	14.6	9.2	14.6	16.0	0.9	13.1	-2.6	12.1	56.0
2018	97.8	-0.9	11.6	15.0	8.8	12.6	17.3	12.3	14.5	-2.6	9.2	74.5
% 1970–2018	-19.9	-106.5	-27.2	0.5	-50.9	41.0	16.2	13.1	32.9	-129.2	135.2	38.0
Tunisia												
1970	108.0	13.9	8.9	3.9	14.9	8.9	6.9	12.9	9.9	18.9	7.9	44.0
1980	114.0	9.0	11.0	6.0	12.0	13.0	11.0	15.0	7.0	19.0	11.0	48.0
1990	120.9	11.2	15.7	9.2	14.0	8.7	10.7	12.5	7.3	19.6	11.9	57.0
2000	118.3	9.5	13.6	11.3	13.4	8.7	10.5	8.3	8.7	21.7	12.4	57.2
2010	129.0	14.6	13.4	13.6	13.1	10.3	12.0	9.1	7.9	21.3	13.9	63.7
2018	117.4	6.7	13.6	9.0	10.9	11.4	11.4	7.4	14.4	21.3	11.4	77.6
% 1970–2018	8.7	-52.0	52.6	131.4	-27.1	27.6	65.4	-42.7	44.8	12.6	44.4	76.3
Uruguay												
1970	147.0	16.9	16.9	17.9	14.9	2.1	18.9	18.9	13.9	12.9	16.9	66.0
1980	135.0	13.0	16.0	21.0	14.0	4.0	19.0	11.0	1.0	12.0	25.0	63.0
1990	153.7	17.7	14.8	17.7	15.1	10.0	18.4	10.3	19.1	12.3	18.3	78.3
2000	153.4	17.9	18.9	18.1	15.0	4.7	19.3	8.5	17.6	14.7	18.6	79.4

(continued)

Table B.1 (continued)

Country	ISP	Educ	Health	Women	Defense	Econ	Demo	Environ	Chaos	Diversity	Welfare	WISP
2010	154.0	13.2	17.8	15.0	14.0	8.3	19.4	9.1	17.4	13.9	25.5	78.5
2018	148.3	7.2	19.0	13.3	11.2	15.9	18.3	10.4	16.9	13.9	22.2	87.2
% 1970–2018	0.9	−57.2	12.2	−25.5	−25.1	656.1	−3.4	−45.2	21.6	7.7	31.6	32.1
Venezuela												
1970	125.0	13.9	16.9	12.9	13.9	12.9	6.9	8.9	13.9	18.9	4.9	55.0
1980	142.0	15.0	15.0	18.0	17.0	11.0	10.0	9.0	24.0	15.0	7.0	63.0
1990	128.6	13.6	10.8	17.4	17.1	7.7	10.5	8.9	19.6	15.1	7.8	63.1
2000	126.7	13.1	13.9	18.4	14.7	6.9	6.4	17.5	9.1	16.3	10.5	58.8
2010	135.0	11.4	12.0	17.1	14.3	7.5	7.1	27.0	8.6	16.0	14.3	59.4
2018	95.3	11.0	9.1	14.0	10.9	−3.1	8.7	7.5	5.0	16.0	16.2	73.8
% 1970–2018	−23.8	−21.0	−46.3	8.7	−21.8	−123.8	25.9	−15.9	−63.9	−15.4	228.9	34.1
Vietnam												
1970	41.0	1.9	9.9	11.9	25.1	2.9	10.9	7.9	2.9	9.9	6.9	28.0
1980	79.0	11.0	7.0	13.0	12.0	9.0	8.0	9.0	−2.0	13.0	−2.0	33.0
1990	57.0	6.1	10.6	11.5	−15.5	13.0	9.0	11.2	0.7	13.0	−2.6	34.2
2000	100.0	14.7	11.1	16.9	11.1	10.1	8.4	9.9	3.7	7.9	6.2	49.4
2010	106.0	9.4	10.5	15.4	10.4	14.7	9.3	9.9	5.0	15.2	6.4	51.7
2018	98.9	10.1	11.0	16.7	10.7	7.3	11.4	8.5	5.1	15.2	2.9	74.8
% 1970–2018	141.3	430.8	10.7	40.5	−57.5	149.8	4.9	7.6	75.0	53.4	−58.2	167.1
Zimbabwe												
1970	78.0	9.9	11.9	3.9	14.9	8.9	4.9	7.9	10.9	6.9	3.1	32.0
1980	67.0	9.0	6.0	12.0	3.0	8.0	2.0	10.0	10.0	9.0	−2.0	29.0
1990	76.6	15.2	8.5	9.8	8.4	8.1	5.5	9.1	4.0	8.9	−1.0	37.2
2000	52.7	15.8	2.5	6.9	4.7	1.4	2.0	12.0	6.2	5.2	−3.9	24.3
2010	57.0	8.2	−0.1	10.0	11.0	−2.5	7.2	13.3	2.8	7.8	−0.6	23.2

2018	21.3	-2.9	-2.2	5.1	9.0	-8.4	1.5	7.0	6.3	7.8	-2.0	51.4
% 1970-2018	-72.7	-129.2	-118.4	29.2	-39.4	-194.2	-68.7	-11.1	-41.9	12.9	-165.0	60.7
Least Developing Countries (N = 41)												
Afghanistan*												
1980	24.0	2.0	6.0	4.0	8.0	7.0	1.0	10.0	2.0	7.0	4.0	4.0
1990	21.4	-4.0	-5.5	-5.0	5.7	6.1	4.7	10.3	-0.2	5.6	3.8	3.3
2000	-12.5	-11.8	-14.8	-7.6	10.0	9.8	-4.9	8.0	-9.7	4.9	3.6	-19.2
2010	-2.9	-7.0	-14.1	-12.0	9.2	16.6	-7.5	8.4	-1.0	7.1	-2.6	-13.9
2018	18.7	10.2	0.3	0.3	8.7	-0.8	-2.1	7.3	-12.4	7.1	0.1	50.9
% 1980-2018	-22.3	408.3	-95.2	-93.0	9.2	-111.2	-308.3	-27.1	-719.8	1.4	-98.5	1171.7
Angola*												
1980	15.0	6.0	2.0	3.0	1.0	1.0	3.0	10.0	2.0	4.0	2.0	5.0
1990	-2.6	1.1	-7.2	1.0	-6.3	6.5	1.4	9.1	-3.7	-2.0	-2.6	-3.2
2000	-34.7	-6.7	-8.4	-2.1	-41.1	5.9	-2.4	11.6	1.7	-2.2	8.9	-9.7
2010	4.0	-3.4	-5.2	-3.7	0.7	6.3	-2.1	11.5	5.1	-2.8	-2.6	-4.0
2018	29.8	11.1	-0.3	0.1	10.5	3.8	-6.7	10.0	7.3	-2.8	-3.2	51.9
% 1980-2018	98.7	84.9	-115.6	-98.1	953.8	280.5	-324.4	0.3	264.6	-170.0	-258.4	938.1
Bangladesh*												
1980	49.0	1.0	1.0	0.1	16.0	4.0	3.0	6.0	15.0	18.0	2.0	18.0
1990	48.6	-1.6	1.1	0.9	16.4	8.9	3.4	-0.7	5.7	17.2	-2.6	18.9
2000	77.5	-1.0	6.4	0.1	14.5	9.2	3.7	5.9	7.9	20.2	10.5	32.4
2010	88.0	1.0	4.0	9.3	14.9	13.1	4.6	8.2	7.1	18.8	6.7	37.8
2018	90.7	11.1	5.6	7.3	8.9	10.2	8.3	7.2	7.3	18.8	5.8	70.0
% 1980-2018	85.0	1014.2	459.9	7237.6	-44.6	155.5	177.3	20.0	-51.0	4.4	191.2	289.1
Benin*												
1970	43.0	1.9	0.1	0.9	13.9	6.9	4.9	6.9	1.1	2.9	4.9	14.0
1980	52.0	3.0	1.0	0.1	16.0	6.0	3.0	11.0	0.1	3.0	9.0	17.0

(continued)

Table B.1 (continued)

Country	ISP	Educ	Health	Women	Defense	Econ	Demo	Environ	Chaos	Diversity	Welfare	WISP
1990	37.2	-0.6	0.6	-9.1	15.8	9.6	1.4	9.7	-2.6	3.1	9.2	8.1
2000	59.2	-6.2	3.2	-2.9	14.7	3.7	-1.3	12.1	12.5	14.2	9.2	19.4
2010	60.0	-2.8	2.4	-5.9	14.3	7.9	-2.2	15.9	12.6	8.6	9.3	18.7
2018	61.7	3.8	-1.1	-4.6	10.8	13.8	-2.4	12.6	14.2	8.6	6.1	55.9
% 1970–2018	43.6	97.5	-1199.9	-610.6	-22.7	99.2	-148.6	82.9	1194.4	195.5	24.4	299.4
Bhutan*												
1995	44.8	0.2	4.6	5.1	18.6	11.3	4.9	9.4	1.3	4.4	1.0	12.7
2000	45.3	-1.1	3.4	-1.8	10.0	13.0	3.5	17.7	-3.4	2.2	1.8	12.8
2010	60.0	8.8	3.1	3.1	9.2	9.5	2.9	16.6	8.3	1.1	-2.6	23.8
2018	69.1	12.3	7.1	3.9	9.0	11.3	8.7	12.1	10.2	1.1	-6.6	64.4
% 1995–2018	54.3	6056.3	54.0	-23.9	-51.4	-0.6	76.8	28.2	685.5	-74.9	-760.2	405.3
Burkina-Faso*												
1970	35.0	2.1	17.1	0.9	15.9	5.9	3.9	18.9	2.1	3.9	5.9	3.0
1980	46.0	-7.0	-10.0	-1.0	14.0	6.0	3.0	11.0	21.0	0.1	9.0	11.0
1990	36.4	-2.9	-5.2	-4.6	14.0	11.3	2.6	10.1	-1.1	2.0	10.0	7.9
2000	29.5	-10.7	-5.4	-3.3	13.6	-0.4	-0.2	13.6	9.4	2.9	10.1	3.1
2010	63.0	-6.9	-0.8	-1.5	14.0	11.2	9.7	12.6	9.5	3.7	11.5	22.8
2018	50.9	1.7	-1.2	-2.5	8.8	10.9	-4.5	11.6	11.9	3.7	10.5	54.5
% 1970–2018	45.3	-21.2	-106.9	-375.3	-44.6	85.1	-215.6	-38.6	464.5	-5.4	77.4	1715.7
Burundi*												
1970	35.0	0.9	10.1	2.1	15.9	6.9	1.9	13.9	-0.1	4.9	1.9	5.0
1980	41.0	-1.0	-5.0	-4.0	13.0	9.0	4.0	19.0	-2.0	3.0	5.0	8.0
1990	56.1	2.3	3.0	-0.7	14.0	7.1	2.8	17.8	-0.2	3.3	6.6	17.5
2000	20.2	-3.7	-3.1	-1.0	3.0	-2.1	3.6	11.5	-4.3	11.1	5.1	3.4
2010	30.0	-1.4	-8.2	2.4	-0.9	6.8	-2.5	11.1	4.5	10.8	7.4	9.6

2018	49.6	9.3	1.7	4.2	9.0	2.2	-5.1	7.6	5.9	10.8	4.0	57.7
% 1970–2018	41.8	923.1	-83.4	101.5	-43.2	-68.7	-367.5	-45.0	-6610.6	120.0	109.9	1053.8
Cambodia*												
1970	48.0	9.9	3.9	2.9	4.9	15.1	12.9	3.9	2.9	13.9	6.9	23.0
1980	41.0	-4.0	-3.0	6.0	12.0	2.0	8.0	8.0	-2.0	16.0	-2.0	12.0
1990	18.9	0.5	-1.6	-0.5	-16.6	12.5	5.4	7.4	-2.2	16.5	-2.6	11.9
2000	76.0	2.0	-2.0	1.4	11.4	12.6	-0.7	15.7	5.4	19.8	10.5	27.7
2010	79.0	3.4	1.7	4.8	12.5	14.3	3.6	16.0	6.1	19.2	-2.6	30.7
2018	78.9	12.1	5.2	5.2	9.0	7.9	5.6	6.5	8.2	19.2	0.1	66.7
% 1970–2018	64.3	21.7	33.5	77.9	82.4	-47.8	-56.5	66.8	180.7	38.0	-99.1	189.9
Cape Verde*												
2000	91.8	1.1	8.9	10.8	14.5	8.0	4.6	11.3	14.4	14.1	6.4	40.4
2010	109.0	13.3	9.7	13.1	15.8	6.5	2.7	9.3	16.0	13.6	8.6	51.3
2018	111.3	12.7	9.7	12.2	10.7	14.3	6.9	10.3	16.9	13.6	4.1	75.0
% 2000–2018	21.2	1054.5	8.4	12.7	-26.0	78.3	51.2	-8.8	17.5	-3.8	-35.6	85.6
Central African Republic*												
1970	34.0	1.1	6.1	2.9	11.9	9.9	4.9	4.9	1.1	0.9	5.9	10.0
1980	40.0	0.1	-2.0	0.1	15.0	7.0	7.0	8.0	0.1	-4.0	9.0	12.0
1990	33.8	-1.7	-1.0	-2.5	16.0	7.3	3.0	7.1	0.4	-4.4	9.5	8.7
2000	24.5	-7.3	-3.4	-6.4	12.0	4.6	2.7	12.6	6.7	-6.5	9.5	2.5
2010	29.2	-9.0	-6.1	-3.7	14.6	1.7	4.2	14.0	6.9	-4.4	11.0	3.3
2018	3.3	-1.6	-13.6	-9.5	9.0	2.4	-0.4	12.0	-0.4	-4.4	9.8	41.4
% 1970–2018	-90.4	-249.3	-323.6	-426.5	-24.1	-75.5	-108.4	144.0	-136.7	-583.5	66.3	314.3
Chad*												
1970	25.0	7.5	10.1	1.1	8.9	4.9	5.9	12.9	10.9	7.1	5.9	3.0
1980	7.0	-8.0	-9.0	-4.0	10.0	3.0	6.0	10.0	0.1	-7.0	8.0	-4.0

(continued)

Table B.1 (continued)

Country	ISP	Educ	Health	Women	Defense	Econ	Demo	Environ	Chaos	Diversity	Welfare	WISP
1990	18.1	-2.1	-8.3	-8.1	16.2	7.8	4.0	9.0	-1.8	-6.5	7.8	-1.7
2000	17.7	-7.5	-7.3	-8.0	15.3	6.4	-1.1	13.0	5.0	-6.4	8.3	-3.8
2010	14.0	-9.9	-6.0	-15.1	14.9	15.0	-3.5	11.9	4.1	-7.8	10.2	-6.7
2018	19.5	8.1	-8.8	-9.8	10.8	2.3	-1.4	12.0	6.6	-7.8	7.5	46.9
% 1970–2018	-22.0	8.2	-187.1	-988.5	21.0	-52.6	-124.4	-7.1	-39.3	-209.9	26.5	1462.0
Comoros*												
1995	46.1	3.3	0.7	0.3	5.0	8.1	2.2	12.4	10.7	6.0	1.9	18.2
2000	56.7	-1.3	5.5	6.0	10.0	5.8	0.0	11.6	7.2	10.1	1.8	22.1
2010	56.0	-1.5	1.3	5.3	9.2	6.2	1.3	15.6	9.9	11.3	-2.6	20.2
2018	74.6	16.2	2.7	5.5	9.0	8.9	1.8	7.8	11.2	11.3	0.1	65.2
% 1995–2018	61.7	388.4	276.4	1745.0	81.0	9.2	-20.4	-36.8	4.6	89.6	-96.8	258.4
Congo, Democratic Republic of the (Kinshasa) [formerly Zaire]*												
1970	43.0	8.9	4.1	2.9	10.9	5.9	4.9	10.9	2.9	6.1	4.9	15.0
1980	55.0	10.0	2.0	7.0	14.0	-2.0	3.0	10.0	1.0	2.0	8.0	21.0
1990	42.4	2.6	1.1	0.9	14.2	3.2	2.7	9.0	1.2	1.7	8.4	13.8
2000	10.0	-1.5	-6.7	-1.8	5.3	7.9	-2.5	11.0	3.9	-0.4	-5.1	-2.3
2010	24.0	-3.5	-8.5	-2.0	10.7	7.6	-2.2	11.1	1.7	1.5	7.9	2.2
2018	44.8	8.7	-2.7	-3.4	8.8	9.2	-2.4	10.4	9.4	1.5	5.3	54.4
% 1970–2018	4.2	-2.7	-165.1	-215.6	-19.0	55.7	-148.1	-5.0	221.9	-75.4	7.4	262.7
Djibouti*												
2000	36.7	0.1	2.1	3.0	5.8	4.4	2.1	11.7	7.5	9.3	1.8	11.7

2010	37.0	3.8	2.2	−2.1	5.2	2.6	2.1	9.4	7.7	8.7	−2.6	14.3
2018	50.9	5.3	4.7	0.2	8.6	−1.8	3.4	8.8	8.1	8.7	4.8	58.9
% 2000–2018	38.4	7274.1	124.3	−92.6	48.6	−141.7	65.9	−24.7	7.4	−6.9	160.0	403.5
Eritrea*												
1995	23.4	0.7	3.8	2.0	5.0	9.9	3.0	9.7	1.8	0.8	1.9	6.3
2000	−50.8	−2.9	0.2	−2.2	−45.8	−0.5	3.6	11.2	−18.2	2.0	1.8	−15.3
2010	−43.0	1.5	−1.0	−0.8	−55.2	5.9	−5.7	10.9	3.8	0.5	−2.6	−6.6
2018	29.6	2.0	5.6	0.9	8.6	−0.9	4.1	9.4	−0.7	0.5	0.1	54.5
% 1995–2018	26.7	191.4	48.5	−57.2	73.1	−108.7	37.9	−2.8	−141.3	−39.3	−96.8	770.9
Ethiopia*												
1970	35.0	6.1	7.1	2.1	13.9	7.9	3.9	16.9	10.9	4.1	0.1	4.0
1980	−8.0	−6.0	−12.0	−3.0	2.0	6.0	2.0	11.0	−2.0	−6.0	1.0	−10.0
1990	−4.2	−2.4	−8.0	−1.6	12.4	7.7	−0.1	−23.4	9.3	−2.0	3.8	1.2
2000	−15.7	−7.6	−8.7	−1.8	−8.1	5.1	−0.1	11.5	−5.5	−2.9	2.4	−12.1
2010	46.0	0.4	−1.0	−2.0	10.1	13.7	1.1	14.2	7.9	−1.7	2.8	14.6
2018	29.2	0.5	1.1	1.0	8.8	3.5	−2.1	11.9	6.5	−1.7	−0.2	51.4
% 1970–2018	−16.6	−92.4	−85.2	−52.7	−36.4	−55.9	−154.0	−29.6	−40.8	−141.5	−310.4	1183.9
Gambia*												
1995	40.3	0.6	4.7	2.2	9.8	7.5	0.8	7.7	4.6	4.2	2.7	14.6
2000	42.9	−2.1	4.2	−2.1	15.0	4.4	−0.3	11.1	7.3	4.2	1.1	12.5
2010	53.0	−1.9	1.0	−2.3	16.4	5.5	0.5	10.5	8.1	11.8	2.9	16.5
2018	47.8	7.9	4.2	−4.5	8.9	0.2	−1.6	9.6	5.8	11.8	5.5	55.9
% 1995–2018	18.7	1272.7	−11.4	−306.6	−9.2	−96.7	−299.9	25.3	27.2	178.5	103.0	282.4
Guinea*												
1970	42.0	0.9	2.1	0.9	7.9	6.9	3.9	10.9	4.9	0.1	6.9	14.0
1980	22.0	0.1	−3.0	−3.0	10.0	2.0	3.0	6.0	−2.0	0.1	9.0	5.0
1990	17.1	−1.2	−10.4	−7.2	13.8	4.6	1.2	5.7	−0.8	1.9	9.5	−1.0

(continued)

Table B.1 (continued)

Country	ISP	Educ	Health	Women	Defense	Econ	Demo	Environ	Chaos	Diversity	Welfare	WISP
2000	30.6	-6.9	-2.8	-6.2	13.9	3.1	0.1	9.2	6.4	4.1	9.7	5.2
2010	36.0	-1.9	1.0	-2.3	16.4	5.5	0.5	10.5	6.0	11.8	2.9	8.7
2018	48.8	7.1	-1.3	-1.4	8.9	8.0	-2.0	10.3	8.4	3.2	7.5	55.8
% 1970–2018	16.1	685.6	-164.3	-251.5	13.0	16.4	-151.0	-5.5	71.0	3100.0	7.9	298.4
Guinea-Bissau*												
1995	27.9	6.6	3.1	2.5	10.7	3.1	1.7	11.1	11.9	2.8	1.9	6.8
2000	14.5	-9.1	-5.6	-8.8	14.5	3.9	2.0	10.9	8.2	-4.1	2.6	-3.8
2010	8.0	-4.7	-6.4	-3.9	5.8	0.2	-3.2	9.4	8.8	4.6	-2.6	-3.5
2018	53.9	9.1	-4.6	-2.8	8.6	6.8	0.6	12.3	9.4	4.6	9.9	56.1
% 1995–2018	93.0	38.4	-246.6	-210.9	-19.6	116.7	-67.3	10.6	-20.7	64.3	419.3	719.0
Haiti*												
1970	72.0	3.9	0.9	4.9	13.9	4.9	7.9	2.9	10.9	19.9	0.9	28.0
1980	68.0	-1.0	5.0	-1.0	16.0	6.0	10.0	8.0	3.0	18.0	3.0	25.0
1990	69.2	-1.7	1.9	6.5	16.4	8.6	9.0	6.1	1.8	18.3	2.3	28.0
2000	56.1	2.6	-3.1	6.3	10.0	0.1	5.2	7.7	4.5	18.0	4.7	22.8
2010	55.0	-3.5	2.7	6.5	9.2	-4.9	5.7	8.6	7.2	19.9	3.3	22.1
2018	63.0	8.3	-4.1	2.5	10.9	-0.4	5.8	7.4	6.0	19.9	6.7	60.5
% 1970–2018	-12.5	112.3	-548.5	-48.3	-21.3	-108.2	-26.9	153.1	-45.3	-0.1	636.3	115.9
Lao*, People's Democratic Republic of												
1980	53.0	10.0	0.1	8.0	12.0	8.0	6.0	10.0	2.0	2.0	2.0	20.0
1990	33.3	2.1	0.1	6.9	0.6	7.8	3.7	9.3	3.6	1.9	-2.6	14.9
2000	52.3	-0.4	-0.7	2.7	6.4	12.4	2.1	9.0	3.4	6.8	10.5	21.0
2010	67.0	-4.7	-6.4	-3.9	5.8	0.2	-3.2	9.4	4.4	4.6	-2.6	27.0
2018	57.8	10.6	1.1	9.1	11.1	5.9	4.9	10.8	6.1	5.6	-7.3	60.9

	9.1	5.5	991.4	13.6	-7.7	-25.7	-19.0	7.6	205.7	180.0	-463.4	204.6
% 1980–2018												
Lesotho*												
1980	93.0	9.0	4.0	11.0	16.0	11.0	7.0	11.0	9.0	15.0	2.0	36.0
1990	77.9	7.5	6.4	13.7	7.9	6.5	6.2	10.9	2.4	19.2	-2.6	36.0
2000	78.0	7.4	2.1	16.1	9.4	1.1	5.1	9.3	8.7	16.1	2.6	36.4
2010	93.0	16.2	4.3	18.0	11.0	-1.4	10.3	9.7	12.1	15.3	-2.6	46.1
2018	70.7	6.9	0.7	4.5	8.9	7.2	8.4	8.3	12.2	15.3	-1.6	63.5
% 1980–2018	-23.9	-23.1	-82.3	-59.5	-44.2	-34.7	19.7	-24.5	35.1	2.0	-179.1	76.4
Liberia*												
1970	68.0	1.1	4.9	1.9	16.9	10.9	8.9	9.9	15.9	1.1	1.0	24.0
1980	53.0	6.0	4.0	1.0	16.0	6.0	5.0	6.0	7.0	1.0	2.0	20.0
1990	33.4	1.5	0.3	-0.4	12.8	3.7	2.8	4.3	5.2	0.7	2.3	11.7
2000	10.9	-3.6	-6.4	-4.6	12.5	-3.0	-0.3	11.5	-4.2	7.3	1.7	-5.9
2010	-11.0	0.3	-2.9	-2.9	-5.4	-6.9	0.9	13.9	-13.1	1.3	3.4	-10.6
2018	50.3	7.0	-2.6	1.3	9.0	10.0	-1.6	11.4	10.4	1.3	4.1	56.1
% 1970–2018	-26.0	539.7	-153.4	-31.3	-47.0	-8.4	-117.7	14.7	-34.6	18.2	310.9	133.6
Madagascar*												
1970	81.0	1.1	5.9	9.9	14.9	7.9	3.9	14.9	8.9	7.9	6.9	30.0
1980	76.0	6.0	5.0	11.0	12.0	4.0	5.0	10.0	1.0	12.0	9.0	31.0
1990	58.3	3.2	1.8	7.4	15.3	1.7	3.0	9.1	5.6	1.4	9.7	23.1
2000	54.9	-3.2	-1.6	4.8	14.7	6.2	-0.3	9.8	10.8	3.7	9.8	19.4
2010	63.0	0.3	0.8	6.1	14.6	7.6	-0.8	10.2	10.5	2.3	11.5	24.4
2018	58.1	7.9	-0.6	0.5	8.7	10.1	-1.4	9.2	11.9	2.3	9.6	59.1
% 1970–2018	-28.2	614.2	-110.4	-94.5	-41.9	27.7	-135.3	-38.5	33.8	-70.9	38.4	96.9
Malawi*												
1970	42.0	1.9	4.1	0.1	17.9	6.9	2.9	8.9	7.9	3.1	1.9	11.0
1980	28.0	-3.0	-7.0	0.1	11.0	7.0	1.0	12.0	0.1	7.0	1.0	4.0

(continued)

Table B.1 (continued)

Country	ISP	Educ	Health	Women	Defense	Econ	Demo	Environ	Chaos	Diversity	Welfare	WISP
1990	47.1	-0.8	3.7	2.9	17.1	5.8	-0.6	12.7	-1.1	6.5	0.9	13.2
2000	37.4	-0.1	-1.8	-3.9	15.9	-0.4	2.3	13.8	10.8	1.6	-0.7	8.5
2010	72.0	3.7	5.4	4.1	15.8	11.1	-0.3	14.9	10.1	5.9	1.0	27.2
2018	52.4	8.2	3.7	-0.7	8.9	8.3	-4.8	10.3	12.2	5.9	0.5	56.8
% 1970-2018	24.8	329.0	-10.6	-775.2	-50.6	19.6	-266.5	15.9	54.2	90.3	-73.0	416.6
Mali*												
1970	45.0	1.9	4.1	1.9	13.9	8.9	2.9	10.9	1.1	2.9	5.9	13.0
1980	35.0	-1.0	-3.0	-4.0	14.0	4.0	3.0	9.0	0.1	4.0	9.0	8.0
1990	29.5	-4.5	-7.2	-3.8	14.2	7.3	0.9	8.5	-0.2	4.3	9.9	4.4
2000	43.1	-9.6	-4.1	-1.2	11.1	2.7	0.9	9.7	12.3	11.3	10.0	12.7
2010	50.0	-4.8	-2.7	-5.8	11.0	10.7	-3.1	10.6	12.6	10.6	11.4	15.7
2018	44.7	-0.1	-2.4	-4.3	9.1	7.8	-5.2	10.0	9.6	10.6	9.6	52.3
% 1970-2018	-0.8	-104.3	-159.4	-326.7	-34.3	-12.9	-279.0	-8.5	774.8	264.3	62.7	302.0
Mauritania*												
1970	63.0	5.9	2.1	1.1	15.9	3.9	6.9	2.9	8.9	14.9	5.9	23.0
1980	21.0	0.1	0.1	1.0	-2.0	-5.0	3.0	1.0	1.0	15.0	9.0	10.0
1990	17.1	2.1	-1.9	-0.5	-16.6	2.7	2.7	2.5	0.8	15.8	9.6	12.9
2000	40.5	-5.3	-2.3	-4.1	10.6	7.0	0.1	6.5	6.2	12.3	9.7	12.4
2010	52.0	-4.8	3.8	2.3	7.0	8.4	-0.9	9.3	8.3	11.7	7.4	20.5
2018	57.4	5.8	1.2	-4.7	9.2	4.8	0.2	9.2	10.0	11.7	10.0	57.7
% 1970-2018	-8.9	-1.7	-41.3	-526.7	-42.1	21.6	-97.8	215.2	12.6	-21.5	69.8	150.7
Mozambique*												
1980	22.0	5.0	6.0	2.0	13.0	3.0	1.0	9.0	21.1	7.0	2.0	2.0
1990	3.0	0.6	-8.7	0.9	4.4	-7.3	3.0	8.8	-2.7	6.7	-2.6	-4.3
2000	27.0	-7.2	-6.2	-2.6	11.1	4.3	0.1	11.5	9.9	4.1	1.8	3.9

2010	41.0	−5.5	−5.5	6.1	15.2	6.2	1.4	10.9	10.0	4.4	−2.6	11.2
2018	44.5	−0.9	−0.8	3.7	10.6	6.1	−2.3	9.1	10.6	4.4	4.1	55.1
% 1980–2018	102.3	−118.9	−113.1	85.3	−18.4	103.0	−329.0	0.7	−50.0	−37.1	105.1	2655.8
Myanmar* (formerly Burma)												
1970	78.0	5.9	8.9	14.9	4.9	11.9	9.9	7.9	1.1	9.9	3.9	36.0
1980	66.0	3.0	10.0	7.0	13.0	5.0	8.0	10.0	0.1	6.0	5.0	27.0
1990	82.2	1.6	8.5	9.6	14.0	11.8	9.4	10.4	1.9	9.9	4.9	36.0
2000	80.0	4.8	5.4	10.9	13.4	11.8	8.2	9.2	1.3	11.1	3.9	35.5
2010	48.0	4.2	3.3	9.3	12.8	11.4	9.6	−11.3	0.7	10.4	−2.6	26.7
2018	69.9	8.4	2.7	2.9	10.6	8.1	9.4	8.7	8.4	10.4	0.3	63.9
% 1970–2018	−10.4	42.6	−69.8	−80.7	115.5	−32.3	−4.6	9.8	665.1	4.9	−92.5	77.4
Nepal*												
1970	49.0	0.1	3.0	5.0	18.0	6.0	7.0	10.0	11.0	5.0	0.1	13.0
1980	57.0	2.0	−4.0	1.0	18.0	6.0	5.0	11.0	10.0	5.0	2.0	17.0
1990	54.3	−0.1	−0.4	−5.7	17.5	10.5	5.6	11.2	8.5	5.3	1.9	17.3
2000	63.0	−2.9	5.4	−2.5	15.6	13.8	2.8	11.9	7.9	9.7	1.2	22.2
2010	53.0	2.2	5.9	3.6	11.6	8.4	2.9	14.3	0.6	−0.1	3.1	19.1
2018	73.1	6.7	7.4	3.6	9.0	11.0	7.3	11.4	10.9	−0.1	5.9	65.2
% 1970–2018	49.1	6604.6	146.2	−29.0	−50.2	83.7	4.9	13.7	−1.0	−102.0	5827.4	401.2
Niger*												
1970	34.0	4.1	10.1	1.1	16.9	6.9	2.9	6.9	8.9	2.9	2.9	6.0
1980	39.0	−2.0	−4.0	−4.0	17.0	4.0	2.0	9.0	4.0	6.0	7.0	8.0
1990	28.6	−2.1	−8.3	−3.6	18.2	4.9	0.3	7.9	0.2	3.7	7.4	3.0
2000	19.0	−13.8	−7.2	−6.6	14.2	0.5	−4.1	12.3	9.4	6.9	7.2	−3.9
2010	37.0	−10.0	−1.5	−10.4	14.3	7.9	−5.1	11.4	4.9	5.9	9.4	9.4

(continued)

Table B.1 (continued)

Country	ISP	Educ	Health	Women	Defense	Econ	Demo	Environ	Chaos	Diversity	Welfare	WISP
2018	34.8	−4.3	0.4	−6.9	9.5	8.9	−6.6	10.1	10.7	5.9	7.1	49.6
% 1970–2018	2.4	−205.3	−96.5	−731.2	−44.1	29.4	−325.4	46.8	20.6	102.7	143.5	726.3
Rwanda*												
1970	62.0	0.9	7.1	3.9	14.9	4.9	2.9	16.9	10.9	9.9	2.9	17.0
1980	62.0	1.0	−3.0	6.0	16.0	8.0	1.0	18.0	1.0	11.0	4.0	18.0
1990	62.9	0.9	1.0	4.9	16.0	6.2	1.0	14.5	0.9	12.7	4.7	21.0
2000	55.6	−0.2	−4.3	5.4	9.7	5.9	4.4	15.2	2.7	14.2	2.5	19.0
2010	63.0	−2.4	−2.6	7.5	9.2	10.1	0.0	11.7	6.6	18.5	4.0	23.6
2018	62.6	1.5	1.6	7.0	10.9	5.9	−1.0	9.6	5.8	18.5	2.9	59.3
% 1970–2018	1.0	65.6	−77.4	80.0	−27.1	20.0	−133.4	−43.4	−47.2	86.7	−1.1	248.7
Senegal*												
1970	76.0	0.9	5.9	2.9	14.9	9.9	5.9	14.9	8.9	3.9	6.9	27.0
1980	57.0	1.0	1.0	−2.0	15.0	4.0	3.0	11.0	14.0	3.0	8.0	18.0
1990	63.0	3.3	1.6	−1.4	15.7	8.9	2.9	10.5	9.8	3.0	8.9	23.7
2000	55.9	−5.6	3.4	0.5	14.2	5.1	0.6	13.7	10.2	5.0	8.8	18.5
2010	60.0	−1.0	3.9	−1.0	13.4	7.8	0.7	12.5	12.1	4.6	7.4	22.1
2018	56.5	−4.1	4.9	1.5	9.0	6.7	−1.5	10.4	16.7	4.6	8.4	58.0
% 1970–2018	−25.7	−549.3	−17.9	−49.9	−39.9	−32.0	−125.4	−30.2	87.1	17.6	20.9	114.7
Sierra Leone*												
1970	77.0	0.9	0.9	0.1	16.9	7.9	8.9	17.9	19.9	0.9	1.9	25.0
1980	46.0	2.0	−3.0	−1.0	17.0	4.0	5.0	13.0	9.0	−2.0	2.0	12.0
1990	25.1	−1.5	−5.4	−2.6	17.5	4.9	1.6	12.7	4.6	−8.0	1.2	1.6
2000	0.0	−6.3	−8.6	−3.9	14.2	−4.1	5.8	8.9	−3.5	−2.2	−0.3	−10.0
2010	23.0	0.9	−11.5	−9.1	14.9	3.6	−3.3	10.7	9.6	5.3	1.8	−0.4
2018	31.4	−2.0	−8.8	−7.4	8.7	10.7	−1.6	11.8	12.1	5.3	2.3	47.5
% 1970–2018	−59.2	−315.4	−1061.8	−7450.1	−48.4	35.5	−117.5	−34.0	−39.2	482.4	22.0	90.1

Somalia*												
1970	59.0	4.9	0.1	4.1	13.9	5.9	4.9	10.9	0.1	19.9	1.9	19.0
1980	36.0	-3.0	1.0	-4.0	8.0	2.0	4.0	9.0	-2.0	19.0	3.0	10.0
1990	20.4	-7.3	-4.4	-6.0	7.9	2.4	0.1	8.7	-3.1	19.4	2.8	0.6
2000	23.4	-6.2	-8.9	-0.7	10.0	2.8	2.5	11.6	-3.3	13.8	1.8	1.2
2010	10.0	0.8	-6.9	-10.7	9.2	1.3	-2.6	7.8	0.7	13.1	-2.6	-4.4
2018	23.2	4.5	-3.3	-9.4	9.9	2.3	-1.5	7.7	-0.2	13.1	0.1	48.0
% 1970–2018	-60.7	-8.1	-3428.0	-328.7	-28.7	-61.6	-130.6	-29.7	-254.0	-34.2	-96.8	152.7
Sudan*												
1970	48.0	0.1	5.9	0.1	9.9	12.9	4.9	7.9	1.1	1.9	4.9	18.0
1980	53.0	4.0	4.0	3.0	13.0	4.0	3.0	10.0	9.0	5.0	-1.0	18.0
1990	41.3	1.7	1.0	-0.7	15.8	3.6	3.1	9.0	5.9	1.9	0.1	12.9
2000	39.1	-3.9	3.0	2.0	9.7	13.4	3.2	9.6	-4.0	5.0	1.2	12.6
2010	30.0	3.2	1.6	3.8	11.0	12.8	3.1	10.4	-22.8	3.9	3.0	6.9
2018	18.0	0.6	2.8	-2.0	11.1	-3.5	-5.3	8.5	3.5	3.9	-1.5	48.8
% 1970–2018	-62.5	509.8	-52.5	-2134.7	11.6	-127.5	-207.4	7.8	214.0	104.2	-130.8	171.2
Tanzania*												
1970	41.0	0.9	1.0	0.9	11.9	8.9	3.9	14.9	7.9	12.1	2.9	12.0
1980	52.0	13.0	2.0	10.0	14.0	6.0	3.0	10.0	1.0	-11.0	2.0	20.0
1990	39.6	4.9	4.8	7.1	14.0	3.8	2.1	9.7	1.6	-11.0	2.6	14.7
2000	57.6	2.8	-0.4	6.5	14.5	5.9	-1.1	15.6	8.7	3.2	1.9	19.6
2010	67.0	-1.3	-1.4	6.6	14.6	13.1	0.2	21.1	10.5	-0.7	4.2	22.1
2018	35.1	-3.4	0.4	8.1	8.8	9.8	-3.2	9.2	8.0	-0.7	-1.9	53.9
% 1970–2018	-14.4	-469.9	-56.2	786.2	-26.2	10.3	-183.1	-38.2	1.1	-105.8	-166.6	348.8
Togo*												
1970	38.0	2.1	2.1	1.9	15.9	8.9	1.9	9.9	1.1	0.9	2.9	9.0
1980	44.0	7.0	2.0	4.0	15.0	1.0	3.0	12.0	0.1	-5.0	6.0	15.0

(continued)

Table B.1 (continued)

Country	ISP	Educ	Health	Women	Defense	Econ	Demo	Environ	Chaos	Diversity	Welfare	WISP
1990	49.0	6.2	4.6	-1.0	13.8	5.7	3.9	12.2	0.6	-3.6	6.6	17.4
2000	45.9	1.4	-0.4	-3.1	12.5	0.9	0.5	12.5	7.3	7.9	6.5	14.1
2010	41.0	-1.4	1.7	-4.2	13.4	0.4	-0.5	12.6	6.4	3.7	8.8	11.0
2018	43.7	1.4	0.4	-0.6	8.6	8.7	-2.0	9.6	11.0	3.7	2.8	54.6
% 1970-2018	14.9	-31.8	-80.6	-130.6	-45.7	-2.9	-206.7	-2.7	904.1	306.6	-4.7	506.3
Uganda*												
1970	43.0	6.9	2.9	0.1	13.9	5.9	6.9	12.9	2.1	7.1	1.9	14.0
1980	49.0	1.0	1.0	7.0	18.0	4.0	6.0	15.0	1.0	-5.0	2.0	14.0
1990	40.1	4.8	0.4	2.0	12.0	3.6	0.6	14.3	5.2	-5.3	2.5	12.4
2000	29.9	2.9	-2.1	4.2	13.1	4.1	-2.3	13.1	5.2	-10.0	1.8	6.9
2010	42.0	1.9	0.6	7.9	11.0	10.6	-5.0	18.4	-0.4	-6.1	3.5	11.6
2018	18.9	-3.6	-1.7	6.1	9.3	5.3	-6.1	11.0	8.9	-6.1	-4.4	48.8
% 1970-2018	-56.1	-151.7	-156.9	5954.6	-32.9	-10.1	-187.9	-14.9	325.9	-185.9	-329.4	248.6
Yemen*												
1995	34.0	6.1	0.3	12.2	6.2	6.6	1.0	8.7	6.4	13.7	1.1	10.6
2000	27.6	4.1	3.2	-6.6	3.6	13.0	-7.4	8.7	4.6	7.7	-3.5	8.2
2010	35.0	8.6	3.2	-4.3	-3.3	10.6	-3.1	9.2	7.3	6.7	0.1	16.1
2018	11.8	-2.9	0.1	-1.4	9.4	-2.1	-0.4	7.3	6.5	6.7	-11.4	47.6
% 1995-2018	-65.4	-148.1	-73.6	-111.7	52.7	-132.7	-136.8	-16.4	1.8	-51.1	-1133.3	348.2
Zambia*												
1970	72.0	7.9	8.9	1.9	16.9	6.9	2.9	11.9	10.9	1.0	2.9	27.0
1980	51.0	9.0	4.0	9.0	-9.0	4.0	3.0	9.0	9.0	8.0	5.0	25.0
1990	61.4	9.8	8.0	5.6	8.4	2.9	1.5	8.6	3.3	8.1	5.1	27.9
2000	62.0	9.7	-2.7	1.8	16.4	3.5	-0.1	12.7	8.2	7.3	5.1	22.1
2010	63.0	1.4	-4.6	3.0	11.0	7.4	1.5	21.0	9.9	6.2	6.6	20.8

World	ISP	Educ	Health	Women	Defense	Econ	Demo	Environ	Chaos	Diversity	Welfare	WISP Md
2018	46.2	−1.2	−2.6	2.8	10.7	7.2	−4.1	10.8	10.6	6.2	5.9	53.8
% 1970–2018	−35.9	−115.6	−129.5	46.5	−36.9	3.8	−242.6	−9.2	−2.9	520.0	103.1	99.3
1970 (N = 104)	M = c. 100.0	M = c. 10.0	M = c. 10.0	M = c. 10.0	M = c. 10.0	M = c. 10.0	M = c. 10.0	M = c. 10.0	M = c. 10.0	M = c. 10.0	M = c. 10.0	40.8
1980 (N = 117)	M = c. 100.0	M = c. 10.0	M = c. 10.0	M = c. 10.0	M = c. 10.0	M = c. 10.0	M = c. 10.0	M = c. 10.0	M = c. 10.0	M = c. 10.0	M = c. 10.0	39.6
1990 (N = 117)	M = c. 100.0	M = c. 10.0	M = c. 10.0	M = c. 10.0	M = c. 10.0	M = c. 10.0	M = c. 10.0	M = c. 10.0	M = c. 10.0	M = c. 10.0	M = c. 10.0	47.8
2000 (N = 162)	M = c. 100.0	M = c. 10.0	M = c. 10.0	M = c. 10.0	M = c. 10.0	M = c. 10.0	M = c. 10.0	M = c. 10.0	M = c. 10.0	M = c. 10.0	M = c. 10.0	49.7
2010 (N = 162)	M = c. 100.0	M = c. 10.0	M = c. 10.0	M = c. 10.0	M = c. 10.0	M = c. 10.0	M = c. 10.0	M = c. 10.0	M = c. 10.0	M = c. 10.0	M = c. 10.0	50.0
2018 (N = 162)	M = c. 100.0	M = c. 10.0	M = c. 10.0	M = c. 10.0	M = c. 10.0	M = c. 10.0	M = c. 10.0	M = c. 10.0	M = c. 10.0	M = c. 10.0	M = c. 10.0	48.0

Countries marked with an asterisk after their names are officially designated by the United Nations as "least developed countries," i.e., countries that are among the socially least developed countries in the world as measured by overall level of social, political, and economic well-being. In the current analysis, these countries are referred to as "socially least developed or developing countries" in order to capture the broad socio-political-economic factors by which they are conceptually designated.[1]

[1] United Nations Office of the High Representative for the Least Developed Countries, Landlocked Developing Countries and Small Island Developing States (2017). Enhancing the participation of the Landlocked States in the implementation of Sustainable Development Goal (SDG) 14. Retrieved July 1, 2018 from http://unohrlls.org/event/enhancing-participation-landlocked-states-implementation-sustainable-development-goal-sdg-14/.

ISP Index of Social Progress, *Educ* education, *Econ* economy, *Demo* democracy, *Eviron* environment, *WISP* Weighted Index of Social Progress

The manufacturer's authorised representative in the EU is Springer
Nature Customer Service Centre GmbH, Europaplatz 3, 69115 Heidelberg,
Germany. If you have any concerns regarding our products, please
contact ProductSafety@springernature.com

Printed and bound by CPI Group (UK) Ltd, Croydon, CR0 4YY

29/04/2026

02099460-0008